T0195175

DICTIONARY OF
VETERINARY
NURSING

For Elsevier:
Content Strategist: Robert Edwards
Content Development Specialist: Nicola Lally
Project Manager: Julie Taylor
Designer: Miles Hitchen
Illustration Manager: Nichole Beard

DICTIONARY OF
VETERINARY
NURSING

Fourth Edition

D. R. Lane MSc, BSc (Vet Sci), FRCVS, FRAgS,
BSc (Hons) AAB&T

Former Senior Examiner in Veterinary Nursing

S. Guthrie PhD, BA, BVetMed, MRCVS, MBA (Open)

Former Chief Examiner RCVS Veterinary Nursing Scheme

S. Griffith MSc, DMS

Former Operations Director of the Queen Mother Hospital
for Animals, Royal Veterinary College
Former Senior Examiner RCVS Veterinary Nursing Scheme

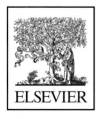

ELSEVIER

Edinburgh London New York Oxford Philadelphia St Louis Sydney Toronto

ELSEVIER

Notices

Knowledge and best practice in this field are constantly changing. As new research and experience broaden our understanding, changes in research methods, professional practices or medical treatment may become necessary.

Practitioners and researchers must always rely on their own experience and knowledge in evaluating and using any information, methods, compounds, or experiments described herein. In using such information or methods they should be mindful of their own safety and the safety of others, including parties for whom they have a professional responsibility.

With respect to any drug or pharmaceutical products identified, readers are advised to check the most current information provided (i) on procedures featured or (ii) by the manufacturer of each product to be administered, to verify the recommended dose or formula, the method and duration of administration, and contraindications. It is the responsibility of practitioners, relying on their own experience and knowledge of their patients, to make diagnoses, to determine dosages and the best treatment for each individual patient and to take all appropriate safety precautions.

To the fullest extent of the law, neither the Publisher nor the authors, contributors nor editors, assume any liability for any injury and/or damage to persons or property as a matter of products liability, negligence or otherwise, or from any use or operation of any methods, products, instructions or ideas contained in the material herein.

Printed in India

Last digit is the print number: 9   8

ISBN: 978-0-702-06635-1

Contents

Preface

The fourth edition of the popular *Dictionary of Veterinary Nursing* appears after a six-year interval, a time when there have been many changes in veterinary nurse education and a greater recognition for animal care assistants.

The Veterinary Nurse Registration Rules were brought into force in December 2014, requiring an approved veterinary vocational qualification and an approved practical training to be undertaken when becoming a veterinary nurse. The Level 6 educational qualification is also available at a number of UK colleges, leading to an Honours degree. The Level 3 Diploma in Veterinary Nursing is a vocational qualification designed to prepare veterinary nurses for professional registration on the Royal College of Veterinary Surgeons' Register of Veterinary Nurses. It is available on either a full-time basis as a stand-alone course, as part of a degree course, or apprenticeship-style alongside a job in veterinary practice.

Veterinary nurses trained outside the UK will continue to have their qualifications assessed against the UK standards as administered by the Royal College of Veterinary Surgeons. Animal care apprenticeships are operated in many locations, and entry-level studies require an understanding of the veterinary words in common use.

This new edition retains its easy-to-use format to provide a quick source of information for those considering entering the profession, for students and for those already qualified. Whether maintaining clinical records, writing reports, completing assignments or looking for data (where the Appendices are of particular value), we hope this dictionary is a practical aide in your daily work.

More than 250 new words have been added, covering topics such as new diseases, chickens, rabbits, other exotics, jurisprudence and business management. Definitions have been updated as required, along with the line drawings, and the Appendices have been expanded. Thus, we hope that anyone working closely with companion animals will find this book relevant and useful.

D. R. Lane, S. Guthrie, S. Griffith

aardvark A rare burrowing animal also known as an earth pig; strictly nocturnal, with a long tubular snout ending in a flexible, pig-like disk. A name favoured by veterinary practices that wish to head alphabetical directory lists.

AAT Animal-assisted therapy. Provision of suitable animals to promote physical, social, emotional or cognitive function in humans; *see also* DELTA.

abaxial The part of the skeleton facing away from the central line of the body or any of its parts; *see also* AXIAL.

abdomen The area between the diaphragm and the pelvis that contains the abdominal viscera.

abdominocentesis A technique for the collection of fluid from the abdomen, by using sterile procedures; fluid can be aspirated from the most prominent part of the abdomen, usually in the midline.

abdominal pump Method of circulatory compression used as an adjunct to chest compression for resuscitation, similar to compression of the chest; it aids oxygen delivery, coronary blood flow and cerebral blood flow but should only be done when a cuffed endotracheal tube has been placed.

abdominal thrust Abdominal compression used in an emergency to relieve airway obstruction; *see also* HEIMLICH MANOEUVRE.

abducens nerve (VI) The sixth cranial nerve, which supplies the lateral rectus eye muscle and the retractor bulbi muscle of the eyeball.

abduct To move away from the median plane or axis of the body; the word is used for abductor muscles, the process of limb abduction, etc.; *see also* ADDUCTION.

Aberdeen suture A method used for stitching small domestic mammals where the suture knot is buried under the skin so that the animal cannot bite it.

abiotrophy Progressive reduction in nervous or ocular function.

ablate To remove totally; a term used in the surgical correction of diseases of the external ear canal.

abortion Termination of pregnancy; the loss of viable fetuses through infection, hormonal failure or mechanical damage, as with a traumatic injury involving fetal membranes; *see also* PREGNANCY.

abrasion An open wound, usually with extensive loss of epithelial tissue, often painful because of exposed nerve endings.

abscess A focus of pus surrounded by inflamed or damaged tissue.

absolute Pure in quality, alcohol 100% strength.

absolute refractory period The time period after an initial stimulus when a cell, such as a neurone, cannot respond to a second stimulus.

absorption The process of transfer across a membrane: examples are taking in nutrients across the wall of the small intestine or reclaiming substances in the kidney.

ABVA The Association of British Veterinary Acupuncturists, founded in 1987. It provides a basic standard for the clinical application of acupuncture.

academic Term used to describe university-level instruction or knowledge; the opposite of practical or applied; *see also* VOCATIONAL.

acanthocytes Red blood cells with a membrane abnormality that allows them to develop multiple, irregular, club-shaped projections from their cell wall surface.

acanthosis A skin disorder where there is an increased thickness of epithelial cells sometimes pigmented with melanin. The increase of pigmented cell layers may be found in the axillae, when it is known as acanthosis nigricans.

acapnia Decrease (strictly, the absence) in the carbon dioxide content of the blood; *see also* HYPOCAPNIA.

acarbose Sugar used in diagnostic work.

acariasis Infestation with surface parasites such as ticks or mites; does not include flea infestation.

acaricide Medical substance used to kill off surface parasites.

accessory carpal bone The most lateral and caudal of the eight small carpal bones; may be the site of fractures in horses and racing greyhounds.

accident An event happening by chance or misfortune; *see also* RTA.

accident book A record book of all accidents/illnesses in the workplace and the actions taken; a statutory requirement to maintain the accident book is part of RIDDOR 2013.

accommodation Process to focus an image on the retina by changing the shape of the lens; the ciliary muscles can flatten or swell the lens at will.

accounts Financial records of a business showing the income, expenditure and profit made.

accreditation The formal recognition of a college/practice's competence by a third party. It provides customers, students and clients with a proven competency measure to make informed choices.

accredited practice A practice that has been awarded accreditation by the RCVS Practice Standards Scheme; accreditation assures the general public that the practice meets core standards of professional veterinary care for the species it treats.

ACE Angiotensin-converting enzyme. In relation to blood pressure control, this enzyme converts angiotensin I (a molecule in the lining of small blood vessels) to the vasoconstricting hormone, angiotensin II. **ACE inhibitors** are drugs that block the action of ACE, allowing peripheral blood vessels to dilate, benefiting heart muscle and lowering blood pressure; *see also* ANGIOTENSIN.

acetabulum Part of the hip joint structure, the recess in the pelvic bone to receive the femoral head. The depth of the socket of the hip joint affects the radiographic interpretation; *see also* VALGUS, HIP DYSPLASIA.

acetylcholine Chemical neurotransmitter synonymous with parasympathetic nerve activity; excess is destroyed by cholinesterase; *see also* ORGANOPHOSPHATE.

acetylcholinesterase Enzyme produced in nerve endings, muscles and erythrocytes; it breaks down acetylcholine in nerve tissue to choline and water.

acetylpromazine A premedicant from the phenothiazine group.

acetylsalicylic acid Pharmaceutical compound used to reduce platelet aggregation; traditional remedy for fever and pain control, commonly known as aspirin, a non-steroidal anti-inflammatory drug.

achalasia Condition affecting the motility of the muscles of the oesophagus; failure of relaxation of the sphincter at the entrance to the stomach; *see also* MEGAOESOPHAGUS.

Achilles tendon The group of tendons that run down to the hock connecting the muscles (gastrocnemius, semitendinosus and biceps femoris) to the point of the hock (tuber calcis).

achlorhydria Absence of hydrochloric acid in the stomach.

achondroplasia Inherited disorder where the bones of the legs fail to grow to their normal size and have a curved or twisted appearance.

achromasia Lack of normal skin pigmentation.

achromotrichia Bleached appearance of the coat owing to a lack of pigment; *see also* VITILIGO.

aciclovir An antiviral substance that inhibits the formation of DNA and has been used to treat or prevent animal herpes infections.

acid Chemical substances with a pH lower than 7, releasing hydrogen ions when dissolved in water.

acidaemia Condition of the blood characterized by low pH. The acid–base balance is the relative amounts of carbonic acid and bicarbonate present; normally the blood will remain slightly alkaline.

acid citrate dextrose (ACD) Anticoagulant mixture used when collecting blood for subsequent transfusion.

acid-fast Term used for those bacteria with capsules that, once stained with carbol fuchsin, resist decolourization by acid alcohol; usually it is mycobacteria that are identified in this way; *see also* ZIEHL–NEELSEN STAIN.

acidosis Disease condition caused by depletion of alkali reserve. May be metabolic (e.g. after diarrhoea caused by shock) or respiratory (when there is decreased respiration and less carbon dioxide is removed from the blood and the normal buffering system cannot function).

acid phosphatase An enzyme usually measured to assess prostate disease but not a satisfactory marker for prostate cancer disease in canines.

acinar Term used for the cells of the pancreas that secrete alkaline fluids. Adjective describing something that resembles a bunch of berries.

acinus Small cavity surrounded by secretory gland cells; in the lung, it is the name for the terminal air sac of the alveolus.

acne Describes a skin condition with many micropustules extending into the dermis; hormonal changes and secondary bacteria are involved; repeat treatments may be needed.

acoustic impedance The boundary between two tissues examined with ultrasound will produce an echo or 'sound reflection'; the main factor that influences acoustic impedance is the density or composition of the tissues.

ACP Acetylpromazine, a drug of the phenothiazine group used for sedation or premedication.

acquired A condition that develops after birth and is not attributable to a hereditary cause.

acral Relates to the limb extremities, including the carpus regions; *see also* LICK GRANULOMA.

acromegaly Growth hormone abnormality that causes a relative increase in the size of the extremities.

acromelanism Deposition of pigment in the body extremities, possibly due to lower temperature at these sites; responsible for the typical Siamese cat pigmentation.

acromion The hook-like prominence at the end of the spine of the scapula bone.

acrosome (of sperm) The hat or covering of the head of the sperm, necessary to supply the enzyme for penetration of the outer wall of the ovum to permit fertilization.

ACTH Adrenocorticotrophic hormone; *see also* CUSHING'S.

actin A protein found in muscle that plays an important part in the process of contraction; *see also* MYOSIN.

actinomycosis Bacterial infection characterized by multiple sinuses that open on the skin.

action (gait) Term used to describe the locomotion of a four-legged animal; often some slight abnormality will be detected that does not amount to lameness.

action potential A change in the electrical potential of the cell across its membrane resulting from movement of sodium ions in increased permeability; of importance in neurotransmission; *see also* NEURONE.

active immunity Immunity produced by the animal in response to the stimulus of an antigen brought into the body.

active principle That part of a drug involved in producing the therapeutic effect.

active transport The transmission of ions or molecules across a cell membrane against the concentration gradient; *see also* SEMIPERMEABLE MEMBRANE.

acupuncture A traditional Chinese system of healing for numerous types of disorders; it depends on the ability to locate acupuncture points of the body and stimulate them by inserting needles; needs a compliant patient.

acute Adjective used to describe a disease of rapid onset, with severe and recognizable symptoms but often a quick recovery following treatment.

acute renal failure (ARF) Sudden failure of kidney function; *see* NEPHROSIS, NEPHRITIS, ANURIA.

acyesis An absence of pregnancy; sometimes the word is used to indicate sterility in a female.

adaption Process of nerve receptors exposed to constant stimulation where the response fails progressively in some receptors.

Addison's disease (hypoadrenocorticism) Hormonal disease caused by an underactive adrenal cortex, with various symptoms and presentations. The acute failure of hormonal secretion is termed an addisonian crisis, requiring urgent treatment for collapse and vomiting. It may be iatrogenic in animals that have long-term steroid treatment suddenly stopped.

additive Substance used to enhance the ability of a feed stuff or similar product to benefit the animal.

adduction Bringing closer to the midline; adductor muscles bring the legs closer together.

adenitis Inflammation of glandular secretory tissue.

adenocarcinoma Malignant tumour involving glandular tissue; may occur in the mammary glands or the intestines.

adenohypophysis The part of the pituitary gland that is glandular; also known as the anterior hypophysis; *see also* PITUITARY.

adenoma Benign tumour of epithelial or glandular tissue, anal adenoma being a commonly occurring example.

adenopathy Enlarged lymph nodes as a result of infection, inflammatory diseases or cancer.

adenosine A nucleotide, part of the structure of DNA and RNA.

adenosine triphosphatase (ATPase) An enzyme used to release energy inside the cell; *see also* MITOCHONDRIA.

adenosine triphosphate (ATP) A molecule involved in the release of energy by the mitochondria within the cell.

adenovirus One of a group of viruses involved in upper respiratory tract infections in animals and birds; *see also* HEPATITIS.

ADH Antidiuretic hormone; *see also* DIABETES INSIPIDUS.

adhesion Abnormal structure connecting two sites, often the result of an inflammatory reaction or trauma; may consist of a fibrous band or a diffuse area of attachment.

adipose tissue Fibrous tissue containing many fat cells; fatty deposits occur after excess nutritional uptake; *see also* LIPOMA.

adjunct An additional drug, treatment or procedure that improves the effectiveness of the primary drug, treatment or procedure.

adjuvant Substance that intensifies an immune response; usually such vaccines have enhanced antigenicity.

adnexa The adjoining parts of a larger organ; the fallopian tubes and the ovaries constitute such a relationship or appendage.

ad libitum Latin term for 'freely', as in a freely available feeding system.

adrenal Situated close to the kidneys, *see also* ADRENAL GLAND.

adrenal cortex The outer part of the adrenal gland, principally secreting glucocorticoids and mineralocorticoids.

adrenalectomy Surgical operation to remove the adrenal gland.

adrenal gland Paired endocrine glands at the proximal pole of the kidneys, secreting adrenaline (epinephrine) and steroid hormones.

adrenaline (epinephrine) Hormone secreted to prolong the actions of the sympathetic nervous system.

adrenal medulla The grey core of the adrenal gland, which produces adrenaline (epinephrine) and noradrenaline (norepinephrine).

adrenergic Applies to the nerve fibres of the sympathetic nervous system that release noradrenaline (norepinephrine) when a signal is transmitted across the synapse. Also describes an agent that acts similarly to adrenaline (epinephrine) as a neurotransmitter.

**adrenocorticotrophic hormone
(ACTH)** Produced by the anterior
pituitary gland. ACTH stimulates the
production of the steroid hormone,
cortisol from the adrenal glands. Used
as a stimulation test in the diagnosis
of hyperadrenocorticism; given
intravenously; blood samples taken
before and after estimate cortisol levels;
see also CUSHING'S.

adrenogenital syndrome Relates to the
abnormal activity of the cortex of the
adrenal gland; known as adrenal sex
hormone dermatosis when skin changes
are present. Sexual changes or some
behaviour patterns are sometimes seen in
neutered animals.

adrenolytic Reverses the activity of the
adrenal gland.

adsorption Process of one substance
becoming attached to the surface of
another substance.

advanced practitioner Qualification
recognized by the RCVS in the UK,
denoting a practitioner who has
knowledge and expertise beyond their
primary veterinary degree but who has
not attained RCVS Specialist status.

adventitious Occurring in an anatomical
place other than the usual one.

adverse event An unwanted and untoward
reaction to a drug.

Aelurostrongylus abstrusus Lungworm in
the cat, associated with loss of condition
and a chronic cough. Intermediate hosts
are the slug and the snail. Diagnosis is
made by looking for larvae in faecal
samples.

-aemia Suffix meaning 'relating to blood'.

aerobe Bacterium that grows best in
culture media with plenty of oxygen
present.

aerobic respiration Customary type
of respiration in the presence of
adequate oxygen; yields carbon
dioxide and water with the production
of energy; *see also* ADENOSINE
TRIPHOSPHATE.

aerophagy (-ia) The habit of swallowing
air while eating; *see also* GASTRIC
DILATION.

aerosol A suspension of particles used as a
method of delivering a liquid substance

as fine particles propelled by a gas
through a fine nozzle.

aetiology The cause of something or the
study of the causes of disease.

afferent Leading in, towards; usually
vessels or nerves that run to the centre.

afterbirth Commonly used word to
describe fetal placenta; includes the
placenta, umbilical cord and ruptured
fetal membranes.

aftercare Nursing attention following an
operation or the convalescent attention of
a medical disease.

agalactia An absence of milk; may be
caused by hormone failure; a febrile
disease with dehydration or emotional
disturbance in a pampered bitch
whelping for the first time; *see also*
MASTITIS.

agammaglobulinaemia The absence of
immunoglobulins in blood.

agar A colloidal protein substance
derived from algae and used to pour
into plates for bacterial cultures and for
electrophoresis.

ageing The process of getting older. Also
a method of estimating the age of horses
using the patterns of eruption and wear
of incisor teeth.

agenesis Imperfect development of the
body or any part of it. An example
is with a bladder of the newborn
puppy seen to be suffering with
urine dribbling and scalding since
birth.

agent A mediator or substance that helps
to produce a chemical, physical or
biological effect. An **anaesthetic agent**
is any substance used medically to
produce general or regional analgesia. A
therapeutic agent is a substance with
a beneficial effect in the treatment of
disease, usually with a specific action to
produce a cure.

agglutination Grouping together or
clumping of cells, widely used in
antibody–antigen measurements and
blood-group typing.

agglutinin Any substance causing
agglutination.

aggression A sign of threatening behaviour
that may go as far as a physical attack on
another animal.

agonal breathing The gasping type of respiration seen in a dying animal.

agonist Drug that stimulates normal tissue activity; may also be a muscle response to cause a specific movement; *see also* ANTAGONIST.

agouti Pattern where the hairs have alternate light and dark bands, usually with black tips, controlled genetically.

agranulocytes The group of white cells with clear cytoplasm that does not take up stain; includes lymphocytes and monocytes.

agranulocytosis A condition where there is a deficiency of neutrophils or granulocytes; *see also* PANLEUKOPENIA.

AIDA Attention, interest, desire, action. Acronym used in classic advertising to describe the behaviour of someone viewing an advert that gets their attention and generates interest in the product or service so that the person desires it enough to take action to buy it.

AIHA Autoimmune haemolytic anaemia; low number of red blood cells because of their destruction by autoantibodies.

air A mixture of oxygen and nitrogen; becomes important in anaesthesia when flows of anaesthetic gases mix with air already in the respiratory tract.

air sacs The main areas for respiratory gas exchange in birds; physiologically equivalent to the lungs.

airway Term used to describe the route of gas exchange between the external environment and the lungs; improved by the insertion of an endotracheal tube in semiconscious and fully unconscious animals.

akinesia Loss of normal motor function which impairs voluntary muscle movement.

Alabama Rot Also called New Forest Syndrome or idiopathic cutaneous and renal glomerular vasculopathy (CRGV); first described in dogs in the USA and now also reported in the UK; exact cause is unclear; the illness begins with skin lesions followed by renal failure, which is almost always fatal.

alanine An amino acid.

alanine aminotransferase (ALT) Enzyme formerly known as SGPT.

alar Wing-shaped; sometimes used to describe the cartilage of the nose.

albinism An inherited lack of pigment in body cells.

albino Animal lacking normal dark pigmentation; cause usually hereditary.

albumin Protein compound found in the blood, in egg white and sometimes in urine.

albuminuria The presence of albumin in urine, which can be caused by kidney disease.

alcohol Organic compound with a hydroxyl element; the main use in veterinary nursing is for skin sterilization and for the preparation of medical compound extracts as tinctures; *see also* ETHANOL.

aldosterone Hormone produced by the adrenal cortex and responsible for the reabsorption of sodium by the kidney tubules. Its secretion is stimulated by angiotensin.

aleukaemia Term used for shortage or deficiency of leukocytes in the blood.

algae, blue–green Cyanobacteria microorganisms; plant-like substances that multiply on wet surfaces or at certain times of the year on surface water. The blue–green forms produce a toxin that can be fatal to animals.

alginate Protein used as a foam to help blood clotting or for wound healing.

algorithm A formula or process for solving a problem step by step.

alignment Word used in orthopaedics to indicate that bone fragments are arranged in correct orientation. **Proton alignment** is the aligning of all the body's hydrogen ions in a magnetic field, permitting an image to be seen (magnetic resonance imaging (MRI)); *see also* PROTON.

alimentary System of the body concerned with digestion and absorption of food; the **alimentary canal** runs from the mouth to the anus.

aliquot Equal-sized subsamples (with no remainder, e.g. 2 is an aliquot of 6); often used simply to describe one sample that represents the whole of the matter.

alkali Substance with a pH above 7 that has the property of neutralizing an acid.

alkaline phosphatase (ALP) Enzyme produced mainly by skeletal muscle and bone that is destroyed by the liver and therefore is frequently estimated as a measure of liver function.

alkalosis State of the body produced by acid losses such as after vomiting. Hyperventilation, by washing out carbonic acid, can produce a similar effect with weakness and loss of consciousness.

allantochorion The outer of the two fetal membranes, relatively tough, which breaks to release fluid early on in the second stage of labour.

allele One of two or more alternative forms of a gene that can occur at a given locus on a chromosome; only one can be present at a time and it exerts a hereditary influence.

allergen A substance, usually protein in nature, which can produce an allergic reaction in a hypersensitized subject.

allergy Hypersensitivity reaction in the body between allergens and antibodies. **Atopic allergy** is a hereditary form of allergic predisposition, most commonly seen as atopic dermatosis; *see also* ATOPY.

alligator forceps Grasping forceps with a long shaft; the points allow the retrieval of foreign bodies or biopsy specimens.

Allis tissue forceps Surgical instrument for holding exposed tissue by tooth-edged, gripping blades with a ratchet handle.

allograft Skin or similar tissue graft from a member of the same species; *see also* XENOGRAFT.

all-or-none law Used in neurology to explain why a group of neurones only responds when a threshold of stimulation is reached; does not permit a partial or graded response.

alopecia Deficiency or complete loss of hair.

ALP Alkaline phosphatase.

alpha First letter of the Greek alphabet, used to denote the first position, e.g.

alpha-amylase, used in the diagnosis of pancreatitis; the **alpha cells** in the pancreas secrete glucagon.

alphaxalone Feline anaesthetic agent.

ALT Alanine aminotransferase.

alternative medicine Various systems for healing, including homeopathy, herbal remedies and aromatherapy that are not part of the veterinary profession's orthodox treatment.

altricial Species born helpless; *see also* PRECOCIAL.

alula The first part of the bird's wing; acts as a free-moving digit; known as the bastard wing.

alveolar Relating to the alveolus; the **alveolar volume** being the volume of the respiratory tract in the terminal portion of the bronchial tree.

alveolus Cavity such as the tooth socket; in birds the sac that is the innermost part of the bronchial tree. The mammary gland may also be described as having an alveolus for gathering milk during lactation.

amacrine Describes neurones in the retina of the eye that lie between the layer of bipolar cells and the ganglion cells and

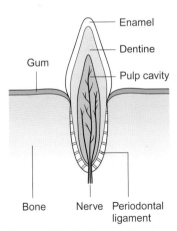

Figure 1. Alveolus. Cross-section of a tooth to show periodontal ligament fibres, which hold the tooth in the socket.

make lateral connections. Named because they have no conspicuous axon.

amastia Congenital absence of one or more of the mammary glands; not uncommon in bitches, where there may be an uneven distribution of teats on either side.

amaurosis Blindness, either partial or total; usually caused by disease of the optic nerve or the brain.

amblyopia Poor sight not caused by any visible lesion of the cornea, lens or fundus of the eye.

Ambu bag A self-inflating bag–mask–valve (BVM) resuscitator; used to provide artificial ventilation to patients who have stopped breathing until they can be connected to a mechanical ventilator, if required.

ambulatory The ability to be mobile; to walk.

amelogenesis The process of laying down of enamel in tooth development.

American Veterinary Medical Association (AVMA) In many ways close to the regulatory function of the RCVS in that it controls education, including nurse technician training (AHTs), in the USA. The BVA of the UK has a more limited interest in veterinary nurse training and employment, other than through the BSAVA.

amine Organic nitrogen-containing substance; appears in many body compounds.

amino acid Nitrogen-containing substance produced during the breakdown of proteins; concerned with growth and repair.

aminoglycosides Group of antibiotics that includes neomycin; used mainly for enteric and gram-negative bacteria. Toxicity may restrict their use in animals to treatment for no more than 5 days.

amitraz Synthetic organic parasitic application considered safer than organophosphorus compounds.

ammonia Compound of nitrogen and hydrogen that has a specific toxic action on brain and other cells; normally converted to urea by the liver. It is a colourless gas that can be turned into a liquid by cooling.

amnion Fetal membrane that forms the innermost compartment to protect the fetus; the amniotic fluid contained in the sac is dark and lubricant in consistency. Injury to or puncturing of the amnion usually leads to premature birth.

amoeba Single-celled microscopic animal.

amorphous Not regularly formed in shape; of diffuse outline.

amoxicillin Antibiotic with broad-spectrum activity, well absorbed from the intestine after oral administration.

amphiarthrosis A cartilaginous joint where both bone surfaces are connected but some degree of movement is possible; *see also* SYNARTHROSIS.

ampicillin Antibiotic administered by mouth or parenterally; active against urinary tract and respiratory infections.

ampoule Container, usually of glass, with a single sterile injection dose.

ampulla Dilated area at the end of a canal such as found in the inner ear of the auditory system; *see also* COCHLEA.

amputation Removal of a leg, part of a leg, dewclaw or tail. Occasionally, part of some other organ is removed surgically.

AMTRA Animal Medicines Training Regulatory Authority The organization given the authority for training qualified and listed veterinary nurses to become persons who can supply all animal medications; listed veterinary nurses will be able to supply POM-VPS and NFA-VPS products in their own right if they are a Suitable Qualified Person (SQP).

amylase An enzyme that catalyses the breakdown of starch into simpler sugar compounds; traces are found in saliva, but the main source of the enzyme is the pancreas.

amyloid A glycoprotein resembling starch that may be deposited in the walls of blood vessels.

ANA Antinuclear antibody.

anabolic Promoting the metabolism to increase tissue growth or muscle mass by the synthesis of protein. An **anabolic reaction** is a chemical process resulting in the formation of energy.

anaemia Decrease in the number of red blood cells below the normal range for the species of animal concerned; *see also* FIA.

anaerobe Bacterial organism that will only grow in culture with limited or no oxygen present.

anaesthesia A state of reduced perception of pain, shown as a loss of sensation or feeling in part or all of the body; *see also* ANALGESIA. **Local anaesthesia** is sensation loss induced in a restricted part of the body where pain is not wanted. **General anaesthesia** is loss of pain over the whole body during unconsciousness of the brain induced by a chemical agent; usually implies muscle relaxation as well. **Dissociative anaesthesia** is a type of general anaesthesia with good analgesia but only superficial sleep. **Regional anaesthesia** is loss of sensation produced by a nerve block or possibly infiltration of a whole field area; includes the injection of an anaesthetic around the spinal cord; *see also* EPIDURAL.

anaesthetic Describing a drug that produces anaesthesia, or when used as an adjective such as the **anaesthetic machine**, describing the use of the apparatus.

anagen Stage of the hair growth cycle equivalent to the active growth stage; *see also* TELOGEN.

anal Relating to the terminal part of the alimentary canal; *see also* PERIANAL, CIRCUMANAL.

anal abscess An infection within the anal sac causing a bulge in the perineum and often sudden, acute pain.

analeptic Substance that reverses an anaesthetic state, stimulating the brain and restoring consciousness.

anal furunculosis Infection with underlying tunnels and ulcers of the skin surrounding the anus; may be difficult to cure.

analgesia Reduced perception of pain, without the loss of awareness.

anal sac One of a pair of small pockets situated ventrolaterally to the anus and opening by a small orifice onto the perineum just outside the internal anal sphincter.

anal sac disease Description of chronic infection associated with excessive secretion of foul-smelling fluid; often seen as an inflammation of the perineum, sometimes with abscess formation.

anamnesis The taking of a history and the collection of relevant facts about a patient.

anaphase The third stage of cell division in both mitosis and meiosis.

anaphylactic shock Peracute response to an antigen in a sensitized animal; characterized by collapse, difficulty in breathing and generalized permeability of the peripheral circulation; *see also* VASCULOGENIC SHOCK.

anaplasmosis A tickborne disease of dogs with symptoms including joint pain, lameness, fever and general malaise. It is considered a zoonotic infection.

anasarca Excessive swelling of the abdomen, the legs and the prepuce with subcutaneous oedema.

anastomosis Joining together or intercommunication between two vessels to form a functioning organ; used surgically after an intestinal obstruction. Physiologically, the word is used to denote the linking of the arterial and venous parts of the circulation.

anatomical dead space The volume of air that fills the space on each inspiration without reaching the alveoli; represents the tracheal, bronchial and bronchiolar space.

anatomy The scientific study of the structure of the body; *see also* HISTOLOGY.

ancillary employees Colleagues working in support roles rather than being primarily involved in direct veterinary care e.g. reception personnel, laboratory technicians, cleaners and practice managers.

anconeal Bone process of the olecranon of the ulna in the elbow; *see also* OSTEOCHONDROSIS.

Ancylostoma Genus of parasitic worm. *A. caninum* is the commonest hookworm of dogs found in the UK; *A. duodenale* is a separate species affecting people.

androgens One of a group of steroid hormones, which includes testosterone, that stimulate the development of male sexual organs.

anechoic In ultrasound examination, a nonresponsive area suggesting a fluid-filled hollow organ or cyst; any organ or structure that produces no echoes compared with adjacent structures; also known as sonolucent (dark).

aneuploidy A condition in which cells have more or fewer chromosomes than the usual number; *see also* HAPLOID, DIPLOID.

aneurysm Disease of the blood vessel wall where there is a dilated area of an artery, vein or sometimes the heart.

angiocardiography Method of studying the circulation of blood in the heart; *see also* ANGIOGRAM.

angiogenesis The formation of new blood vessels.

angiogram Graphic depiction of the blood in circulation using a contrast medium given intravenously and a rapid series of X-rays; useful for diagnosing conditions such as portosystemic shunts.

angioma Tumour made up of blood vessels.

angiopathy Disease of blood vessels – veins, arteries and capillaries.

Angiostrongylus vasorum Lungworm of the dog; rare in the UK.

angiotensin Hormone regulating systemic and renal haemodynamics, often controlling the blood pressure. Angiotensin I and II are most common, but others up to angiotensin VII have been studied for the cause of hypertension.

angiotensin-converting enzyme (ACE) inhibitor Drug used to treat raised blood pressure and heart failure. It works by preventing the conversion of inactive angiotensin I to the powerful vasoconstrictor, angiotensin II. Administered by mouth, usually as a once-a-day dose.

angiotensinogen Inactive form of angiotensin produced in the liver; activated by action of renin to form angiotensin I.

angiotribe Instrument used in the control of bleeding, similar to a strong pair of artery forceps.

angulation Refers to the carriage of the leg of the dog, especially the hindleg of breeds such as the German shepherd where overstraightness or extreme flexion is a bad show point; the angulation of the shoulder joint is also studied.

anhydrosis The inability to sweat.

anhydrous Without water; used to refer to chemical substances heated to drive off water.

Animal and Plant Health Agency Executive agency overseen by DEFRA that safeguards animal and plant health for the benefit of people, the environment and the economy.

Animal Health and Veterinary Laboratories Agency (AHVLA) UK government body now called The Animal and Plant Health Agency, see also ANIMAL AND PLANT HEALTH AGENCY.

Animal Welfare Act 2006 Comprehensive legislation for farmed and nonfarmed animals introducing a 'duty of care' for persons involved in the animals' management.

anion Negatively charged particle; will move towards the positive electrode (anode) when an electric current flows.

anisocoria Unequal size of the pupils of the eye; often indicates a central (brain) injury.

anisocytosis Unequal cell size, as seen in blood smears after some disturbance in erythrocyte formation.

ankyloblepharon Disease of the eyelids where the edges stick together. Normal occurrence in the newborn kitten and puppy up to 10 days of age.

ankylosis Natural fusion together of a joint end; *see also* ARTHRODESIS.

annulus fibrosus Circular ligament surrounding the nucleus pulposus of the intervertebral disc.

anode The positive electrode to which negative ions transfer in the X-ray tube head (from the cathode) when high-voltage current acts.

anodyne Medication reputed to dull pain; *see also* ANALGESIA.

anoestrus Cessation of reproductive activity; forms the quiet part of the oestrus cycle. The word may also be used to denote anovulatory sexual quiescence; *see also* INFERTILITY.

anogenital Refers to the perineal region; a developmental error is to have a cleft or common opening, similar to that of the bird; *see also* CLOACA. The **anogenital distance** is the distance between the anus and vulva in the female or anus and penis in the male; distance is greater in the male than the female and is a useful indicator for sexing kittens, hamsters, mice, etc.

anomaly Something that stands away from the normal; may include deformities or lethal genes.

anorchism Absence of visible testes, may be unilateral; *see also* CRYPTORCHID.

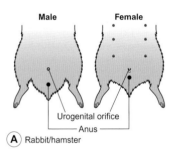

A Rabbit/hamster

Male   Female

Urogenital orifice
Anus

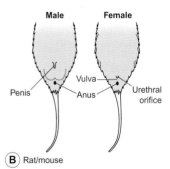

B Rat/mouse

Male   Female

Penis   Vulva
Anus   Urethral
orifice

Figure 2. Anogenital distance. Redrawn with permission from Aspinall V. Clinical procedures in veterinary nursing. Edinburgh: Butterworth-Heinemann, 2003.

anorectal Involving the area within the rectum and up to the external orifice, includes the location of the perianal sacs.

anorexia Loss of appetite; may be used to include partial inappetence or any situation where an owner notices that an animal is not rapidly ingesting its food. Pets should be weighed to ascertain how serious the problem is; rarely is it a psychological problem of the animal.

anoxaemia Reduced oxygen tension in the blood.

anoxia Absence of oxygen in the tissues; a serious condition that may first be recognized by cyanosis and frequent, deep respirations.

ANP Atrial natriuretic peptide; used as a biochemical measure of heart disease.

antagonist A counteracting agent such as the reversal of a sedative drug. The term is also used to describe a muscle that has an opposite action to an agonist muscle.

ante Before (from L.); opposite of post (e.g. **antemortem**).

antenatal Before birth.

anterior The part nearest the front of the animal; *see also* CRANIAL and ROSTRAL.

anterior pituitary gland The most active hormone-producing area of the brain; seven individual hormones identified; *see also* HYPOPHYSIS.

anteversion Forward tilting of bone, as found in hip dysplasia.

anthelminthic Medication used to kill or expel worms; may be described as broad-spectrum in action or sometimes specific for cestodes only.

anthrax Bacterial infection; the cause of death in animals eating contaminated carcass meat; zoonotic infection but responsive to penicillin if used early enough; vaccination is possible using a spore vaccine.

anthropomorphism The attribution of human thoughts, feelings or physical attributes to an animal.

anthropozoonoses Diseases that can be passed between humans and animals; *see also* ZOONOSIS.

anti- Indicates something against or counteracting (rather than beforehand).

antiadrenergic Medication that opposes the effects of the sympathetic nervous system,; includes beta-blockers.

antiarrhythmic Medication used in the treatment of heart disorders to stabilize the heart's rhythm; may also be used to describe a substance that prevents cardiac arrhythmia.

antibacterial Substance that kills or stops the growth of bacteria.

antibiotic Substance that is produced by microorganisms, or synthesized as a derivative, to kill or inhibit the growth of bacteria or fungi.

antibody Natural substance synthesized in the body in lymphoid tissue (B lymphocytes) in response to exposure to an antigen; it has a specific effect on antigens, neutralizing them or rendering them harmless. Antibody formation is frequently used in the diagnosis and assessment of allergies and immune status; *see also* ANTIGEN.

anticholinergic Medication that inhibits parasympathetic activity, especially acetylcholine; *see also* PARASYMPATHOLYTIC.

anticholinesterase Medication that inhibits the action of the enzyme acetylcholinesterase; allows the nerves to transmit abnormal impulses, as after nerve gas poisoning.

anticoagulant Agent used to reduce blood clotting, also used as a rodenticide in pest control; *see also* POISONS.

antidiuretic hormone (ADH) Hormone produced by the posterior pituitary gland, involved in fluid regulation of the body, increasing water and salt resorption by the kidneys. It is destroyed by the liver; *see also* DIABETES INSIPIDUS.

antidote Substance that reverses or neutralizes a toxic substance in the body.

anti-emetic Medication to suppress or stop vomiting; may act centrally or on the stomach wall.

antifungal Destructive to fungal infections; may be a chemical agent or natural immunity by the body.

antigen Substance that, under suitable conditions, stimulates an immunological response and reacts with antibodies.

antihistamine Drug used to inhibit the effect of histamine released in the body. Used to control allergic reactions, particularly skin pruritus, but sometimes also used for their anti-emetic and sedation effects.

antihypertensive agents Drugs to lower blood pressure; include angiotensin-converting enzyme (ACE) inhibitors, calcium antagonists, alpha-1-antagonists, beta-antagonists and diuretics.

anti-inflammatory A substance or action that reduces inflammation.

antimicrobial Substance with effect against all microorganisms, including viruses; *see also* ANTIBIOTIC.

antioxidant enzymes Substances that neutralize free radicals and help to prevent damage to tissues. Pathways exist in the body that are largely genetically determined; *see also* VITAMIN E.

antiparasitic Substance that destroys either external or internal parasites or both.

antiseptic A skin disinfectant; includes any substance that inhibits the growth or spread of bacteria and is not harmful to animal tissues.

antiserum A serum that contains antibodies.

Anti-social behaviour, Crime and Policing Act 2014 Legislation that can be used in the control of dangerous dogs in England. *See also* DOG CONTROL NOTICES.

antispasmodic Substance used to reduce painful spasms, usually of smooth muscle, in the treatment of bladder or intestinal diseases.

antitoxin Substance effective against specific toxins; was used to describe the serum injected to prevent tetanus after a contaminated wound was treated.

antitrochanter Ridge of bone dorsal to the acetabulum that helps support and articulate with the femur.

antitussive Cough suppressant; often acts centrally.

antiviral Agent effective against viruses.

antrum Describes a cavity such as the distal area of the stomach, next to the pylorus. **Pus in the antrum** refers to an infection of the maxillary sinus of the head.

anuclear cells Those seen during vaginal cytology that indicate that large keratinized cells are present and mating or insemination can take place with a high rate of success.

anuria Failure of the kidneys to produce urine.

anus Terminal orifice of the alimentary canal; *see also* ANAL SAC.

anvil Used to describe one of the three bones of the middle ear; *see also* INCUS, STAPES, EAR, MIDDLE EAR.

anxiety Nervous state; symptoms in dogs and cats include destructive chewing, vocalization and inappropriate defaecation and urination.

anxiolytic Medication used in the treatment of animal conditions such as separation anxiety. 'Sedative' drugs such as diazepam and temazepam are used in human dentistry for patients experiencing fear and similar medication has been used for veterinary purposes in animals. Clomipramine may be effective as an alternative treatment in dogs.

aorta Major blood vessel arising from the heart's left ventricle, running through the thorax and into the abdomen; arteries carry the blood on further through the body.

aortic valve Known as the semilunar valve, a valve in the proximal aorta preventing backflow of blood into the left ventricle of the heart.

APC Abbreviation for the human tablet medication of 'aspirin, phenacetin and caffeine', which is less favoured for veterinary pain relief.

aperient Used to describe a mild laxative or one used for moderate purgation.

apex The very tip of a tooth root or the point of the heart. **Apical** is used also for the cranial lung lobe.

APHA Animal and Plant Health Agency, an executive agency sponsored by **DEFRA.**

aphakic crescent The appearance of the eye that indicates that the lens has partially luxated; seen best with the ophthalmoscope; a 'half moon' or crescent of bright reflectivity shows where the lens has moved from and the retina reflects the light back.

apheresis The process of collecting whole blood from a donor or patient, filtering out one or more individual components and then returning the filtered blood back into the donor or patient.

aplasia Lack of development of cells or an organ, as in **aplastic anaemia**; a nonregenerative condition; *see also* HYPOPLASIA.

apneustic centre Controls inspiration as one of three respiratory centres located between the pons and the medulla; *see also* RESPIRATORY CENTRES.

apnoea Temporary cessation of breathing; the patient should be monitored closely.

apocrine One type of glandular tissue, found in the hair follicle as a sweat gland; equivalent to the sweat glands in the hairy parts of the human body associated with pheromones; *see also* SEBACEOUS GLAND.

aponeurosis Tendinous sheet formed where muscles join together, as in the tendinous portions of the abdominal transverse and oblique muscles that form the midline; *see also* LINEA ALBA.

apophysis Projection from a bone; also describes the pineal gland adjacent to the pituitary gland.

apoptosis The controlled, programmed death of cells, a natural process in the body.

appendicular That part of the skeleton that is away from the spine and brain; includes all four legs.

appetite The level of desire to eat food. The ingestion of food is controlled by many factors, including blood sugar level.

apposition Placed close to, as in fracture repair, so that fragments can come into contact for better repair.

appraisal Formal method of monitoring an individual's progress against previously agreed-upon criteria, usually performed by the 'line manager' or next most senior person.

apterium The bare skin in the spaces between bird feathers.

aqueduct A canal containing fluid such as the **aqueduct of Sylvius** in the midbrain connecting the ventricles.

aqueous General term for a watery state.

aqueous flare Streaks or misting of the aqueous humour through an increased protein (antibody) level; may be seen after corneal ulcer repair.

aqueous humour Clear fluid that occupies the space between the cornea and the lens; loss of fluid through corneal injury can have serious consequences for vision.

Arachnid Group of insects; includes eight-legged spiders, mites and ticks.

arachnoid The middle of the three membranes encasing the brain and spinal cord, so named because it was thought to resemble a spider's web.

aradicular hypsodont Condition where the tooth continues to grow throughout life and never develops a true root with a closed apex; found in guinea pigs and rabbits.

arboreal Types of animals living in trees.

arbovirus One of a group of viruses that includes those that multiply in arthropods and then infect bitten animals.

arcus An arch shape; important in eye examination as an early stage of cataract lens degeneration.

area centralis Part of the fundus or the place on the retina first seen with the ophthalmoscope; may show the earliest signs of hyper-reflectivity in a degenerative eye.

area postrema The part of the brain that is involved in vomiting reflexes; *see also* CHEMORECEPTOR TRIGGER ZONE.

areflexia Loss of reflex activity, as found after major injury to the spinal cord or nerve section.

areola A small area (from L.), often pigmented; the different-coloured part of the iris that surrounds the pupil of the eye. Also describes the brownish area surrounding the nipples of the mammary glands.

areolar connective tissue Loose, spongy tissue found subcutaneously; also found between and surrounding the internal organs.

arginine Amino acid, important because the cat cannot synthesize it for the hepatic urea cycle; this can lead to ammonia reaching the brain if the cat has anorexia.

ARMD Autosomal recessive muscular dystrophy, an inherited condition found in Labradors at 3–6 months of age; can be confirmed by muscle biopsy.

arnica Commonly used homeopathic remedy, derived from the plant known as leopard's bane. Used in the treatment of sprains and strains, bruises, etc. Accidental and surgical injuries may benefit from arnica used two or three times a day.

aromatherapy Favoured medication in complementary medicine treatments, with essential oils being inhaled or applied directly to the skin.

arrectores pilorum Muscles used to straighten up the hairshaft, as invoked by the frightened cat or dog wishing to appear larger than normal.

arrhythmia Loss of the normal regular heartbeat; the condition of sinus arrhythmia is considered a good feature on auscultation when the vagus nerve accelerates the beat on inspiration and slows or suppresses it on expiration; also referred to as dysrhythmia.

arsenic Poisonous substance formerly used as a preservative and as a herbicide.

artefact An artificial product; a blemish on an X-ray plate is an example (also spelled **artifact**).

arterial Relating to the high-pressure circulation system of the blood.

arteriole One of the smallest end-vessels of the arterial circulatory system that connects to the capillary bed.

arteriosclerosis A disease of the inner lining of arteries caused by the build up of deposits, which leads to narrowing of the vessels. In the horse this can lead to rupture of the affected artery.

artery Elastic-walled blood vessel into which blood is propelled from the heart; contains oxygenated blood, the exception being the pulmonary artery.

artery forceps Instrument used to control bleeding from blood vessels that have been incised or damaged, especially during a surgical procedure. A versatile instrument adapted for many other uses in veterinary nursing.

arthritis Complex condition previously described as joint inflammation; may be immune-mediated, infective or the result of trauma; *see also* OSTEOARTHRITIS, DEGENERATIVE JOINT DISEASE.

arthrocentesis Aspiration of the joint by puncturing the capsule with a needle to remove fluid.

arthrodesis Surgical fusion of a joint, obliterating the joint space and removing all movement.

arthropathy Disease of a joint, often degenerative; *see also* DEGENERATIVE JOINT DISEASE.

arthroplasty Surgical remodelling of a joint, as used for total hip replacement.

arthroscope Surgical equipment used to inspect or perform surgery on a joint through a very small opening in the joint capsule.

articular Relating to the moving surfaces of a joint.

artificial insemination Method of introducing live sperm into the vagina, cervix or uterus of the animal to promote conception or to control infectious disease (e.g. *Brucella canis*).

artificial respiration Form of life support either by intubation and bag compression, or less effectively, mouth-to-nose assisted breathing or thorax compression techniques.

arytenoid Word used to describe the cartilage of the larynx to which the muscles that alter the shape of the vocal cords attach.

ascarid Roundworm group that includes *Toxocara* and *Toxascaris* species.

ascites Fluid accumulation in the abdominal space, greater in quantity than and of different composition from normal peritoneal fluid.

ascorbic acid Commonly known as vitamin C; synthesized by all animals, except the guinea-pig, which must have a dietary source.

asepsis Usually applied to surgical procedures performed without any infection present. There are rules for nurses on the maintenance of asepsis; *see also* STERILE.

ASIF Method of fracture fixation using compression plates and screws and equipment devised by the Association for the Study of Internal Fixation.

aspartate aminotransferase (AST) An enzyme used in amino acid transamination; one of the liver enzymes; measured to estimate muscle damage, e.g. in cardiac infarction, formerly known as SGOT.

aspergillosis Fungal infection, particularly in the nasal cavity as a chronic discharging state, caused by *Aspergillus fumigatus*.

asphyxia Starvation of oxygen through restriction of inspired air reaching the lungs; suffocation.

aspiration Term used for the withdrawal of fluid to examine the contents; used for diagnosis of or as a temporary solution for a distended mass.

aspiration pneumonia Inflammation of the lung substance caused by inhaled foreign matter, usually stomach contents, that lodges in the bronchioles and alveoli.

aspirin Synthetic compound; the first discovered antiprostaglandin; used to lower the cohesiveness of blood platelets. Toxicity may be a problem in cats unless very low doses are used.

assessment Used as a first-stage nursing procedure to inform the veterinary surgeon, categorize priority of treatment or plan the nursing care; *see also* TRIAGE.

assimilation Body process for converting nutrients absorbed into the body into useful substances such as fat, protein, glucose, etc.

AST *See* ASPARTATE AMINOTRANSFERASE.

asteroid hyalosis Eye condition seen with the ophthalmoscope, as if there were many tiny stars shining in the vitreous;

sometimes thought by the owner to be a cataract.

asthenia Weakness, lack of strength, debility.

asthma A condition induced when narrowing of the airways produces respiratory distress accompanied by coughing and wheezing. Considered to be an allergic disorder, it may also be induced by emotional stress and air pollutants such as diesel exhaust droplets. **Cardiac asthma** is a term used for respiratory distress and exhaustion after minimal exercise caused by advanced cardiac disease, usually left ventricular dilation and failure.

astragalus One of the small bones that make up the hock joint (proximal row).

astrocyte Brain cell of ectodermal origin; in neoplasia, astrocytomas may be benign or malignant.

asymmetry Unequal placing, often a congenital defect of the body but normal in reference to the location of the kidneys. Externally, small changes of symmetry may be of great significance in identification and recognition of an individual.

asymptomatic A word used to describe a disorder that exists but exhibits no detectable signs.

asystole Serious heart condition when the heartbeat is absent; the ECG has a 'flat line'; *see also* CARDIAC ARREST.

ataractic Medication that produces a state of calmness and freedom from anxiety, similar to the state produced by a tranquillizer.

atavism Condition described in hereditary disorders when a very remote ancestor exhibited a similar disorder.

ataxia Unsteady walking; shaky or unbalanced gait; may indicate a cerebellar disorder.

atelectasis Collapse or failure of part of the lung to expand.

atheroma Lipid degeneration of the walls of the arteries.

atlantoaxial joint The joint between the first and second cervical vertebrae; area for subluxation with severe consequences; *see also* ODONTOID, TETRAPLEGIA.

atlas First cervical vertebra, which articulates with the occipital condyles at the atlantooccipital joint.

atom The smallest particle that forms an element; *see also* MOLECULE.

atomic number In chemistry, the number of protons or electrons present in an atom.

atomize The process of reducing to small particles; *see also* NEBULIZER.

atonic Diminished or absent muscle tone; used to describe bladder and colon dysfunction.

atopy Hereditary tendency to develop allergic signs, especially skin disease, epiphora and secondary bacterial infection of the abdomen and feet. Canine atopy involves IgE; such animal patients are described as atopic; trigger is often an inhaled allergen; may be confirmed via intradermal skin testing.

atraumatic needle Round-bodied surgical needle used for suturing soft tissue and external sites where there is the risk of the skin tearing if put under tension.

atresia The absence at birth, or the closing caused by trauma, of one of the body orifices.

atresia ani Lack of a perforate anus. Seen in newborn animals that initially seem to thrive but then suck less and develop bulging of the perineum below the tail.

atresia of nasolacrimal ducts Absence of satisfactory tear drainage; leads to epiphora and face staining; sometimes only the lower of the two ducts is closed.

atrial Relating to the first chambers of the heart; *see also* FIBRILLATION.

atrial fibrillation An arrhythmia of the heart caused by the contractions of the atria being disorganized and irregular.

atrial natriuretic peptide Hormone produced in the atrium of the heart as a response to overdilation; assists fluid loss.

atrioventricular (A–V) Relates to both heart chambers on the left or the right side, or both; *see also* A–V.

atrium One of the large cavities of the heart into which the veins pour blood, named after the central room of a Roman house.

atrophy Condition of wasting of a normal-sized organ; may result from disuse, faulty nutrition or hereditary atrophy; *see also* RETINAL ATROPHY.

atropine Natural product, now synthesized, that acts in a similar way to the sympathetic system response through its action in blocking acetylcholine. May cause long-term dilation of the pupils when applied to the cornea; used to reduce saliva production when injected as a premedicant.

attenation Common communication system in insects where sensory hairs are used in olfactory and tactile message giving.

attenuation Method of reducing virulence; the weakened organism can then be used as a vaccine.

atypical An unexpected response; pneumonia caused by *Mycoplasma* is a so-called atypical pneumonia.

audit cycle Continuous process of setting clinical standards, observing practice, comparing performance against standards and implementing changes to improve quality of patient care.

audition Sensation of hearing.

auditor Professional person conducting an audit, e.g. financial auditors may examine and certify practice accounts on an annual basis and clinical audits may be carried out to improve ways of working and standards of veterinary care.

auditory Relating to hearing or the ear anatomy and physiology; the ear connection with the pharynx is known as the **auditory tube**.

auditory brainstem response (ABR) A test to measure hearing ability; *see also* BRAINSTEM AUDITORY EVOKED RESPONSE.

auditory canal Connection between the pinna of the ear and the tympanic membrane before reaching the middle ear cavity.

auditory nerve The eighth cranial nerve, most involved in balance and hearing; *see also* CRANIAL NERVE.

auditory ossicles Three small bones of the middle ear; *see also* MALLEUS, INCUS, STAPES.

aura Earliest stage of the epileptiform convulsive attack; detected in humans by some trained assistance dogs, but most pet owners will not be able to discern it in their own animal starting a fit.

aural Relating to the ear.

aureus Golden or yellow-coloured.

auricular cartilage The stiffening part of the external pinna, including the funnel-shaped structure leading down to the middle ear.

auriscope Instrument for inspecting the external auditory canal.

aurotrichia Inherited disorder of miniature schnauzers where golden patches appear in the coat of the thorax and flanks.

auscultation The art of listening for noises in the thorax or abdomen, produced by gas or liquids, that helps make a diagnosis.

autoagglutination The clumping together of blood cells, caused by the presence of antibodies in the serum.

autoantibody Substance produced by the body that reacts to some antigenic constituent of the body's own organs or tissues.

autoclave Metal chamber constructed to withstand high pressure that allows sufficient heat sterilization to take place to destroy spores as well as bacteria.

autoimmune One of a group of disorders where the autoantibodies destroy or damage perfectly normal functioning tissues; a mistaken protective response treating the tissue self protein as a foreign antigen.

autologous graft Usually a skin graft removed from one area of the body and attached to another area with a skin defect.

autolysis Self-destruction of cells; thus a fixative or freezing of samples is required for histopathological examination; see *also* LYSOZYMES.

autonomic nervous system The part of the nervous system that controls all body functions and responses that are not under conscious control; *see also* SYMPATHETIC, PARASYMPATHETIC.

autophagy Autophagocytosis, the breakdown of cells due to lysosome actions.

autopsy Alternative name for the postmortem examination performed on a dead animal; compare this with BIOPSY.

autosomal Term used in genetics for hereditary factors carried on chromosomes other than the X and Y sex chromosomes; such factors will not be sex-linked.

autotransfusion (of blood) Technique to collect spilt blood during a procedure, filter it and transfuse it back into the animal's vein.

Australian bat lyssavirus Virus found in flying foxes and fruit bats; zoonotic disease that is a notifiable disease in Australia.

A–V Abbreviation for atrioventricular. **A–V valves** lie between the atrium and the ventricle to prevent regurgitation of pumped blood. **A–V bundle (bundle of His)** is made of Purkinje fibres and conducts electrical impulses from the S–A (sinoatrial) node. **A–V node** is part of the heart's mechanism for setting off each contraction or beat; *see also* S–A NODE, MITRAL, TRICUSPID.

avascular Lack of blood supply; seen in the fundus at the final stage of retinal atrophy or in the normal anatomy of the cornea to enable clear vision.

avermectin An injectable anthelminthic, usually safe in very small mammals using appropriate dose rates; *see also* ANTHELMINTHIC.

avian Relating to birds.

avian infectious bronchitis Respiratory disease of birds caused by a coronavirus, resulting in breathing difficulties, kidney damage and poor eggs; a vaccine is available.

avian influenza Form of viral influenza affecting birds, and a notifiable disease; humans may contract the disease from close contact with infected birds; there is world concern that the virus could mutate to allow human-to-human transmission, triggering a flu pandemic.

avian tuberculosis *Mycobacterium avium* infection causing chronic wasting; clinically affected birds should be culled.

avirulent In an infectious agent, lacking ability to produce disease and therefore able to be used to stimulate immunity as a vaccine.

AVMA American Veterinary Medical Association.

AVM-GSL Authorized veterinary medicine – general sales list; list that includes medications that may be supplied by any retailer as there are no restrictions on its supply.

avulsion Tearing away; trauma from road-traffic accidents being the most frequent cause of such injuries.

axial Central part of the skeleton based on the spinal cord, pertaining to or relative to the 'axis line'. The axial surface of the digit faces the axis, the abaxial faces away from the axis.

axial skeleton The main structural support for the whole skeleton, consisting of the skull and spine. Ribs and sternum are also considered axial; *see also* APPENDICULAR.

axilla That part of the body between the thorax and the forelimb, commonly called the armpit.

axis 1) The second cervical vertebra, notable because of its weak odontoid peg structure. **2)** The centre line of the body or organ, often used in anatomical descriptions.

axolemma A nerve axon's cell membrane.

axon A long structure of the nerve tissue that helps to conduct the electrical impulse to the nerve endings. May be sheathed in myelin produced by the Schwann cells to allow quicker transit of the nerve impulse.

axonopathy, progressive Disease mainly of the Boxer breed, characterized by ataxia and weakness of the hindlegs.

Ayres Design of T-piece anaesthetic circuit.

azathioprine Cytotoxic medication used as a cortisone-sparing agent; acts as an antimetabolite and synthetic purine analogue to block incorporation of natural purines into DNA; will affect the normal metabolism of all cells.

azotaemia Presence of excess nitrogen-containing compounds in the blood (a more correct description than URAEMIA).

azygos Unequal; the word is used for the vein that drains blood from the cranial abdominal skin across the thorax to join the right vena cava or empty directly into the right atrium.

Babesia Parasite that lives for part of its life cycle in the erythrocytes. There are separate species for the dog and cat, as well as for cattle. Usually spread by tick bites, the disease babesiosis in dogs is characterized by fever, haemolysis and jaundice.

bacillary typhlitis *See* TYZZER'S DISEASE.

bacillus, *pl.* bacilli Organism of the genus *Bacillus*; can be used to describe any rod-shaped bacterium.

Bacillus Gram-positive, rod-like bacteria known for their spores that can persist for years. *B. anthracis*, the cause of anthrax in all species, may cause death in foxhounds and other animals that feed on an infected carcass.

bacitracin Antibiotic used mainly for skin infections, reputedly named after Mary Tracy, a patient who had a wound contaminated with the soil organism *Bacillus subtilis*. The bacteria produced an antibiotic substance subsequently developed for clinical use.

backbone The name given to the spinal column; composed of individual vertebrae; it extends from the base of the skull to the tail tip.

back-cross Term used in breeding that implies the mating of an offspring to one or another of its parents. It is a test for breeding a heterozygote to a homozygote so that the subsequent litter can be studied.

backflow The flow of fluid in the wrong direction, e.g. blood flowing back through a faulty valve in the heart.

background radiation Additional radiation experienced by the whole population, caused by natural isotopes, radiation from outer space and previous earth-based nuclear accidents.

Backhaus towel clamp Clip used for fixing drapes to the patient during an operation.

backscatter Radiation risk to attendants during radiographic procedures, as radiation can be deflected more than 90° from the main X-ray beam; the risk is increased with metallic objects or dense bone deflecting the ionizing radiation.

back-up routine Saving a copy of computer records; should be done at least daily and the files stored safely in case of computer theft or malfunction.

bacteraemia The invasion of the bloodstream by living bacteria; a sign of infection.

bacteriocidal Able to kill bacteria.

bacteriostatic Preventing the growth or increase in numbers of bacteria.

bacterium, *pl.* bacteria A group of microorganisms that lack a distinct nucleus; most bacteria have a rigid cell wall or capsule. The capsule is associated with virulence and protects the organism against phagocytes; some antibiotics work by dissolving this capsular wall, e.g. penicillin and cephalosporins.

bacteriuria Bacteria in urine.

Baermann technique Laboratory procedure to detect motile worms such as *Angiostrongylus vasorum* larvae.

Bain system Anaesthetic circuit based on fresh gases passing up a central tube to the patient and exhaled gases passing down an outer sleeve; allows for a degree of rebreathing and low respiratory resistance; *see also* COAXIAL.

balanced anaesthesia The use of a combination of narcotics, analgesics and muscle relaxants to produce a satisfactory level of anaesthesia that allows the surgeon to operate and causes minimal damage to the patient.

balanitis Inflammation of the penis; the glans may become red and sore from repeated licking.

balanoposthitis Inflammation of the penis and prepuce, often associated with a green or yellow discharge from a dog's prepuce; disease of young intact males.

baldness *See* ALOPECIA.

ball-and-socket joint *See* ENARTHROSIS.

balloon catheter A sterile catheter with a bulb at the end that can be inserted into a tube or blood vessel and inflated with air or sterile water to occlude or dilate it.

ballottement Diagnostic test using the finger tips to palpate for an object floating in fluid; may be used with caution during examination late in pregnancy.

Baluchi Alternative name for the Afghan hound.

bandage A roll of material used for wrapping round the body either to support or to compress, as in the case of haemorrhage and limb oedema. Bandages are also used to keep dressings closely applied to the skin surface; *see also* COTTON CONFORM, FIGURE-OF-EIGHT, PLASTER OF PARIS, ROBERT JONES.

band cells Immature leukocytes (neutrophils) with characteristic curved nuclei.

BAOS Brachycephalic airway obstruction syndrome; *see also* TRACHEOTOMY.

BAR (bright, alert, responsive) Case note indicating that an animal has a normal level of consciousness and awareness.

barbiturates Group of drugs that induce sleep; may be used in anaesthesia and are commonly used in overdose strength as a method of euthanasia. Thiopental sodium is the most frequently used barbiturate for routine induction of anaesthesia.

Barden test Manipulation of the hip joint under deep sedation or anaesthesia to assess the degree of hip dysplasia/joint laxity; *see also* ORTOLANI SIGN.

Bard–Parker Surgical instrument name; known as a term for a scalpel handle, but there are also forceps described with this name.

barium Radiopaque material used in contrast radiography. A chemical element that is usually used in its sulphate form; can be mixed with food or poured into the mouth as a suspension.

Barlow's disease Hypertrophic osteodystrophy; *see also* OSTEODYSTROPHY.

Barlow's sign A test for congenital hip luxation first used in newborn children. Heard as a click on flexing and abducting the joint; has been used to indicate hip dysplasia in puppies; *see also* HIP DYSPLASIA, ORTOLANI'S SIGN.

baroreceptor Specific sensory nerve structures to detect changes in blood pressure, etc.; *see also* HYPERTENSION.

Barr body Contracted X chromosome of the female: the sex chromatid; *see also* CHROMOSOME.

barrier cream A water-impervious cream used to protect the skin.

barrier nursing A term used in infectious disease nursing to describe isolation of the patient, using separate utensils, ensuring scrupulous attention to hands, clothing disinfection, etc.

basal energy requirement (BER) The amount of energy used by an animal when it is resting completely in a cage and kept at normal body temperature.

basal metabolic rate (BMR) The amount of energy required for the maintenance of respiration, heartbeat, peristalsis, body muscle tone, glandular secretions, etc.; *see also* BASAL ENERGY REQUIREMENT.

basal narcosis Term that was used in anaesthesia to indicate that a narcotic had been given before inducing general anaesthesia.

base pairs complex nitrogen-containing bases that form specific crosslinks to hold the helical chains together in DNA; *see* DNA.

bases Chemical structures that are the opposite of acids, often alkaline when in solution.

basket cells Seen in blood smears as indistinct cells with pale eosinophilic nuclear material lacking shape; indicates blood sample has degenerated or has been over-chilled or that excessive pressure was applied when the slide was made; *see also* SMUDGE CELLS.

basophil Granular leukocyte with granules in the cytoplasm that stain with basic dyes; basophils are capable of ingesting foreign proteins and producing heparin and histamine.

basophilia Increased uptake of basic dye; may indicate some toxic change in the leukocyte.

beak Structure formed of keratin that, together with the beak bone, makes the structure on the bird's head used for feeding and for attack. Beak trimming is necessary if there is any malformation, lack of wear or parasite infestation.

beam Term used in radiography positioning to show the direction of X-rays, e.g. horizontal beam.

becquerel SI unit used to measure the radioactivity of a source; it has replaced the curie.

bed sore (decubitus ulcer, pressure sore) Can develop on the elbows of larger breeds of dog; any excessive or prolonged pressure on the skin when the dog lies on a hard surface is the commonest cause. Other sites of the body, such as the hocks or the ischium, may also be affected.

bee Insect with a sting that can cause injury to dogs or cats as an acute skin reaction.

behaviour The way in which an animal performs; patterns of behaviour are the subject of much psychological study, and the modification of behaviour has become a specialized science.

benchmarking A systematic process to measure and compare an area of business activity or performance against professional standards or other similar organizations. This helps a business or organization understand where improved performance may be required.

benign Not harmful, the opposite of malignant; when applied to tumours indicates that a full recovery is likely.

benzalkonium chloride Quaternary ammonium compound (Quat), used as a surface disinfectant with detergent properties.

benzathine penicillin *See* PENICILLIN.

benzimidazoles Group of anthelminthics more often used in large- than in small-animal practice.

benzodiazepines A group of sedative compounds (includes diazepam) used for sedation and behaviour modification.

benzoyl peroxide Preparation used on the skin for its keratolytic properties and for its antibacterial effect on staphylococci; may cause adverse reactions in some dogs, so should be used with care.

berus Latin name of the common adder/viper, *Vipera berus*.

best practice Clinical practice that is proven through research and evidence to produce desired results.

beta cells Pancreatic cells that produce insulin; *see also* DIABETES.

beta-blocker Drug that blocks the action of adrenaline (epinephrine) at organs with a beta-adrenergic receptor. This effect is used in the heart to decrease contractility and rate, cause vasodilation of arterioles and improve the airway by relaxing bronchial muscles.

betamethasone A synthetic steroid preparation with great potency if used on the skin surface; orally the duration of effect may not be to the animal's benefit.

BEVA British Equine Veterinary Association.

bicarbonate A salt containing hydrogen, carbon and oxygen that can be easily broken down by the body to provide an alkali reserve. Bicarbonate is one of the extracellular buffers that can take up excess hydrogen ions, and with the help of the enzyme carbonic anhydrase, will produce waste products of water and carbon dioxide, both of which can be excreted easily by the body.

biceps muscle The two-headed muscle; the dog, cat and horse have such a muscle in the foreleg as well as the hindleg. **Biceps brachii** is a shoulder extensor and elbow flexor muscle on the cranial surface of the humerus. **Biceps femoris** is an extensor muscle lying caudolateral to the femur.

bicipital Adjective for the shoulder region's biceps brachii muscle or tendon, e.g. bicipital rupture, after an injury.

bicuspid Heart valve with two cusps that is found on the left side of the heart between the atrium and ventricle; also known as the mitral valve; *see also* MITRAL.

b.i.d. Dispensing instruction for a medicine to be given twice a day. (L. *bis in die*.)

bifida Congenital abnormality; condition when the dorsal processes of the spine fail to fuse; *see also* SPINA BIFIDA.

bifurcation Branching into two forks, for example: the division of the trachea into the right and left main bronchi.

big head *See* MILLER'S DISEASE.

bijou bottle Small sample bottle.

bile Clear, orange fluid produced in the liver that is stored in the gall bladder. Strongly alkaline, it has an important role in the emulsification of fats as an aid to their digestion; *see also* BILIOUS VOMITING SYNDROME.

bile duct The tube that connects the gall bladder to the duodenum. Many small ducts unite to form the main bile duct. The cystic duct leads from the gall bladder to form the common bile duct.

bile pigments Breakdown products that cause the dark colour of bile; *see also* BILIRUBIN, BILIVERDIN.

bile salts Products that break the surface tension of fats, allowing for ease of digestion and absorption.

bilious vomiting syndrome Condition in some dogs that vomit first thing in the morning; believed to be the result of an empty stomach collecting acid and perhaps bile reflux. Usually treated by dietary change, feeding carbohydrate in the late evening.

bilirubin One of the bile pigments produced by the breakdown of haem from the blood; it normally circulates in the plasma and is processed by the liver. Bilirubin is yellow and gives colour to the faeces.

biliverdin A green-coloured bile pigment converted to bilirubin in the liver.

bioavailability The portion of a drug that is available at the site (tissue) where its action is required. Drugs given by mouth may have a low proportion of their content absorbed into the circulation.

biodegradable An important feature whereby a chemical product can be broken down by natural means such as enzymes or bacteria.

biological value (BV) A measure of the availability of proteins; it is the percentage of absorbed nutrient that is utilized and not lost immediately by excretion.

biopsy Taking living tissue from the body, usually for microscopic examination for the purpose of diagnosis or to assess cancer risk after tumour removal.

biosecurity Procedures and measures taken to prevent the introduction or spread of diseases in plants or animals.

biotechnology The science of biology when used for manufacturing and commercial purposes.

biotin A member of the vitamin B group. Rich sources of the vitamin are egg yolk, yeast and liver, and it is unlikely that deficiency would occur with normal feeding.

bisecting Dividing into two parts, e.g. **bisecting angle** in dental radiographs.

bistoury knife A surgical instrument of historic use, consisting of a long narrow blade used for lancing abscesses and opening up sinuses.

BKD Bacterial kidney disease; in trout, characterized by bulging eyes, swollen abdomen, pale gills and haemorrhage at the base of the gills.

bladder A stretchable hollow bag that stores fluid, most commonly referring to the storage organ of the urinary tract; it is lined by transitional epithelium and has a smooth muscle wall that allows for great distension. The outer

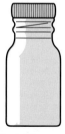

Figure 3. Bijou bottle.

layer is the peritoneum; *see also*
CYSTOCENTESIS.

bland Description used for a mild,
non-irritant substance such as a 'bland
ointment', e.g. K-Y® jelly used when
clipping up the eyelids to prevent hairs
falling on the cornea.

blast cells Immature cells; usually applied
to those of the bone marrow and those
that would not normally appear in
the peripheral circulation; *see also*
MYELOBLAST.

bleeding *See* HAEMORRHAGE.

bleeding time A measure of the ability
of the blood to clot: an incision is
made in the gum or skin and the time
taken for the blood to stop flowing is
measured in minutes; often used as a
quick test for thrombocytopenia and
haemophilia.

blepharitis Inflammation of the eyelids;
the upper or lower eyelids may be
affected at the edges; often seen as dry,
yellow crusts.

blepharospasm Spasm of the orbicularis
muscle of the eyelid, often the result of
a foreign body or corneal injury.

blindness Inability to see; may not be
easily detected if a dog or cat has lost
its vision slowly; *see also* NIGHT
BLINDNESS.

blind spot Optic disc or area at the back
of the eye where the optic nerve
emerges – called the blind spot
because there are no rods or cones
in this region; also the area behind an
animal where it cannot see – this area
is larger in a forward-looking predator
and relatively small in a prey animal
with a wide area of monocular vision to
each side.

blister Fluid-filled skin lesion, larger in
size than a vesicle.

blister disease A disease of snakes
where blisters arise between
gastrosteges; possibly associated
with a damp environment, see
GASTROSTEGES.

bloat Condition of a distended abdomen,
either the result of gorging food or from
an accumulation of gas in the stomach;
see also GASTRIC DILATION,
TYMPANY.

block *See* HEART BLOCK.

blood Fluid tissue that circulates
throughout the body in the arteries,
capillaries and veins. Consists of
a liquid component called plasma and
a cellular component that gives the red
colour.

blood bank Store of whole blood, red
cells or plasma collected from donors
for use in recipient patients requiring
blood replacement therapy. Veterinary
blood banks have to be authorized and
conform to regulations, and are subject to
inspections.

blood–brain barrier The division between
the body circulation and the brain
substance; it is only slightly permeable
to electrolytes and other ionic solutions.
Many therapeutic substances with large
molecules cannot readily reach the brain
for this reason.

blood clot A solid mass formed from
the elements of the blood either within
the blood vessel or elsewhere; *see also*
THROMBOSIS.

blood collection The process of taking
blood from a donor (approximately
450 ml from a dog, 50 ml from a cat)
for the creation of blood products for
transfusion into other animals.

blood donor An animal from which blood
is collected (with voluntary consent from
owner) to be transfused into one or more
other animal recipients.

blood group The antigenic structure of
the surface of erythrocytes means that
a first transfusion of blood can be given
without risk, but subsequent transfusions
may result in haemolysis and even death.
Cross-matching blood and obtaining
recent information about the blood
groups of dogs and cats reduces this
hazard.

blood 'poisoning' The presence of
bacteria or their toxins in the circulating
blood, usually associated with severe
illness.

blood pressure (BP) The pressure of
the blood inside the walls of the main
arteries. The highest BP is recorded
during systole (**systolic blood pressure**)
and corresponds to ventricular contraction.
The lower **diastolic blood pressure**
occurs as the heart relaxes and fills.

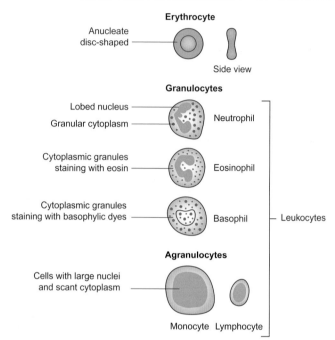

Figure 4. Blood cells: erythrocytes and leukocytes.

blood products Any part of the blood collected from a donor and used for transfusion to a recipient. This can be whole blood, packed red blood cells, plasma or platelets.

blood urea nitrogen (BUN) The urea content of serum or plasma, as measured by the nitrogen content; a marker for the renal clearance of nitrogenous waste; elevated as a result of dehydration, renal disease or urinary tract obstruction; reduced because of malnutrition or portosystemic shunts; somewhat outdated and superseded by other renal markers.

blue eye A popular description of a corneal opacity caused by oedema of the interstitial cells. Particularly associated with the Afghan hound breed when live CAV 1 virus was first used for vaccination against hepatitis, but blue eye may occur in a dog recovering from a hepatitis virus infection.

blue–green algae Cause of poisoning in dogs that have bathed in or drunk from stagnant pools. Poisoning is most likely in warm weather after the sudden growth of the algae, and the dog may show signs within 20 minutes of swallowing some of the water; *see also* ALGAE.

blunt dissection A method used by surgeons to separate fascial planes with minimal haemorrhage. Unless used with skill it could cause tissue damage and shock.

B lymphocyte Lymphocytes that develop from stem cells in haemopoietic tissue – fetal liver and spleen, and the bone marrow. B lymphocytes are involved in the production of antibodies and secrete immunoglobulin (Ig) molecules. They are independent of the thymus gland lymphocytes; *see also* LYMPHOCYTES.

BOX 25

BNP Brain natriuretic peptide; hormone used as a biochemical measure of heart disease, first recognized in the pig's brain but principally secreted by the heart.

body bag Also called cadaver bag; description of any disposable container used for dead animals; *see also* WASTE.

body cavity Refers to those areas within the body lined with serous membrane. The peritoneal cavity, the thoracic cavity and the pericardial cavity are all potential spaces but only contain a minute quantity of fluid between the viscera in the healthy animal.

bogspavin A fluid swelling of the tibiotarsal joint in horses due to the increased production of synovial fluid, which has many causes, e.g. infection, poor conformation, concussion or nutritional deficiency.

bolus injection Method of giving intravenous medication in a concentrated mass; used also in contrast radiography when giving an opaque substance.

bonding In psychology, developing a close but selective relationship. Important in puppy and kitten socialization; *see also* IMPRINTING.

bone Hard, rigid tissue that forms the internal skeleton of mammals; *see also* ENDOCHONDRAL OSSIFICATION.

bone marrow Vascular tissue mixed with fat; the soft contents of the long bones; has the important function of producing platelets and red and white cells for the blood.

bone spavin Hard bony swelling, often around the hock of the horse; *see also* SPAVIN.

bony labyrinth Tunnels in the temporal bone that contain the sensitive organs of hearing and balance; *see also* INNER EAR.

booster vaccine Method of increasing immunity by administering vaccine after the initial vaccination course has been completed. Essential for vaccines using a killed antigen, such as *Leptospira,* and in general use for most dog and cat vaccines on a once-a-year basis, although some animals have longer-lasting immunity.

borborygmus Noises from the abdomen associated with gas or fluids passing into a larger hollow area of the intestinal tract; *see also* BOWEL NOISES.

Bordetella Bacteria associated with respiratory-tract infections of the dog and cat. *B. bronchiseptica* is considered to be one of the causes of kennel cough and infectious bronchitis.

Borna disease Fatal neurologic disease in horses and sheep caused by a virus and has been associated with psychiatric disorders in humans. Discovered in southern Germany and is a notifiable disease in Australia.

Borrelia burgdorferi A tick-borne spirochaete; cause of acute arthritis; *see also* LYME DISEASE.

botulism Poisoning, usually fatal, from ingestion of animal matter contaminated with *Clostridium botulinum*. An acute toxaemia.

bovine spongiform encephalopathy (BSE) Prion disease that affected many cattle in the late 1980s and early 1990s but may have caused a similar condition of spongiform encephalopathy in cats. Dogs were never known to be infected, although many consumed raw offal.

bowel clamps Surgical instruments with a fine, long non-cutting and non-crushing blade used to isolate a length of intestine before incision. Various surgeons have given their names to these: Doyens, Gillman, etc.

bowel noises Caused by increased peristalsis and liquids squirting from the small intestine into the gas-containing large intestine; *see also* BORBORYGMUS.

Bowie–Dick indicator tape Tape used to seal up plastic instrument packs; it has heat-sensitive markings that change to dark brown at 121°C; however, it does not show whether the inside of a pack has reached the required temperature for the required time to be sterilized.

Bowman's capsule The envelope, two cell layers thick, that encloses the tuft of capillaries in the nephron that constitutes the glomerulus.

Box turtle An imported species (*Terrapene*), mainly from America;

requires little water in its living space and is essentially carnivorous. The African box turtle is *Terrapene carolina.*

Boyle's law Quoted in anaesthesia; essentially it means that as the pressure of a gas is reduced, the volume of the gas increases, assuming that the temperature is not altered.

brachial plexus The nerve centre for the foreleg, originating from the sensory branches of the last four cervical and first two thoracic nerves; it is located medial to the shoulder joint and can be damaged after some chest injuries.

brachycephalic Description of the short-faced, wide-head condition seen in the boxer, King Charles spaniel and pug dogs, etc. The condition of the skull bones may cause obstruction of the nasal passages and other airway obstructions; the lower lip folds may become moist and chronically infected.

brachycephalic airway obstruction syndrome (BAOS) A condition of short-nosed dog breeds where the airway is restricted by narrow nares and the nasal cavity, a long soft palate, an overlarge tongue base or a narrowed trachea.

brachydont Tooth type found in some dogs and cats where there is a short crown-to-root ratio, but there is a true root present.

bradycardia Slow heart rate, often associated with hypokalaemia.

bradypnoea Slow but regular breathing.

braided suture Multifilament plaited material used in suturing and said to hold a firmer knot. May be absorbable or non-absorbable. The wick-like effect can be a problem, limiting its use as a skin suture.

brain The encephalon comprises all of the nervous system within the cranium. It contains fluid ventricles and is divided into the fore-, mid- and hindbrain.

brain death Cessation of neurone function; indicated by loss of pupil response and other reflexes and slower breathing.

brainstem The base of the brain responsible for connecting the higher centres to the spinal cord; includes the pons, medulla oblongata and thalamus.

brainstem auditory evoked response (BAER) Test used to assess hearing in dogs and people; assessing hearing acuity (in the sedated pet) by measuring electrical activity in the brain.

brainstorming Method of generating new ideas and solutions to a problem, often done in small groups where all members are encouraged to contribute spontaneously to the discussion.

branchial The position in the neck where, in the embryo, the fish gills might have arisen; a cyst may develop at this site in dogs, filled with saliva; it is thought to represent the branchial arches of the embryo.

breath hydrogen test Measurement of the hydrogen gas produced by gastrointestinal bacteria. After dosing with a sugar, expired gases are collected using an anaesthetic mask and measurements are made with a breath hydrogen analyser. Repeat samples taken over several hours help to distinguish between gastric *Helicobacter* infection and small intestine and colon bacterial overgrowth.

breech birth Term used to describe posterior presentation of the fetus (puppy or kitten) when the legs remain flexed and forward rather than the 'normal' hind toes first, followed by the tail and then the rump.

breeding The animal's pedigree or the physical act of mating; *see also* CROSS-BREEDING.

breeding season Those times in the year when an animal can be mated; *see also* SEASON.

breed standard A specification laid down by a Kennel Club committee to which a pedigree dog must conform. *See* www.the-kennel-club.org.uk.

bridge A marker used in animal training when a reward is given when a required behaviour is performed.

brille Also known as an eyecap or spectacle, a transparent layer of skin that protects the eye when no eyelid exists, as in snakes and lizards.

brisket Part of the body at the base of the neck composed of fat and connective tissue that extends between the front legs.

bristle feathers Sensitive, thin, bare-shafted feathers that have a tactile function.

broad ligament The suspensory ligament of the uterus; *see also* MESOMETRIUM.

broad-spectrum antibiotic One that has a wide range of activity against many bacteria; *see also* ANTIBIOTIC.

broken down 1) Dog breeder's terminology for the bleeding that indicates the onset of pro-oestrus. 2) A term used to describe a horse or dog with sudden-onset lameness, often caused by tendon injury.

bronchial Adjective relating to some conditions of the bronchi.

bronchiectasis Medical condition, the result of chronic dilation of the bronchial tubes frequently associated with a secondary infection.

bronchiole A very small branching tubular continuation of a bronchus each tube subdivides until the terminal bronchiole, where air then moves into the alveoli via the alveolar ducts.

bronchitis Inflammation of one or both bronchi; may be caused by inhaled particulate irritants, dust, spores, pollen or smoke but is equally often caused by viral or bacterial infections. The signs of repeated coughing and increased bronchial sounds on chest auscultation are characteristic.

bronchodilator Substance that increases the width of the airway in the lungs by increasing the lumen or preventing a spasm of the constricting smooth muscle.

bronchoscope Endoscope designed to examine the lining of the lower respiratory tract; it can also be used to obtain samples by aspiration or by washing and to remove inhaled foreign bodies.

bronchospasm Disorder caused by contraction of the muscles of the smaller bronchioles, possibly because of an inhaled irritant substance. Bronchospasm may occur in the anaesthetized animal; *see also* ASTHMA.

bronchus, *pl.* **bronchi** One of the larger airways entering the lung from the trachea; some smaller bronchi supply the lung lobes.

brood patch Area of bare skin on a bird's ventrum that allows it to pass heat easily to eggs during incubation; the feathers regrow after the eggs have hatched.

broodiness Natural tendency of a bird to sit upon eggs to incubate them until they hatch; this is advantageous in the wild but laying birds sitting in the nest box on infertile eggs will lose condition; discouraged by moving the broody hen to a separate enclosure with food and water but no nesting materials.

Browne's tubes Sealed glass tubes used during autoclaving to confirm that sterilization in the centre of the pack is adequate; a colour change from orange–brown to dark green occurs with heat; tubes for temperatures of 121–134°C can be selected. Tubes for hot-air-oven monitoring can also be used.

brown fat Fat deposited in connective tissue that is more easily mobilized; it is important in young and in hibernating animals for heat production and as a rapid release form of energy stores.

brown hypertrophy of the cere Overgrowth of the base of the budgerigar's upper beak; hyperplasia of the keratin may be caused by parasites and will lead to breathing difficulties and weight loss.

Brucella canis Gram-negative bacterium often considered to be one of the causes of abortion in dog kennels.

bruising The effect of trauma with discoloration and haemorrhage of affected tissues; where there is a blood clotting disorder, bruises may develop from very trivial injuries. Colour changes in bruises are the result of the breakdown of the haemoglobin; *see also* CONTUSION.

bruit A sound similar to a murmur, usually less noticeable, and the result of blood being forced past a small, constricted area of the vascular system.

Brunner's glands Found in the duodenum, producing digestive enzymes.

brush border Surface area of small intestine where enzyme activity and absorption take place; *see also* VILLUS.

BSE *See* BOVINE SPONGIFORM ENCEPHALOPATHY.

buccal Adjective used to describe the mouth cavity towards the cheek.

buccal mucosal bleeding time (BMBT) A simple test for bleeding disorders in dogs where the gum is cut, and the time for the blood to stop flowing is measured; *see also* VON WILLEBRAND'S DISEASE.

buccal stomatitis Inflammation of the cheek mucosa.

buccinator muscle One of the cheek muscles.

buck male rabbit

bucket handle tear Common meniscal injury where the meniscal cartilage of the stifle develops a tear shaped like a bucket handle.

bucket muzzle Form of restraint in the dog used to prevent biting but one that is loose enough not to restrict breathing.

Bucky grid A moving grid used in radiography to control secondary scatter but avoiding the parallel lines on a plate where a stationary grid has been used. (Sometimes called Potter–Bucky grid.)

buffers Reagents used to combat acidity or alkalinity.

buffy coat Used in haematology as a rough measure of platelets and white cells; seen in a centrifuged blood sample as a layer above the red cells.

bulbar conjunctiva The portion of the outer layer of the eyeball that covers the white sclera.

bulbo-urethral gland A pair of small glands that lie between the prostrate gland and the perineum, responsible for part of the ejaculate of the male. Not found in the dog.

bulbus glandis The swelling at the base of a dog's penis caused by vasodilation; its function is to retain the penis in the vagina as part of the 'tie'.

bulla Blister, usually can be seen to contain serous fluid.

bullous (*adj.*) Used to describe skin with many large blisters or in the lung condition of emphysema where there are air-filled cavities present; *see also* PEMPHIGUS.

bumblefoot Infection of the footpad of a bird caused by *Staphylococcus* spp.; may respond to antibiotics but may need surgical curettage.

BUN *See* BLOOD UREA NITROGEN.

bundle of His Specialized fibres that conduct the electrical impulse across the heart; also called the A–V (atrioventricular) bundle.

bunny-hopping A term used to describe a dog's movement when both hindlegs are advanced together, often indicating abnormal gait with hip dysplasia or some spinal disorder.

buprenorphine A semisynthetic opiod used as an analgesic lasting 6–8 hours.

bur (burr) A surgical instrument used to enlarge a cavity or to debride a bone.

burn A severe injury to tissue caused by dry heat, chemicals, radiation or electricity. Injuries are characterized by necrosis, peeling of skin, etc. Fluid loss may be anticipated; treatment for shock should be given along with pain relief, and attempts should be made to prevent infection of the burn. *See* SCALD.

bursa, *pl.* bursae A small fluid-filled sac occurring in tissue, often the result of repeated injury or friction.

butorphanol A synthetic morphine-like substance used both as an analgesic and to suppress coughing.

butyrophenones A group of drugs used for pre-anaesthetic medication, not licensed for animal use at present.

cachexia Condition of weight loss, general bodily decline and weakness. Muscle loss is most noticeable on the temporal muscles of the skull and can be a sign of progressive diseases such as neoplasia.

cadaver The body of a dead animal.

caecotrophs The material resulting from fermentation in the caecum of the rabbit, wrapped in a mucus coating and different from faeces.

caecotrophy Process of extending the period for cellulose breakdown adopted by rabbits, where the soft faeces are removed from the rectum and ingested to pass through the alimentary tract a second time to produce hard, dry pellets of faeces.

caecum The proximal part of the large intestine. Relatively narrow in the dog and cat but enormous in the rabbit for fermentation in the digestion process.

caesarean section Surgical birth of a fetus by means of an incision through the abdominal wall and then an opening into the uterus.

cage paralysis Muscular weakness in hamsters usually caused by a lack of exercise.

calamus Central shaft of the bird's feather.

calcaneus One of the bones of the tarsus; a square structure in the proximal row of the bones that forms the point of the hock.

calcar Bone area distal to the head of the femur where the bone spike should be excised in an excision arthroplasty.

calcification The process of depositing calcium salts in the tissue; *see also* HYPERPARATHYROIDISM.

calcinosis cutis Calcium deposited in the epidermis, characteristic of hyperadrenocorticism. The skin is usually thin and hairless and nodules can be felt with the finger tips.

calcipotriol May cause poisoning by accidental ingestion, as it is found in human skin creams.

calcitonin Hormone secreted by the parafollicular cells of the thyroid gland. It reduces blood calcium levels and limits calcium uptake from bone.

calcitriol Hormone produced in the kidneys that assists absorption of calcium from the intestine.

calcium Chemical element required in the food as it is an important constituent of bones, teeth and blood; nutritional diseases are more common in the young, growing animal. Calcium is important physiologically for muscle contraction so calcium-channel blockers are used in the treatment of heart arrhythmia.

calcium oxalate Crystalline salt found in the urine, associated with acidic urine where there is an excessive excretion of oxalates. This may be a metabolic defect in some breeds; *see also* UROLITHIASIS.

calculus, *pl.* **calculi** Any unusual deposit of mineral salts as found in the bladder (**urinary calculi**) but may also occur in the kidney (**renal calculi**), the prostate or the teeth (**dental calculus** or tartar).

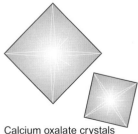

Calcium oxalate crystals are typically pyramidal or octahedron-shaped

Figure 5. Calcium oxalate crystals.

Calicivirus A virus of the cat commonly associated with 'cat flu' signs.

calling Popular term for the breeding season of the cat; oestrus is associated with a raucous cry in some cats.

callus 1) Tissue laid down during the repair of fractures; eventually becomes organized into harder, denser bone. **2)** Callus also refers to the hard leathery skin on the elbows of larger breeds of dog, the result of pressure sores or of friction.

calor (L. heat); one of the four classic signs of inflammation. *See also* DOLOR, RUBOR, TUMOR, INFLAMMATION.

calorie Measure of food value defined as a unit of heat necessary to raise the temperature of 1 g of water through 1°C (strictly from 14.5 to 15.5°C). Now replaced in food value measurement by the joule. (1 cal = 4.1855 joules.)

calvaria Anatomical term for the dermal bone roof of the skull, fused with cartilage bone walls and floor to form a brain case.

Calvé–Perthes disease Disease of the hip; *see also* LEGG–CALVÉ–PERTHES DISEASE.

Campylobacter Gram-negative motile microorganism that grows best in microaerophilic to anaerobic conditions. *C. jejuni* is a cause of infectious diarrhoea in dogs that has zoonotic implications.

Campylobacter upsaliensis *See* UPSALIENSIS.

canal Passageway; used anatomically: alimentary, auditory, nasolacrimal, semicircular, etc.

canaliculi A narrow passageway used, as in **bone canaliculi**, for the histological structure of bone, or as in **bile canaliculi**, from liver to bile ducts.

canal of Schlemm Structure in the eye that permits drainage of aqueous humour from the anterior chamber of eyeball.

canal of Volkmann Structure of long bone that permits a blood supply to enter to the bone marrow by a nutrient artery.

cancellous Description of open bone tissue of the medullary cavity as opposed to compact CORTICAL BONE.

cancellous bone Less dense bone with an open trabecular structure and large sinusoids containing bone marrow, as found in vertebrae, flat bones and the ends of long bones.

cancer Abnormal growth of tissue; implies neoplasia and usually means a malignant tumour.

***Candida* (thrush)** Yeast-like fungal infection, not common in dogs and cats; *Candida* spp. were sometimes called *Monilia* in humans.

canine Relating to the dog.

canine distemper (CD) A viral infection; *see also* DISTEMPER.

canine hip dysplasia (CHD) *See* HIP DYSPLASIA.

canine tooth The corner tooth of the mouth with the longest point, used in carnivores for skin penetration and gripping prey. The four deciduous canines are replaced by permanent canines in the growing animal.

canker 1) Term applied to ear disease in dogs; implies overgrowth of tissues; may be seen in advanced chronic otitis. **2)** Term used to describe overgrowth of the frog in the equine hoof.

cannabis A Schedule 1 drug (S1) recognized as an addictive drug in the Misuse of Drugs Act 1971; has some medicinal properties and may be the cause of small-animal poisoning, either accidentally or after deliberate experimental use on pets.

cannibalism One animal eating another of the same species; can occur with some species, e.g. hamsters where a mother may eat her young if she is disturbed and stressed.

cannon The third and biggest metacarpal bone in the horse.

cannula A tube for insertion into a body opening; a **lacrimal cannula** for the tear ducts or an **intravenous cannula** that will then occupy the lumen of the vein.

canthotomy Incision of the canthus for greater exposure of eye structures during surgery.

canthus The angles at the corners of the eyelids known as the **nasal (medial)** and **temporal (lateral) canthi**.

capacitation Part of the reproductive process where the sperm in the ovarian tubes finally mature to allow fertilization of the ova to take place.

Capillaria Parasitic nematodes mainly found in birds. Species of *Capillaria* also affect small rodents and fish.

capillary Very small, one cell thin-walled blood vessels that allow the exchange of oxygen and solutes within the tissues.

capillary refill time (CRT) Test used for quick assessment of shock or circulatory failure; pressure applied to the gum causes blanching, and the time until the gum is pink again is measured in seconds.

capnograph A piece of equipment that measures and produces a continuous graph of the amount of carbon dioxide in expired gas from a patient. It is useful in assessing the adequacy of ventilation and to diagnose circulatory problems.

capsid The protein coat of a virus.

capsule 1) The membrane-like sheath that encloses some anatomical structures, a **joint capsule** being an example; also used to describe the covering of some neoplasms. **2)** Used in pharmacy for a small gelatine container for some medications. **3)** The outer protective layer of bacteria, which may be attacked by antibiotics.

capsulotomy (lens) Technique used in cataract surgery of the eye so that an intracapsular lens extraction can be performed by first incising the outermost layer, which then remains to keep the vitreous in place.

captopril Medication used in cardiac disease, one of the ACE INHIBITORS.

caput The head of; used anatomically as in **caput epididymidis**, the head of the epididymis.

carapace Dorsal shell of groups of animals such as turtles, tortoises and crustaceans; see PLASTRON and SCUTES.

carbamate Toxic substance found in garden herbicides and fungicides.

carbaryl An insecticide with less toxicity than other similar synthetic preparations.

carbohydrate Chemical compounds of great nutritional importance containing carbon, hydrogen and oxygen; they can be stored in the body as glycogen, or if excessive amounts are fed, fat will be laid down.

carbolic acid A phenol, formally used as a kennel disinfectant, but because of its toxicity, now limited to laboratory use to disinfect glassware. Classified as a corrosive poison.

carbon dioxide Gas, the result of the oxidization of carbon compounds, that is found in exhaled breath in higher concentration than in air; *see also* RESPIRATION.

carbonic anhydrase An enzyme found in red blood cells and of importance in removing carbon dioxide from the tissues. Inhibitors of carbonic anhydrase are used in the treatment of glaucoma to reduce aqueous formation; the action on the eye is entirely separate from any diuretic effect.

carbon monoxide Gas with poisonous properties causing damage to the central nervous system and asphyxiation. Birds are particularly sensitive to such toxic fumes, as produced by smouldering matter or gas fires where there is insufficient room ventilation.

carboxyhaemoglobin The product of carbon monoxide poisoning where the blood appears cherry red; usually fatal as tissues become starved of oxygen; *see also* CARBON MONOXIDE.

care pathways The written planned patient care processes to take place within an agreed timeframe by a multidisciplinary team.

carcass (carcase) disposal Legal requirement in the UK is that bodies must be treated as clinical waste materials and handled as semi-hazardous substances. A dispensation allows the body to be treated as the legal property of the owner, allowing burial of pets of all sizes in the owner's garden.

carcinogen Substance that causes neoplasia or cancer. Hazardous substances may be labelled carcinogenic and adequate precautions must be taken in their handling.

carcinoma A malignant neoplasm.

cardia The part of the stomach near the opening from the oesophagus, distal to the cardiac sphincter.

cardiac Relating to the heart.

cardiac arrest The cessation of the heart's action as a pump, a 3-minute emergency requiring well-planned action; *see also* RESUSCITATION.

cardiac centre The nerve centre of the brain situated in the medulla oblongata that controls blood flow and pressure by receptors from the autonomic nervous system.

cardiac cycle One complete contraction and relaxation cycle of the heart.

cardiac massage A method of resuscitation during cardiac arrest by surgical opening of the chest and manual massage of the heart.

cardiac sphincter A band of muscle found at the proximal opening to the stomach where the oesophagus joins and controls emptying of the oesophagus and filling of the stomach; *see also* VOMITING.

cardiac tamponade An effusion of blood or other fluid in the pericardial space surrounding the heart causing excessive pressure on the heart muscle. The heart shadow on radiograph is enlarged and the heart sounds are muffled.

cardinal signs Traditionally the most important clinical signs: pulse, temperature and respiration rate.

cardiomyopathy Degeneration of the heart muscle so that the heart fails progressively as a pumping organ, usually accompanied by dilation of the heart.

cardiopulmonary arrest (CPA) Cessation of both the heartbeat and respiration.

cardiopulmonary cerebral resuscitation (CPCR) *See* CARDIOPULMONARY RESUSCITATION.

cardiopulmonary resuscitation (CPR) The nurse's action is to follow the ABC (airway, breathing, circulation) routine of clearing of the airway, ventilation of the lungs, preferably with oxygen and then chest compression and massage of the heart area to maintain circulation; *see also* RESUSCITATION.

cardiovascular Adjective used to describe conditions of both the heart and the blood vessels.

cardiovascular centre Nerve centre of the brain situated in the medulla oblongata that controls the blood pressure by nerve receptors of the cardiac and vasomotor centres.

cardioversion A method of using defibrillation or drugs (or a combination of both) to convert an abnormal heart rhythm into a normal rhythm.

caries Disease of the teeth with erosion of the enamel and pitting of the dentine.

carina 1) The pointed keel of a bird's breast. **2)** A part of the bronchus dorsal to the heart; can often be identified on radiographs of the chest.

carminative Medical substance used to relieve flatulence and colic.

carnal Pertaining to the body; fleshy.

carnassial tooth Upper fourth premolar tooth (three-rooted) and the lower first molar tooth in the dog, used together as a pair of shearing cutters. In the cat, the upper third premolar and the lower molar are developed for the same purpose.

carnivore An animal that feeds on flesh, primarily by preying on other animals.

carotid Describes anything near the carotid arteries, the main blood vessels to the brain on either side of the neck.

carotid body Chemoreceptor area at the bifurcation of the common carotid arteries that can influence the medullary respiratory centre.

carotid sinus A dilated area at the base of the internal carotid artery containing blood pressure receptors. The **carotid sinus reflex** is a reflex induced by stimulating the upper neck area that slows the heart.

carpal Adjective for the area of the foreleg known as the carpus; it is equivalent to the wrist; *see also* CARPUS.

carprofen Non-steroidal anti-inflammatory drug having its effect via COX-2 inhibition; used short-term for post-operative pain relief and long-term in the management of chronic conditions such as osteoarthritis.

carpus A group of small bones situated between the distal ends of the ulna/radius and the metacarpus.

carrier Implies an animal that has a low-grade infection but is still capable of infecting other animals. It may also be used for a heterozygous animal carrying recessive genes.

car sickness Motion sickness, more common in dogs than cats; if medication is required in cats it is best to use chlorpromazine.

cartilage Dense connective tissue, found chiefly at joints and between bones.

cascade prescribing Use of a veterinary drug licensed specifically for the species being treated; if no suitable preparation is available, a drug licensed for another animal species may be used instead; drugs licensed for human use can only be used in animals if there is no specific veterinary preparation; written owner consent must be obtained before any human formulations can be given.

cash flow The movement of money within a company due to its business activities over a specified time period; the difference between opening and closing balances.

cassette Word used to describe a specific container, such as those used in radiography, often with intensifying screens with a pressure pad to ensure close film contact.

cast In veterinary work, a method of external support using a mouldable material, e.g. a fibreglass or **plaster cast** used in fracture repair; *see also* PLASTER OF PARIS.

castration Surgical (or chemical) removal of the testes, used to prevent breeding and undesirable social behaviour. The word can be used to describe the neutering of both sexes, but in the UK it is restricted to the male animal. It is considered that the operation involves entering a body cavity, although the scrotum is external in dogs and cats.

catabolic reaction Chemical reaction with the breakdown of molecules, often with the release of energy.

catabolism Process of breakdown of cells, a negative metabolic state.

catalase Enzyme responsible for many chemical reactions in the body that produce oxygen and water.

catalyst Substance that promotes or alters the rate of a chemical reaction. The catalysts of biochemical processes are known as enzymes.

cataract An opacity of the lens or its capsule; described as congenital or acquired, also as central, cortical, post-polar, etc.

catarrh Discharge of mucoid material from a surface, often the result of inflammation.

catecholamine Substance released at nerve endings that helps to combat stress.

cat flu Upper respiratory tract infection caused by a variety of bacteria and viruses.

catgut Was an absorbable ligature or suture material produced from sheep intestine prepared in a sterile manner, now little used; *see also* CHROMIC CATGUT.

cathartic Traditional term for a substance that induces defaecation.

catheter A flexible tube introduced into the body for administering fluids or withdrawing unwanted fluid or laboratory specimens. **Intravenous catheters** and **urethral catheters** are the two most common types used in veterinary medicine.

cathode The negative electrode of the X-ray tube head from which electrons are emitted.

cation A positively charged ion, e.g. metallic ions, etc.

cat scratch disease (CSD) Infection of a wound in humans following a scratch from a cat; occurs worldwide; *Bartonella henselae* is involved, but the exact mode of transmission is not fully understood; kittens under 12 months are often involved in the spread of infection; a regional lymphadenopathy occurs 3–14 days after the scratch or bite.

cauda equina Anatomical structure at the distal end of the spinal cord in the lumbar region.

cauda equina syndrome A condition of the lumbosacral articulation characterized by incoordination of the hindlegs; it may be painful, and there is often incontinence as the nerve control is damaged.

caudal Relates to the tail of the animal so is most commonly used when describing the posterior or 'backwards' direction in anatomy.

caudal oral stomatitis Inflammation of mucosa rostral to the oropharynx.

caudocranial Describes the radiographic positioning when the main beam is directed from the rear end towards the head end, used in stifle joint X-rays, etc.

caudolateral Describes the position used in surgery to enter the elbow joint, as for an un-united anconeal process operation.

cautery A method of controlling haemorrhage or removing excess tissue by burning. Often an electric current, a hot instrument or a chemical agent such as silver nitrate is used.

CAV Canine adenovirus. **CAV 1** is the virus causing infectious canine hepatitis.

cava A hollow place, as in **vena cava**.

Cavia **(cavies)** One genus of the rodent family, commonly seen as guinea pig pets for children; noted for its inability to manufacture vitamin C and for a gestational period that is as long as that of a dog.

cavy Guinea pig, *Cavia porcellus*.

CBC Complete blood count.

The abbreviation is frequently used when haematology tests are requested for a blood sample.

CD *See* CONTROLLED DRUG.

CDR Controlled Drugs Register; *see* MISUSE OF DRUGS ACT 1971.

CDRM Chronic degenerative radiculomyelopathy, a degenerative disease of older dogs; may be immune mediated.

cell The basic structure of the living organism.

cell-mediated immunity Protection against infection that involves cytotoxic T lymphocytes.

cell membrane Lining of the cell just within the outer wall; important function is to control the passage of substances into and out of the cell.

cellulitis Skin infection in the deepest layers of the skin, seen also as furunculosis of dermis and subcutis. Often seen in cats when bites have introduced bacteria into the subcutaneous space.

cellulose One of the components of dietary fibre from plants; insoluble and poorly fermentable. The main function is to delay food transit in the cat and dog and to help to form a firm defaecation product. Herbivores can digest cellulose in their adapted large intestines or ruminant stomachs; *see also* RABBIT, CAECOTROPHY.

Celsius Unit of temperature measurement, similar to centigrade.

centigrade Measurement of temperature from original metric unit system.

central nervous system (CNS) The portion of the nervous system that includes the brain and spinal cord.

central progressive retinal atrophy (CPRA) Form of retinal dysplasia characterized by dark pigment accumulating in the retina, leading to loss of central vision. Genetic in origin, the disease was first identified in the Briard but CPRA affects many large breeds, and it is now thought that a dietary cause (low levels of vitamin E) contributes to the appearance of the disorder; *see also* DYSPLASIA, RETINA.

Central venous catheter Also known as a central line, a catheter that is placed into a large vein, usually the jugular in the neck, to administer fluids and drugs, to obtain blood or to measure central venous pressure.

central venous pressure (CVP) Pressure measured in the jugular vein; can be used to study the flow of blood back to the heart and is important in monitoring shock.

centre of ossification During the formation of bone, will arise in the cartilage as two or as many as seven separate centres; the area where bone formation starts.

centrifuge A laboratory device to rotate liquids, such as blood or urine, at high speed, to separate out the more solid constituents from the liquid ones.

centriole Two cylindrical structures found in cell cytoplasm near the nucleus and the Golgi apparatus.

centripetal Tending towards the centre; word used in describing conjunctival overgrowth in the rabbit.

centromere Temporary attachment of the chromatids during cell division.

centrosome The part of the cytoplasm containing the centrioles.

centrum The body of a vertebra.

cephalic Relating to the head end of the body.

cephalic vein A vein located on the craniomedial aspect of the forelimb; commonly used for administration of intravenous drugs or to collect blood samples.

cephalosporins A group of broad-spectrum antibiotics that are active mainly against Gram-positive bacteria.

cerclage Encircling a bone with a loop of wire, as in fracture stabilization.

cere The firm bulge at the base of a bird's beak. Useful in sex discrimination of

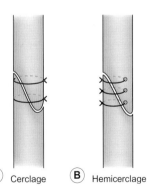

(A) Cerclage   (B) Hemicerclage

(A) Wire wrapped round outside of bone to compress fracture line

(B) Wire anchored through one cortex to compress the fracture line

Figure 6. Cerclage wiring. (a) Cerclage wiring; (b) hemi-cerclage wiring.

budgerigars as it is light brown to pink in females and blue in males.

cerebellum Part of the hindbrain; the cerebellum is responsible for involuntary control of balance, posture and coordination of movement.

cerebrocortical Relating to the cerebrum (forebrain).

cerebromedullary cistern A store for CSF at the caudal brain region; *see also* CISTERNA MAGNA.

cerebrospinal Relating to the brain and spinal cord.

cerebrospinal fluid *See* CSF.

cerebrum The largest part of the brain, often called the 'cerebral hemispheres'.

ceroid Waxlike. An inherited storage disease with yellow–grey discoloration of the skin is known as **ceroid lipofuscinosis**.

cerumen Waxy secretion of the glands of the outer ear.

ceruminolytic A substance used in ear cleaning to dissolve wax.

ceruminous glands Glands in the lining of the outer ear that secrete CERUMEN.

cervical Relating to the animal's neck or the neck of the uterus.

cervical lymphadenitis Bacterial infection by *Streptococcus zooepidemicus* affecting the cervical lymph nodes of guinea pigs; the swellings may burst to discharge pus.

cervix Narrow portion of the uterus where it joins the vagina.

cestode Parasitic worm that is flat and has no alimentary tract – tapeworm.

cetaceans Group of sea mammals that includes the harbour porpoise and bottlenose dolphin; both are found off the UK coast.

Chagas disease Caused by *Trypanasoma cruzi* spread by bites, mostly by insects *Triatominae* or 'kissing bugs'. Although mainly a disease of Latin America, it is notifiable in Australia.

chalasia Relaxation of a body opening such as the cardiac sphincter; *see also* MEGAOESOPHAGUS.

chalazae Structure that restrains the yolk inside the egg during development.

chalazion (meibomian cyst) Swollen sebaceous gland in the eyelid.

chameleon Small reptile kept as a pet; has the ability to alter its body colour.

channelling Effect when soda lime settles in an underfilled canister in a rebreathing circuit so that the exhaled gases can pass through without contacting fresh soda lime and thus without resorbing carbon dioxide.

charting (records) The keeping of clinical records; in veterinary nursing helps the veterinary surgeon understand the patient's progress.

Cheatle's forceps Long-handled forceps stored in disinfectant and used to transfer sterile equipment; *see* FORCEPS.

cheek teeth A collective term for the premolar and molar teeth in horses and rabbits.

cheilitis Inflammation of the lips.

cheilorrhaphy Surgical repair of the congenital defect of a hare lip.

Chelonia Members of the reptile family of chelonians.

chelonian Reptile of the order *Chelonia*, turtles and tortoises.

chemoreceptor A cell or group of cells that responds to a specific chemical compound, e.g. the taste buds and receptors in the mucous membrane of the nose.

chemoreceptor trigger zone (CRTZ) Found on the floor of the fourth ventricle of the brain; connects to the vomiting centre and relates to the vestibular apparatus. The zone is susceptible to a variety of stimuli, including bloodborne substances such as toxins; usually results in reflex vomiting.

chemoreceptors Sensory receptors for changes in chemical consistency, pH, etc.

chemosis Oedema of the conjunctiva, often causing the eyelid to bulge outwards.

chemotherapy The treatment of illness by chemical means, particularly relevant to cancer therapy.

cherry eye Prolapse of the nictitans gland of the third eyelid; *see also* NICTITANS GLAND.

Cheyletiella Group of surface-feeding mites, noted for excess skin scaling in dogs ('walking dandruff'); also found on cats and rabbits and a cause of pruritic vesicles in humans.

Cheyne–Stokes respiration Type of automatic breathing seen in respiratory failure where the patient inhales air deeply followed by a period of shallow or invisible chest movement. The breathing pattern is repeated periodically at short intervals. It occurs particularly in states of coma and just before death.

CHF Congestive heart failure (not 'chronic').

Chick–Martin test A traditional test for the efficiency of antiseptics and disinfectants.

chief cells Found in the stomach layers, responsible for pepsinogen production.

chigger Name for larval mites of the genus *Trombicula*, also known as harvest mites.

chin acne *See also* HEAD GLAND DISEASE, PYODERMA.

chipmunk Squirrel-like creature sometimes kept as a domestic pet.

chitonaside Product from sea shells that has a moisturizing effect when incorporated in skin dressings and makes the active principle effective for longer.

Chlamydia *See* CHLAMYDOPHILA.

chlamydiosis Disease caused by organisms of the genus *Chlamydia* or *Chlamydophila*; in birds, known as psittacosis or ornithosis. Also causes chronic conjunctivitis in cats, and in sheep is a cause of abortion. The human eye disease trachoma has *Chlamydia trachomatis* as its causal agent, and there is also a sexually transmitted human infection of importance, but it is not related to the feline disease; *see also* CHLAMYDOPHILA, PSITTACOSIS.

Chlamydophila A genus of bacteria that are extremely small and can live within the cell. Various strains of *Chlamydophila* (formerly *Chlamydia*) *psittaci* are the cause of psittacosis in psittacine birds (parrots, parakeets) and mammals. Feline pneumonitis is caused by *Chlamydophila felis*; bacteria are transmitted by inhalation of infectious droplets and by ingestion, as when coat grooming occurs; *see also* CHLAMYDIOSIS, PSITTACOSIS.

chloramphenicol Antibiotic effective against a wide range of organisms, now most widely used as a topical application, e.g. as an eye ointment.

chlorhexidine An antiseptic used in solution as an effective skin disinfectant before surgery.

chlorine An extremely pungent and toxic gas; however, used in the form of liquid 'bleach', can be a very effective disinfectant.

chlorpromazine One of the phenothiazine antipsychotic drugs; has been used as a mild 'tranquillizer' in dogs and cats as an alternative to acepromazine. It is an effective antiemetic for cats, especially when travelling.

chlortetracycline Antibiotic effective against many bacteria but used mainly for oral medication or in the form of eye ointment.

choanae A funnel-shaped structure; used to describe the area at the back of the pharynx where the paired openings lead from the nasopharynx.

choanal slit Main nasal passage communicating with the oropharynx.

chocolate agar Heated blood agar used in bacteriology to culture fastidious pathogens such as *Neisseria* species. The heat treatment breaks down haemoglobin and gives the agar the brown colour.

chocolate poisoning Accidental poisoning of pets as a result of overeating chocolate. Sickness and diarrhoea are usual, with elevated liver enzyme levels, but rarely there are more severe effects on the heart; *see also* THEOBROMINE.

cholangitis Inflammation of the bile duct.

cholecalciferol Alternative name for vitamin D_3.

cholecystokinin Hormone secreted by the crypts of Lieberkühn in the small intestine; affects the production of bile and of pancreatic juice.

cholemesis Vomiting of bile.

cholesterol Steroid found in animal fat, present in the blood and frequently measured during biochemical screening tests. Elevated blood levels (hypercholesterolaemia) are associated with thyroid disease but diet influences the sample collected.

choline Basic compound involved in the transport of fat in the body; phospholipids and acetylcholine are two products for which it is needed. At one time it was listed as part of the vitamin B group but no longer, as it can be synthesized by all animals from serine. It may be given as an oral supplement in the treatment of liver disease.

cholinergic Describes those autonomic nerves that release acetylcholine as the neurotransmitter; also used to describe drugs that mimic the actions of acetylcholine; *see also* PARASYMPATHOMIMETIC.

cholinergic synapse Any nerve junction where acetylcholine plays a main role in transmission.

cholinesterase An enzyme that splits acetylcholine into acetic acid and choline. With any organophosphorus poisoning, the enzyme is inhibited, and the effects are muscle fibre contraction with tremors; often sickness and diarrhoea follow initial increased salivation.

chondral Adjective used for cartilage.

chondrocyte A mature cartilage cell.

chondrodystrophy A disorder of cartilage formation.

chondroma Benign tumour of cartilage.

chondroprotective agent Drugs used to treat arthritis, having a direct effect on repair of articular cartilage.

chordae tendineae The 'strings' in the ventricles that stop the A–V heart valves from everting.

chorea Rapid involuntary movements, often most noticeable in the jaw muscles; usually considered to be a sequel to canine distemper infection; *see also* FITS.

chorioallantois The fetal membranes that lie outermost, and therefore, may be described as the first 'water bag', as it is the amnion that lies closest to the fetus.

chorionic gonadotrophin Hormone produced by the placenta during pregnancy; may be collected from urine. After refinement it may be injected as a source of luteinizing hormone.

choroid The middle coat in the eyeball, richly supplied with blood vessels; contains the sensory receptor cells and associated pigment cells.

choroid hypoplasia A congenital disease of collie breeds where defects in the development of the eye may cause loss of vision; *see also* COLLIE EYE ANOMALY.

choroid plexus Brain structure that secretes cerebrospinal fluid (CSF). A compact mass of pia mater, blood vessels and ependyma that protrudes into the lumen of the fourth ventricle.

Christmas disease (haemophilia B) Hereditary disease of specific dog breeds and short-haired cats with a blood-clotting defect. Carrier females exist that can be identified by blood testing.

chromatid Found in the nucleus of the cell during division; each chromosome forms two identical chromatids.

chromic catgut Natural product used in suturing; prepared from sheep intestine and hardened by immersing in chromic acid to delay its breakdown (and loss of strength) when in the animal's body.

chromosome One of the thread-like strands in the nucleus that carry genetic information. Composed of two coils of DNA.

chronic degenerative radiculomyelopathy (CDRM) Progressive wasting disease of the hindlimbs, usually affecting the German shepherd breed; of unknown cause; *see also* RADICULOMYELOPATHY.

chronic disease One that has been present for some time and does not immediately progress to cause the death of an animal.

chronic obstructive pulmonary disease (COPD) Respiratory difficulty in the horse caused by allergens (usually in hay) – also known as 'heaves' or 'broken wind'. Symptoms include 'heaving' to force air out of the lungs at the end of exhalation, coughing, exercise intolerance, nasal discharge and weight loss. The abdominal muscles of affected horses may become enlarged because of the 'heaving'. Repeated episodes of inflammation of the airways due to allergens cause oedema and permanent thickening of the airways, making respiration more difficult. Treatments include changing the environment to prevent contact with allergens, e.g. turn out to grass or the use of hypoallergenic bedding, and the administration of anti-inflammatory medication such as corticosteroids and bronchodilators such as clenbuterol.

chronic pulmonary osteoarthropathy Seen as hard swellings above the toes of all four legs. A disease state of bony enlargement as a result of reduced oxygen supply after certain chronic lung diseases. Known also as hypertrophic pulmonary osteopathy.

chronic renal failure (CRF) May represent the end stage of a number of diseases affecting the kidneys.

CHV 1 Canine herpes virus 1; *see also* HERPES VIRUS.

chyle Milky fluid, the product of digestion in the intestines, which is carried in the lacteals to the thoracic duct.

chylomicron Large conglomerate of fats and protein in the blood; transports fat digestion products from the small intestine to the tissues after meals.

chylothorax The presence of chyle in the pleural space, often the result of traumatic damage to the thoracic duct or neoplasia of the mediastinum.

chyme The semiliquid product of digestion in the stomach, a mixture of food, saliva and gastric secretions that passes through the pylorus into the duodenum; normally has a low pH.

chymosin Enzyme produced in the stomach of the young animal to aid milk digestion.

cicatrix Contracted area, as seen when a wound heals leaving a scar.

ciclosporin Immunosuppressive compound (also called cyclosporin(e) or cyclosporin A); a cyclic oligopeptide able to block activated T cells; *see also* T CELLS.

cilia Fine, hair-like processes that cells can use to waft away mucous material. The word is also used for the eyelashes; *see also* ECTOPIC CILIA.

ciliary body An important part of the eye that supports the lens and contains muscles; these squeeze the contents and help the lens to focus. The ciliary body connects the choroid with the iris and produces the aqueous humour for the anterior chamber of the eye.

cimetidine A histamine H_2 receptor antagonist, used in tablet form to reduce the acidity of the stomach. Allows certain drugs to reach the small intestine that would be damaged by a low pH.

ciprofloxacin Antibacterial agent, effective mainly against Gram-negative aerobes; used in gastrointestinal and urinogenital infections. The ability to penetrate intracellularly makes it suitable for treating chlamydial and pseudomonal infections.

circadian rhythm Pattern of sleep followed by activity with associated physiological responses. The protein melanopsin produced in cells in the retina is involved in carrying information to the brain centre.

circle system An anaesthetic rebreathing system in which oxygen as the carrier and anaesthetic gases are delivered to the patient and carbon dioxide is removed.

circulation The passage of blood around the body.

circulatory shock Develops from circulatory insufficiency as the result of a fall in cardiac output; dilated capillaries with pervious walls lead to inadequate perfusion of the peripheral tissues.

circumanal (perianal) glands Sebaceous glands situated just outside the anus in a ring; *see also* ANAL ADENOMA.

cirrhosis A liver disease characterized by loss of normal hepatic cells and fibrosis causing scarring of the liver lobes.

cisterna magna Dilated area of the subarachnoid space at the base of the skull between the cerebellum and the medulla oblongata.

CITES Convention on International Trade in Endangered Species.

CJD *See* CREUTZFELDT–JAKOB DISEASE.

CK Creatinine kinase.

clavicle The collar bone; only of importance in the domestic cat. The dog has a tendon band but no bone.

clean-contaminated (wound) Description of a surgical wound that was sterile but has become contaminated. One example is the accidental leakage of the intestinal contents during an enterotomy.

clearing time During the development of a radiograph (X-ray) plate, the milky appearance of the plate after it is put in the fixer should become 'clear' after 30 seconds, but the plate should be left longer to fix.

cleft palate A fusion failure seen in the newborn animal. Newborn kittens and puppies should always have their mouths examined for congenital defects; the defect in the palate may allow milk to reflux down the nose while feeding; *see also* HARE LIP.

clindamycin Synthetic antibiotic used for treating contaminated wounds and for oral infections.

clinical Anything associated with the study and management of sick animals.

clinical audit A cyclical process of measuring clinical performance against agreed standards and implementing changes to improve quality of patient care.

clinical competence The skills and ability to provide clinical care safely and effectively without the need for supervision.

clinical effectiveness Understanding whether clinical actions are producing desired results. Collecting evidence of what works well can then be used to improve patient outcomes.

clinical governance The overall system for improving the quality of patient care.

clinical guidelines Recommendations on clinical care supported by the best available evidence from clinical research.

clinical negligence Failure of a vet or nurse to carry out their duty of care to a patient effectively.

clinical protocol The use of clinical evidence to design documented guidance systems for members of the clinical team to achieve best practice.

clinical record The record of the health of an animal kept by a practice; may be paper-based or held on computer.

clinical supervision Provision of guidance and support by an experienced and skilled professional for a less experienced professional or student to enable the supervisee to gain greater skills, knowledge and understanding of accountability in veterinary practice.

clinical trial A research study that, with owner's consent, enrols animals to take part in procedures, receive medication, use products, etc. to measure their effectiveness.

clinical quality indicators Specific quantitative measures that are used to assess and appraise the quality of clinical and support functions that affect patient outcomes so that quality can be improved.

Clinical Waste Regulations Legislation to regulate the disposal of undesirable materials. The Control of Pollution Act, Collection and Disposal of Clinical Waste Regulations and Environmental Protection Act should all be consulted.

clitoris Area of cavernous erectile tissue lying within the vulval cleft; the female equivalent of the penis in the male.

cloaca The external orifice of birds and reptiles; fulfils the dual function of excretion and reproduction.

clone Replica produced by artificial division of the DNA as a form of asexual reproduction; all clones contain the same genetic material.

closed-angle glaucoma The type of raised intraocular pressure caused by a shallow anterior chamber of the eye and a narrowed junction between the cornea and the iris, resulting in obstruction to the normal fluid outflow.

closed wounds Those where the skin surface is unbroken; *see also* CONTUSION, HAEMATOMA, RUPTURED SPLEEN.

Clostridium Group of bacteria characterized by their ability to survive for long periods away from the animal by forming resistant spores. They can cause serious illnesses such as tetanus, botulism poisoning and bacterial endotoxaemia.

clot A solid mass of blood (or lymph); the final result of coagulation.

cloxacillin Broad-spectrum antibiotic, one of the semisynthetic penicillins.

Cnemidocoptes Parasite of birds. One species, *C. pilae*, causes scaly beak in budgerigars.

CNS Central nervous system.

coagulase Enzyme produced by staphylococci; an antigenic substance often found in more pathogenic strains and related to thrombus formation in infected tissues.

coagulation Process of stopping bleeding by the clotting of blood.

coagulation disorders A general term for any condition of prolonged

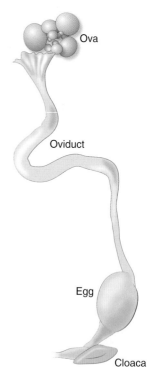

Figure 7. Chicken Reproductive System.

bleeding caused by an impaired clotting mechanism, includes von Willebrand's disease, DIC and haemophilia.

coagulopathy A disorder of blood coagulation; *see also* DIC, HAEMOPHILIA.

coaption The bringing together of tissue surfaces to aid healing.

coaxial Used to describe one tube running inside another; used in anaesthetic circuits with low resistance to expiration; *see also* LACK, BAIN SYSTEM.

cobalamin The vitamin B_{12} compound notable for containing the metal cobalt. Its measurement is used to assess absorption from the small intestine; *see also* MALABSORPTION.

Coccidia Single-cell organisms characterized as Sporozoa; they can live parasitically inside gut epithelial cells. Other species affect the liver cells. Can cause diarrhoea in rabbits and poultry, and sometimes also in puppies and kittens. Infection is through ingesting faeces, as resistant oocysts can remain viable in the soil for months.

coccidiosis Disease caused by multiplication within the body of minute protozoal parasites. *Eimeria* are a common cause of diarrhoea in the domestic rabbit. Treatment is by medicating the drinking water and improving hygiene. *Isospora* (or *Levineia*) are two species that infect dogs; another two species affect cats; uncommon except in puppies, kittens and immunosuppressed adults.

coccygeal Referring to the tail area.

cochlear Relating to the spiral tube in the inner ear known as the cochlea.

Code of Practice for the Promotion of Animal Medicines Code of practice that all UK manufacturers of veterinary medicines have to comply with; the Code is overseen by the National Office of Animal Health (NOAH).

Code of professional conduct The RCVS Code of Professional Conduct that identifies veterinary nurses' professional responsibilities.

Codman's triangle One of the radiographic features of an osteosarcoma, where areas of osteolysis and periosteal proliferation may outline a triangular shape.

coefficient of inbreeding Mathematical expression that predicts the likelihood of homozygosity occurring in offspring.

coefficient of relationship Mathematical expression of the relatedness of two individuals.

coeliotomy Incision into the abdomen; *see also* LAPAROTOMY.

coffin joint Foot joint of the horse between the second and third phalanges and the navicular bone.

cognition Mental facility to recognize and reason; an animal's first reaction is to investigate; subsequent processing of the information depends on the individual.

coitus Sexual union through the penis being inserted into the vagina to promote the release of semen for the intra-abdominal fertilization of eggs by the sperm; *see also* REPRODUCTION.

colectomy Excision of the colon is rare, but subtotal colectomy is sometimes a preferred treatment in chronic constipation of the cat when the ileocaecal junction is preserved.

Colibacillosis *See* Escherichia coli.

colic Abdominal discomfort, usually arising from the gastrointestinal tract; acute colic

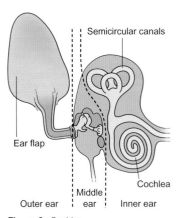

Figure 8. Cochlea.

in the horse is an emergency condition, which can have many causes such as intestinal obstruction, parasitic infestation and intestinal strangulation. Common types of colic are obstructive, flatulent and spasmodic; *see also* PAIN.

colitis Inflammation of the colon, a medical condition often associated with excessive mucoid faeces, sometimes alternating with periods of normal faecal output. Severe cases show tenesmus and blood; *see also* COLONIC INFLAMMATORY DISEASE.

collagen Protein substance that supplies strength to fibres in the body.

collateral A side branch of an anatomical structure. **Collateral ligament**, *see* LIGAMENTS.

collecting duct Found in the kidney between the distal convoluted tubes and the renal pelvis.

collie eye anomaly (CEA) A congenital, hereditary, bilateral eye condition of collie breeds where the choroid is hypoplastic; may result in blindness from a retinal haemorrhage; now most frequently found in the Shetland sheepdog; *see also* RETINAL DYSPLASIA.

collimation Coning down the X-ray beam to only the area of interest.

collimator Device for coning down the primary X-ray beam to only the area of interest.

colloid solution A solution in which small particles are permanently suspended. Colloidal particles will not pass through a semipermeable membrane; *see also* SEMIPERMEABLE MEMBRANE.

coloboma Defect of structure, often a pit; when applied to the eye it means a developmental defect in the wall of the sclera so that the choroid bulges through it. Eyelids lacking shape may be described as having a palpebral coloboma.

colon Part of the large intestine stretching from the caecum to the rectum; plays an important role in the absorption of water and salt. Particularly well developed in herbivores such as the rabbit.

colonic inflammatory disease Disease of the colon may be of a chronic

inflammatory nature and there are many possible causes; neoplasia and motility disturbances are separate diseases.

colorimeter Laboratory instrument for measuring fine colour differences.

colostrum The first fluid available to the newborn animal. Rich in proteins, it carries maternal antibodies and is replaced by the milk from the lactating animal's mammary glands.

colour Doppler imaging (CDI) A form of ultrasound used to show blood flow.

colposuspension Surgical technique used in the treatment of urinary incontinence: the bladder neck is attached to the prepubic tendon of the linea alba.

coma State of deep unconsciousness from which the patient is unable to be roused.

comedo, *pl.* comedones Blocked sebaceous glands often contaminated by skin bacteria; *see also* ACNE, HYPOTHYROIDISM.

commensal An organism that lives off another without causing harm to either.

comminuted fracture Injury where the bone is broken into many small pieces, as after impact with a high-speed vehicle or a crushing injury.

communicable disease A disease that may pass from one animal to another by direct contact, via an object such as a brush or through a vector such as an insect bite. All communicable diseases are transmissible, unlike metabolic diseases.

Community Protection Notice An option open to the police in England to control a dog through its keeper such as requiring a muzzle to be worn or kept on a lead when out of the home.

compact bone Found in the long bones for strength; dense arrangement of the haversian system increases durability but can still fracture when force is applied.

compensatory hyperdynamic shock In shock, there is an immediate rise in the heart rate, with both arterial and venous constriction that helps to increase the circulating blood volume and raises the blood pressure. Unfortunately, this response may not last, and treatment for shock with fluid therapy and other measures is needed and would be more suitable.

competitive advantage The benefit that one product or service has over its competitors, often based on a key attribute or unique proposition that people will value.

competitor A rival business or product.

complete blood cell count (CBC) Abbreviation frequently used when haematology is requested for a blood sample.

compound Any substance consisting of two or more elements chemically combined.

compounding The mixing of drugs by a veterinarian or pharmacist to meet the specific needs of a patient, e.g. mixing two injectable solutions or adding a medication to a topical paste.

compress Pressure pad applied to an open wound to stem bleeding; after a sprain or strain, a **cold compress** can be used to prevent swelling.

compulsive behaviour A ritualistic behaviour pattern such as tail chasing, flank sucking (particularly in the Dobermann pinscher), wool sucking (Siamese cats) and fly biting.

computed tomography (CT) scan Axial tomography, a method of studying deep structures by looking at 'slices' of the body with scanning X-rays.

concentration gradient Increased specific gravity as in renal filtration; may require active transport to overcome.

conception The start of pregnancy, following fertilization of the ovum.

conch (*pl.* conchae) Bony structure found in the nasal cavity, *see* TURBINATES.

concussion Trauma to the CNS causing a limited period of unconsciousness. Usually a head injury following an RTA is the cause.

conditioned response In behavioural terms, the intended response is elicited by a specific cue or situation. The conditioned response involves learned behaviours rather than fixed actions (instinctive behaviour).

condyle A rounded prominence on a bone, forming part of an articular surface.

cones, retinal Receptor cells in the retina more associated with colour vision,

although this does not necessarily apply to animals.

confidentiality Tacit agreement between an owner and a practice that privacy will be respected; clients have the right to see all computerized case records for their animal and details cannot be given to a third party without the client's consent.

conflict of interest A situation where there is the possibility of a clash between a person's or organization's self-interests and other professional or public interests.

congenital Describes a condition present at birth; it may be hereditary or develop after some injury during pregnancy.

congestive heart failure A serious condition where the pumping action of the heart is no longer adequate to maintain the circulation; signs are dilated veins and enlarged heart chambers; *see also* MYOCARDIUM.

conjunctiva The surface lining of the eyelids and covering of the sclera up to its junction with the cornea.

connective tissue Tissue systems to support and bind together other specific tissues.

consensual light reflex The constriction or dilation of the pupil of the eye opposite to the eye that is being stimulated (by light changes).

consent form A legal document that details the procedures to be carried out on an animal and the possible risks involved, which is signed by the owner, to give permission prior to proceeding.

constipation Faeces retained in the rectum and large intestine; hard lumps may be difficult to pass and straining may alert an owner to the problem. May be diet-related or caused by a painful prostate or pelvic injury.

consultant A fully trained specialist who accepts responsibility for diagnosis and advises on treatment; *see also* SPECIALIST.

contact inhibition The anticancer mechanism when a cell stops dividing when it comes into contact with another cell.

contagious disease Originally only a disease spread by direct animal-to-animal contact; today the term is often used for any communicable disease.

continuing education A lifelong learning process that involves attending courses, reading books and journals, etc. to stop the qualified person from 'stagnating'; *see also* CONTINUING PROFESSIONAL DEVELOPMENT.

continuing professional development (CPD) The requirement for all veterinary staff to undertake regular training to update their knowledge; can be through formal courses, attending congresses, etc.; 105 hours of CPD over 3 years are required for UK veterinarians and 45 hours over 3 years are required for RVNs.

continuity of care Once an animal has been accepted as an inpatient by a veterinary surgeon, responsibility for the animal remains with that veterinary surgeon or practice until another veterinary surgeon or practice accepts the responsibility.

continuous quality improvement A proactive approach to ensuring the likelihood of positive clinical outcomes using a Plan, Do, Study, Act cycle.

contract of employment An agreement between an employer and employee that sets out the terms and conditions of employment, commonly detailing pay, holidays, working hours, etc; once in force, it can only be changed with the agreement of both parties; written contracts are recommended as they prevent potential misunderstanding.

contrast media In diagnostic imaging, techniques such as radiography, CT or MRI, a substance used to highlight an organ or structure; positive contrast is provided by barium and iodine compounds; negative contrast is provided by air.

Control of Substances Hazardous to Health (COSHH) A set of regulations in the UK for safe and healthy working conditions.

controlled drug Specified category of POM-V (Prescription Only Medicine – Veterinary) drug; consists of five groups or schedules, but only four have veterinary application as a veterinary surgeon has no authority to possess

drugs from Schedule 1. It is a legal requirement to adhere to the Misuse of Drugs Act 1971 and the Misuse of Drugs Regulations 1985, regulations relating to the purchase, storage and recording of the use of controlled drugs. Prescribing veterinarian needs to include their RCVS membership number on any prescription for Schedule 2 or 3 drugs.

contusion Injury to tissue by a blunt object – similar to a bruise; the skin usually remains unbroken.

Coombs' test Test on blood used in the detection of primary autoimmune disease. Detects immunoglobulin G and/or M on erythrocytes in the sample. Positive results may also be found with other red cell membrane disorders such as anaemia, and with drug administration.

coprodeum Part of the cloaca in birds, separated by a mucosal fold from the urodeum.

coprophagia Undesirable habit of eating faeces, often acquired kennel behaviour owing to attractive food residues. The rabbit has a similar process to digest cellulose in the food but then the soft faecal pellets are taken directly from the rectum into the mouth; *see also* CAECOTROPHY.

copulation The act of sexual union; the word usually is only applied to animals; *see also* COITUS.

coracoid Bone in the shoulder joint of birds that runs from the keel to the shoulder.

corium Part of the skin equivalent to the dermis.

cornea Surface of the eye that is transparent to light as it totally lacks blood vessels and is composed of layers of parallel tissue: epithelium, stroma and Descemet's membrane.

corneal lens A protective soft contact lens placed over the cornea at the front of the eye to act as a bandage in dogs with corneal erosion to allow healing.

corneal sutures Must be very fine and with low irritancy; Ethilon 4/10 to 10/0 may be favoured.

cornification Hardening or keratinization of skin surface; may be excessive in some disorders such as seborrhoea.

corn snake *Elapae guttata* a member of the Colubridae family; has only a right lung and no caecum nor pelvic spur.

coronary arteries Blood vessels just below the pericardium supplying the heart muscle.

coronary band Found at the base of the nail in the epidermis or around the top of the hoof; the tissue of the coronary corium and perioplic corium, which together provide nourishment to the horn of the equine hoof.

coronavirus Single-stranded RNA virus associated with feline infectious peritonitis and with diarrhoea in dogs.

coronoid process There are two such bony prominences of importance in animals. One is found on the mandible near the temporomandibular joint. The other site is the medial coronoid process of the ulna, where the heads of the radius and ulna articulate with the humerus; *see also* OSTEOCHONDROSIS.

corpus callosum A band of fibres that connects the two cerebral hemispheres, found in the brainstem (diencephalon).

corpuscle Small cell or body; *see also* ERYTHROCYTE.

corpus luteum Literally 'yellow body', a structure found in the ovary after ovulation, responsible for hormone production (progesterone).

corpus spongiosum Part of the penis characterized by its vascular beds, which allow the penis to stiffen prior to mating; forms the bulb proximally and the glans distally.

cortex The outer part of a structure; variously applied to the forebrain, the filtering part of the kidney and the hardest part of the bone.

Corti, organ of The sensory region within the cochlea used in hearing assessment.

cortical bone Compact bone covered by periosteum.

cortical cataract Lens opacity that is first seen at the edge of the lens but then spreads across the capsule, causing loss of vision.

corticosteroid Steroid hormone produced by the adrenal cortex or synthesized in the laboratory.

corticotrophin-releasing hormone Hormone from the hypothalamus that controls secretion of ACTH by the anterior pituitary; *see also* ACTH.

cortisol Naturally occurring hormone produced by the adrenal cortex; *see also* HYDROCORTISONE.

coryza Profuse discharge from the mucous membrane of the nose, applies especially to birds.

cotton conform bandage Type of open-mesh, flexible bandage that makes applying dressings to limbs of the dog easier than using white open-wove (WOW) bandages.

cough Expulsive effort originating in the thorax; usually a reflex action to expel mucus or foreign matter but may be caused by unusual pressure on the airways, e.g. cardiac cough from a dilated atrium.

counterconditioning A process of training an animal to respond to another stimulus so that it engages in a behaviour that is incompatible with the previous undesirable behaviour, e.g. barking at the postman.

coupage A physiotherapy manoeuvre used to assist the removal of fluids from the thorax; a chopping action of percussion over the ribs; from the French word *couper*, to cut.

covalency Bonding of atoms to form a molecule.

cow hocks An abnormal conformation of the horse seen when the hocks are too close together.

cow pox Viral infection that sometimes affects cats as a spreading papular eruption.

coxa plana Flattening of the head of the femur, one of the radiographic signs of damage to the epiphysis.

coxa vara Deformity of the hip joint with a change in the angle of articulation.

coxitis Inflammation of the hip joint.

CPK Creatine phosphokinase. Three isoenzymes occur, found in skeletal muscle, cardiac muscle and the CNS. Used to measure muscle damage, may increase tenfold.

CPR Cardiopulmonary resuscitation; an emergency procedure to use when breathing stops, as well as in circulatory failure; known as the 3-minute emergency; *see also* CARDIOPULMONARY RESUSCITATION.

cramp A general term applied to painful muscle spasms.

cranial Closest to the head or the cranium.

cranial nerves Twelve pairs of nerves that originate in the nervous tissue of the brain and extend through the cranium to reach their targets: **I** Olfactory nerve; **II** Optic nerve; **III** Oculomotor nerve; **IV** Trochlear nerve; **V** Trigeminal nerve; **VI** Abducens nerve; **VII** Facial nerve; **VIII** Vestibulocochlear nerve; **IX** Glossopharyngeal nerve; **X** Vagus nerve; **XI** Spinal accessory nerve; **XII** Hypoglossal nerve.

craniocaudal Means in simple terms 'from the front to the rear'. Used as the direction of entry of the X-ray beam as when examining the elbow joint.

craniomandibular osteopathy A specific disease of the West Highland white terrier breed as an autosomal recessive condition but also seen in Scottish terriers, other terriers and rarely in large breeds such as the Pyrenean mountain dog and the boxer. Known also as 'lion jaw', it is a nonneoplastic proliferation of bone that may affect the joint, causing difficulty in opening the mouth owing to a symmetrical enlargement of the bones of the mandible; other skull bones may also be affected.

cranium The dome of the skull, and the other bones that surround the brain.

crash trolley Trolley containing equipment and drugs for emergency resuscitation; all clinical staff should know where the trolley is and how to use the equipment.

creatine A nonprotein substance synthesized by the body from amino acids.

creatinine A product of creatine metabolism and constantly formed in muscle; it can be measured in the blood as a reliable indicator of renal function; normally there is a constant excretion of creatinine in the urine.

cremaster Muscle found in the spermatic cord, responsible in the male rabbit for retracting the testes into the abdomen outside the breeding season. Most other domestic animals have very restricted voluntary control of this muscle.

cremation Disposing of a body by burning; considered environmentally sound; *see also* CLINICAL WASTE REGULATIONS.

crenation Appearance of erythrocytes often seen after slow air drying of films or from shrinkage when blood is placed in a hypertonic solution.

crepitus Grating feeling or noise when broken bone fragments move across each other or roughened cartilage. Similarly, a sound is heard with the stethoscope when there is a dry lung inflammation; also known as crepitations.

Creutzfeldt–Jakob disease (CJD) Human disease of spongiform encephalopathy; the 'new form' variant has been related to the ingestion of beef products. Characterized by a very long incubation period of 10 years or more. The main effect of control regulations for pets is that raw, hard beef bones are no longer freely available for dogs to chew, as a result of perceived disease risks.

CRF Chronic renal failure.

crib biting When a horse grips an object (often the top of their stable door) in order to stretch its neck and gulp air. The gulping is called wind-sucking; both crib-biting and wind-sucking are considered to be stable vices.

cricoid A ring structure; usually means one of the cartilage structures that make up the larynx.

Crimean Congo haemorrhagic fever A tickborne viral disease common in East and West Africa; may affect animals and is zoonotic, having caused a recorded death in the UK, notifiable in Australia.

critical care unit (intensive care unit, ICU, CCU) Area set aside specifically for nursing high-dependency, critically ill patients.

crop An enlargement of the distal oesophagus of a bird that stores food, allowing it to soften and swell prior to entering the glandular proventriculus.

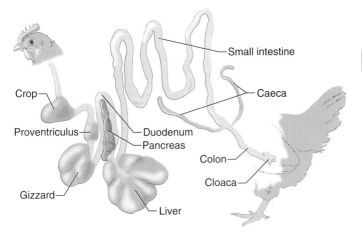

Figure 9. Chicken Digestive System.

cross-breeding Indicates an out-cross of two different strains of the same species; this will help to reduce the effect of recessive genes that may be harmful in close breeding.

cross-matching A test necessary for determining the compatibility between donor blood and recipient blood before transfusion; the clumping of red blood cells indicates incompatibility.

CRRT Continuous renal replacement therapy; a treatment used for patients with acute renal failure often due to poisoning or septic shock.

cruciate Shaped like a cross; usually applied to the ligaments between the femur and tibia: the anterior and posterior cruciate ligaments.

crura (of diaphragm) Bands of fibromuscular tissue that arise in the lumbar vertebrae and attach to the central tendon of the diaphragm.

crush cage Wire cage with a movable wall, often used to restrain feral patients.

cryosurgery Method of surgical treatment using an intensely cold source to freeze tissue.

cryotherapy The application of cold to an area of the body, which decreases the flow of fluid to the tissues and slows the release of chemicals that cause pain and inflammation.

crypt A blind pit, used anatomically, as in the crypts of Lieberkühn of the intestine.

crypto- Meaning 'hidden', usually combined with another word.

cryptorchid Usually indicates that at least one testis has not descended into the scrotum, but strict definition would mean that both testes are hidden in the abdominal cavity.

Cryptosporidium Coccidia-like parasites that may enter drinking water supplies, affecting humans and house pets; *C. meleagridis* causes disease in birds.

crystalloid Substances of inorganic origin dissolved in water, commonly used to describe the 'salts' group of intravenous fluids. The other group of replacement fluids are known as colloids.

crystals Aggregation of molecules in solution, looked for in centrifuged urine. The sediment may normally contain crystals, depending on the urine pH.

CsA Ciclosporin A; used as suppressor of immune cell activation in autoimmune and allergic diseases; *see also* CICLOSPORIN.

CSF Cerebrospinal fluid. A protective fluid layer that surrounds the spinal cord and brain and circulates nutrients within the brain ventricles.

CT *See* COMPUTED TOMOGRAPHY.

Ctenocephalides The commonest genus of fleas of the dog and cat.

culpability Responsibility or accountability for a fault, error or accident.

cupula Found in the semicircular canals of the inner ear as a jelly-like substance; a balance control; *see also* ENDOLYMPH.

curette Surgical instrument shaped like a long-handled spoon used for cleaning out diseased tissue from a wound, obtaining cancellous bone graft, etc.

cushingoid Describes any disorder with signs of increased thirst, muscle weakness, pendulous abdomen and hair loss that is not caused by hyperadrenocorticism.

Cushing's disease Hyperadrenocorticism; may be caused by an adrenal cortex tumour or overstimulation by the pituitary gland; *see also* PDH.

cusp A small flange as seen in a tooth or the tricuspid heart valve's structure.

cutaneous Relating to the skin surface.

cutaneous trunci reflex Used to test spinal nerve reflexes; *see also* PANNICULUS.

cutdown, venous Method of introducing a cannula into a vein by making a small skin incision immediately above the vein; a hypodermic needle or a scalpel blade may be used.

cuticle The outermost covering: sometimes used to describe the skin, the outermost part of the hair shaft, part of the nail, or in birds, the eggshell covering.

cutis Alternative skin name; *see also* DERMIS.

CVA Cerebrovascular accident; usually an intracranial haemorrhage or a haemorrhage onto the brain surface following injury.

CVO Chief Veterinary Officer. The head of the Department of Food Rural

Affairs and Agriculture (DEFRA) for all veterinary matters.

cyanocobalamin Vitamin B_{12}.

cyanosis Bluish appearance of the skin, tongue or mucous membranes caused by insufficient oxygen reaching the tissues. An alternative term used is 'dusky', and remedial action is urgent; *see also* RESUSCITATION.

cycloplegia Term used in eye disease where the pupils do not constrict with light; the paralysis may be the result of medication or nerve injury when there is fixed dilation of the pupils; *see also* MYDRIASIS.

cyclophosphamide Cytotoxic agent effective in neoplasia treatments, especially proliferative lymphoid tumours.

cyclosporine *See* ciclosporin.

cyesis Pregnancy; *see also* PSEUDOCYESIS.

Cynicomyces A genus of yeasts found in the rabbit's caecum and necessary for digestion of fibre.

cyst Defined as a fluid-filled cavity; some are called **retention cysts**. The **prostate cyst**, which causes prostate enlargement, is one example, but this may only account for 5% of prostate disease in the dog.

cystic endometrial hyperplasia Condition of the lining of the uterus that may develop in metoestrus; *see also* PYOMETRA.

Cysticercus tenuicollis Larval stage of the tapeworm of the dog, *Taenia hydatigena*, found in offal of sheep, pigs and wild ruminants, on which dogs may feed.

cystine calculi One of the more common types of calculus in dogs as they form in acidic urine; may cause obstructions. They are 'stones' produced by errors of the metabolism of cystine and lysine.

cystitis Inflammation of the bladder, may be caused by bacterial infection or irritation from calculi.

cystocentesis Procedure to puncture the bladder via the abdominal wall with a sterile needle or cannula in order to obtain a urine sample.

cystogram A picture of the bladder taken with X-rays, usually involves a positive or a negative contrast agent; *see also* PNEUMOCYSTOGRAM.

cystopexy Procedure to fix the bladder wall to the abdominal wall; may help to draw the vagina out of the pelvic canal and contribute to the control of urinary incontinence.

cystoscopy Endoscopic examination of the urinary bladder.

cystotomy Surgical procedure to open up the bladder; first involves a laparotomy incision.

cytokines Substances that are involved in the inflammatory response and are part of cell-mediated immunity.

cytology The study of the cell structure.

cytopathic Toxic substances that work at the individual cell level causing disease and cell death.

cytoplasm The substance of the cell other than the nuclear material and the organelles; *see also* PROTOPLASM.

cytoplasmic droplets Structures along the tail of immature sperm, either distal or proximal. Immature sperm are usually the result of some testicular insult.

cytotoxic An agent that destroys the cells; may be used in neoplasia treatments.

Czerny–Lambert An inverting suture at one time much in favour for repair of intestinal incisions as the suture material passed through the mucosa only.

dacryoadenitis Inflammation of the lacrimal gland of the eye.

dacryocystitis Inflammation of the lacrimal sac, usually occurring when the duct draining the tears to the nose is blocked; *see also* LACRIMAL GLAND.

dactyl Relating to a digit or toe.

Dangerous Dogs Act Act of Parliament introduced in 1991 that was designed to stop people from keeping specific breeds of dogs traditionally used for fighting; relates also to the Wildlife and Countryside Act 1981, as any dog found disturbing livestock can be legally shot.

Dangerous Wild Animals Act Act of Parliament from 1976 prohibiting the keeping of any dangerous animal unless a licence has been issued by the local authority; the premises and the animal will be inspected by a veterinary surgeon accompanied by an environmental health officer prior to licensing, and there is an annual relicensing inspection; a list of animals considered dangerous is available.

DAP Dog appeasement pheromone.

darkroom Area set aside for developing radiographs and reloading radiograph cassettes, usually a lightproof room.

dartos The muscle under the skin of the scrotum that causes it to wrinkle and helps to contract the size of the scrotal sac.

Data Protection Act European legislation allowing individuals to have access to records about themselves; an individual must give consent for his/her personal data to be stored electronically.

Day One Competences The essential skills, stipulated by the RCVS, that a veterinary nurse or surgeon must have mastered by graduation.

DCM Dilated cardiomyopathy; *see* CARDIOMYOPATHY.

DCRV Double chambered right ventricle. A rare congenital heart disease of dogs.

DDSP Dorsal displacement of the soft palate. A dynamic obstruction of the horse's airway that may occur during exercise, often associated with a small epiglottis.

deadly nightshade Garden and hedgerow weed that has berries containing atropine, which could cause death if eaten in any quantity.

dead space 1) Surgical term used to describe a poorly apposed gap in the tissues that is likely to fill with serum or blood and then become infected. **2)** In the respiratory system, it represents the part that contains air but does not exchange oxygen and carbon dioxide at the alveolar level.

deafness Total or partial loss of hearing in one or both ears. Obstruction in the external canal and loss of sensory nerve routes (sensorineural deafness) are the two most frequent causes; *see also* BRAINSTEM AUDITORY EVOKED RESPONSE.

deamination A process of metabolism in the liver when protein from the diet is used to produce new amino acids or to provide energy and ammonia is released; normally the liver converts the ammonia to urea for excretion by the kidneys.

death, signs of Absence of heartbeat, no respiratory movement, dilation of pupils with loss of eye reflexes, loss of corneal reflex, glazing of the cornea, body cooling and eventual rigor mortis in 12 hours.

debility Weakness, loss of body strength; multiple causes of this condition; *see also* ANAEMIA.

debridement Cleaning up a wound by removal of contaminating foreign matter and devitalized tissue, healing then takes place by granulation if coaptation is impossible; *see also* WOUNDS.

debulking procedure Technique used in tumour surgery to remove the majority of the neoplastic mass to make the remainder more suitable for chemotherapy or radiotherapy.

decerebrate rigidity A severe neurological sign seen after a head injury that often indicates a midbrain lesion. Signs in the unconscious patient are of a change in posture with the fore- and hindlegs and the neck held in extensor rigidity.

deciduous Something that falls off or sheds; most commonly used for temporary dentition (milk teeth), which fall out early in life.

declawing Onychectomy involves the removal of the claw and the terminal phalanx; it is generally discouraged but has been used to prevent furniture injury by an active cat. The paws are usually bandaged for the first 24 hours postoperatively.

decompression Applied to acute neurological situations, raised pressure of fluid on the brain being an example of a need for urgent surgical or medical attention.

decubital ulcers A skin ulcer produced by prolonged lying down; usually affects the point of the elbow where there is little soft tissue between the bony prominences and the skin.

decussate Crossing, especially in a Y-shape.

decussation The point at which two or more objects in the body cross over; applies especially to nerve tracts; *see also* OPTIC CHIASMA.

deep pain sensation Pain measured by the animal's attitude and behaviour; not always easy to assess but is an important prognostic indicator in spinal injuries. A test for deep pain is to crush the base of the nail with artery forceps.

defaecation Act of passing faeces through the anus from the rectum; involves both conscious expulsion and involuntary peristaltic movement to fill the rectum.

deferent 1) Vessel or nerve that conducts away from the centre. 2) Relating to the vas deferens in the male reproductive system.

defibrillation Use of a defibrillator to restart or correct cardiac contractions.

defibrillator Electrical equipment used in ventricular fibrillation to give a controlled electric shock to restore normal heart rhythm in cases of cardiac arrest. Can also be used to rectify atrial fibrillation.

deficiency Anything caused by a lack of a substance; deficiency diseases result from insufficiency of some essential nutrient in the diet; *see also* RICKETS, TAURINE.

definitive host Point in the life cycle of a parasite where the sexual stage of the infecting organism occurs.

DEFRA Department of Environment Food and Rural Affairs.

degenerative joint disease (DJD) Progressive condition leading to erosion of cartilage and new bone deposits around the joint; *see also* ARTHRITIS.

degloving injury Major injury after accidents when the skin is peeled back from the subcutaneous tissue with loss of associated blood supply. Skin flaps may be non-viable and have to be removed before surgery involving skin transplantation techniques; *see also* AVULSION.

deglutition Swallowing. Birds have a special swallowing mechanism that allows the crop to fill even when the head is down for floor feeding.

degranulation Loss of granules as a part of the secretory process. Mast cells release histamine.

dehiscence Splitting open, often after trauma; a surgical wound that opens.

dehydration A reduction in the total body water content and the signs associated with deficiency of water in the tissues and circulation, caused by diseases, shock or inadequate fluid intake.

delayed suture Method for dealing with contaminated wounds where, after debridement and coaptation of tissues, the skin is left open to granulate before being closed by suturing once the tissues have cleaned; *see also* DEBRIDEMENT, THIRD INTENTION HEALING.

delayed union Term used for a bone fracture that heals more slowly than expected.

delegation The passing of authority and responsibility for a task from one person to another; effective delegation is a key management skill.

delirium Disordered mental state, shown as excessive behaviour when an animal is handled but returning to previous state if left alone.

delivery Term to denote activity in parturition.

delta Fourth letter of Greek alphabet having the form of a triangle D. The delta cells of the pancreas secrete somatostatin; *see also* SOMATOSTATIN.

DELTA Society in the USA that has great influence in human–companion animal interactions.

deltoid A muscle of the shoulder joint that has two heads; a large muscle named because of its triangular shape.

demi- Prefix denoting 'half of'.

***Demodex* spp.** Ectoparasitic mites that inhabit hair follicles and may cause little irritation. Each species is specific to the host. In immunosuppressed and growing animals, the parasites cause a pruritic response with hair loss and sometimes secondary bacterial infection; *see also* PUSTULE.

demulcent Substance used to protect and soothe mucous membranes, relieves irritation by coating the surface; milk and honey are used in first aid.

demyelination Degenerative process of nerve tissue where the myelin sheath is destroyed or removed.

denature Remove a principle or alter a protein structure; the change in a protein, through heat or enzyme activity, which can alter its biological activity.

dendrite Tree-like arrangement of branches from a nerve cell, involved in nerve conduction.

denervation Interruption of the nerve supply to the muscles or section of a nerve that conducts sensation to the CNS.

dens Tooth or tooth-like structure. The second cervical vertebra has a cranially projecting process known as the dens.

dental Relating to the teeth; may be used to describe a nurse or a hygienist.

dental abrasion A condition in horses where there is wearing of the teeth

caused by a tooth rubbing against an object, as in crib-biting.

dental attrition A condition in horses where there is wearing of the teeth caused by teeth rubbing against other teeth.

dental formula A shorthand way of writing the number of teeth, detailing the number of upper and lower incisors, canines, premolars and molars on each side of the jaw.

dentigerous cyst A cyst of dental origin, causing a local swelling on the jaw.

dentine Sensitive calcified tissue forming the bulk of the tooth; it is covered by the outer enamel and there is a central pulp cavity; *see also* TOOTH.

dentistry The profession of caring for, repairing and repositioning teeth.

dentition Normal teeth in the dental arches of the mouth; may be deciduous or permanent.

deoxyribonucleic acid *See* DNA.

de Pezzer catheter A mushroom-shaped tip gives the name; sometimes used for tube gastrotomy.

depigmentation Loss of normal colour, seen in some skin diseases. Internasal depigmentation is common in dogs in the winter months; *see also* VITILIGO.

depolarization Reversal of the electrical potential across a membrane as a result of the movement of charged ions; part of the transmission of nerve impulses.

dermal Relating to the skin.

dermal adhesive A special type of glue that is used to hold edges of skin tissue together while the wound heals; can be used instead of sutures in some wounds and can reduce the likelihood of scarring.

Dermanyssus gallinae Poultry mite that occurs in many aviary-reared birds, known also as red mite; it can cause severe anaemia in the host.

dermatitis Any inflammatory condition of the skin, especially from some outside influence such as bacteria, parasites, fungi and mechanical damage.

dermatology The scientific study of skin disease.

dermatome 1) Instrument for taking split-thickness skin grafts. 2) Area of skin innervated by a single spinal nerve.

dermatomycosis Fungal infection of the skin; *see also* RINGWORM.

dermatomyositis Disease syndrome characterized by muscle weakness and dermatitis.

Dermatophagoides A genus of very small mites that feed on household dust and are now considered one of the most important causes of skin allergies in dogs.

Dermatophilus congolensis Gram-positive parasitic bacterium that causes dermatitis; infection often arises acutely in horses after heavy rain – hence the colloquial names of rain scald and mud fever.

dermatophytosis Fungal infection of the skin; *see also* RINGWORM.

dermatosis Any non-specific disorder of the skin.

dermis The true skin layer, lying immediately beneath the epidermis; it contains blood vessels, lymphatics, nerve endings, glands and hair follicles; *see also* CORIUM.

dermoid cyst A cyst containing curled round hair, sebum and skin debris; often found along the back or on the head, representing the fusion sites of the embryo's ectoderm. A congenital condition where hairs grow from the cornea or bulbar conjunctiva onto the eye surface.

descemetocele A bulging of Descemet's membrane of the eye that may appear when the overlying corneal layers are eroded, as in a deep corneal ulcer; requires urgent attention.

Descemet's membrane The innermost lining of the cornea; this structure is important in the healing of corneal wounds.

descenting Surgical removal of the perianal scent glands of the ferret; not performed in the UK but still performed in some countries; removal does not stop the 'must' smell as this comes from skin glands.

desensitization 1) Medical procedure to reduce an allergic response by giving small but progressively increasing doses of antigen by injection. 2) In behavioural therapy, systematic exposure to an adverse stimulus beginning at a low intensity that provokes only a mild response then gradually increasing the intensity; used to reduce anxiety, to habituate an animal to a lower-intensity stimulus (e.g. noise of telephone bell, etc.); *see also* NOISE PHOBIA, HYPOSENSITIZATION.

desflurane A volatile liquid anaesthetic gas administered with oxygen for induction and maintenance of anaesthesia. It is a fluorinated methyl ether that has the most rapid onset and offset time of any of the other volatile anaesthetic gases.

desquamation Sloughing of epidermal cells.

detrusor Smooth muscle of the bladder that contracts to expel urine.

develop Chemical process that converts grains of silver halide to black silver particles on a film that has been exposed to X-radiation.

developer Solution used as a reducing agent in the first stage of radiographic film processing; consists of either phenidone-hydroquinone or metol-hydroquinone.

Devil facial tumour disease A cancerous infection of the mouth and face caused by the bites of Tasmanian devils, a small, wild rodent found in Tasmania; notifiable disease in Australia.

devitalization Loss of blood supply to tissue; seen especially after trauma and makes the tissue non-viable.

dewclaw Vestigial first digits that still have a function in racing dogs when cornering at speed; hind dewclaws are better removed when the dog is young, although the tendency now is to leave the front claws, unless, as in some terrier breeds, the claw grows in a half circle, penetrating the flesh.

dewlap The loose fold of skin hanging below the neck of rabbits, etc.

dexamethasone A synthetic analogue of cortisol with a potent anti-inflammatory action; available as oral, injectable and topical preparations; may produce polyuria/polydipsia. Sudden withdrawal of the drug after long-term use may predispose to Addison's disease.

dextran Used in fluid therapy, it consists of a polymer of glucose with side chains to prolong the osmotic action. A large molecule, it remains in the circulation and is not lost via the kidneys. Used as a plasma expander and useful if plasma is not available.

dextrose saline Crystalloid solution used in fluid therapy mainly to replace water and chloride deficits as the strength of the isotonic solution does not allow sufficient glucose to be provided as an energy source.

diabetes insipidus A condition characterized by polyuria and polydipsia, the production of urine with a low specific gravity and without glucosuria. It is most commonly caused by defective antidiuretic hormone (ADH) secretion by the pituitary gland; also a less common nephrogenic form where the kidney is insensitive to ADH. Diagnosis is based on a water-deprivation test and response to ADH.

diabetes mellitus Metabolic disease where carbohydrate, fat and protein metabolism is defective owing to a failure to produce or respond to insulin. Diagnosis is based on elevated fasting plasma glucose levels, and if these exceed the renal threshold, glucose will be present in the urine. The most common form in animals is type I diabetes mellitus, where B cells in the islets of Langerhans of the pancreas fail to produce sufficient insulin; treatment for this form of the disease includes regular administration of insulin and other hypoglycaemic agents, and diet. Type II (non-insulin-dependent) arises when the body fails to respond to secreted insulin; *see also* INSULIN.

diagnosis The art and science of determining the cause of illness by considering the patient's signs and symptoms, the history provided by the owner, together with such laboratory tests and imaging techniques as needed.

dialysis Form of filtration where mineral salt molecules diffuse through a semipermeable membrane. **Peritoneal dialysis** involves use of the peritoneum as a semipermeable membrane: isotonic fluid is injected into the abdomen and then withdrawn – solutes may pass from the bloodstream into the fluid and hence be removed from the body.

diapedesis The outward passage of blood cells through the capillary walls into tissue spaces.

diaphragm Muscular structure that divides the thoracic cavity from the abdominal cavity; there are tendinous parts nearer the abdominal floor and important entry points for major conducting structures that need to pass from one cavity to the other, such as the aorta and oesophagus.

diaphragm, ruptured An abnormal tear in the diaphragm, usually after abdominal trauma; the tear may allow abdominal viscera to enter the thoracic cavity, causing rapid breathing, collapse and death if untreated; *see also* HERNIA.

diaphysis The shaft of a long bone; consists of a tube of hard cortical bone with a marrow cavity.

diarrhoea Rapid passage of soft faecal matter from the intestines to the exterior; the passage of abnormally soft or liquid faeces is accompanied by fluid and electrolyte losses (particularly bicarbonate and potassium).

diarthrosis Joint articulation where there is free movement between the bone ends through the joint capsule and supporting structures; *see also* SYNOVIA.

diastole The part of the contraction cycle of the heart that represents the relaxation of the atria and ventricles and the time when they are filling again with blood.

diastolic blood pressure The lowest blood pressure, measured when the heart is in the relaxed phase of the cardiac cycle. See also BLOOD PRESSURE.

diathermy Method of using high-frequency electric currents to elevate the temperature of a small area of tissue so that blood coagulates; at a higher frequency it can be used to cut tissue. A type of diathermy is also used to deliver moderate heat for physiotherapy purposes in the treatment of deep-seated pain.

diathesis Haemorrhage, as seen in many blood clotting disorders.

diazepam A sedative and anxiolytic; may be used as a premedicant prior to general anaesthesia and is also used to control epileptiform seizures; when given intravenously it can be used to stimulate the appetite in cats; *see also* EPILEPSY.

DIC Disseminated intravascular coagulation. A serious disorder where activation of the coagulation and fibrinolytic pathways leads to the formation of thrombi in small vessels and an increased tendency to haemorrhage; associated with some viral infections, neoplasia, heat stroke and liver disease; the prognosis is very poor.

dicoumarol Potent anticoagulant; may be found in mouldy hay fed to smaller pets.

diencephalon The thalamus and hypothalamus; a relay station between the forebrain and the brainstem, it controls autonomic and endocrine functions.

diet Mixture of foods that the animal eats; the diet should meet the minimum nutritional requirements for that animal and specific diets may be advisable for certain disease states.

dietary hypersensitivity Allergy to a component of the diet, where certain foods precipitate responses varying from severe gastroenteritis to skin rashes; the basis of treatment is to feed an elimination diet that is bland and contains a 'novel' protein source which the animal is unlikely to have come into contact with before; other elements can then be added one at a time, to identify the allergen.

differential white cell count Laboratory technique where the white blood cells are counted manually on a thin blood smear or using an automatic processor; the relative numbers of neutrophils, eosinophils, basophils, lymphocytes and monocytes are obtained to assist in diagnosis.

diffusion The random movement of particles in a solution or gas so that they eventually become evenly distributed.

digestibility Amount of food in the diet that can be absorbed and not lost in the faeces.

digestible energy (DE) Measure of the proportion of food consumed that is available as energy as opposed to the amount lost in faeces, etc.

digestion Process of breaking down complex dietary substances into smaller particles and constituents that can be absorbed through the intestinal wall.

digital extensor muscles Group of muscles running on the cranial aspect of the fore- or hindlimb that will extend the toes during locomotion.

digital flexor muscles Group of muscles running on the caudal aspect of the fore- or hindlimb that act to flex the toes and push the animal forwards.

digital radiography Radiographic technique where the image is recorded electronically; a computer is used to set the exposure and a digital image is produced. This is now the most common method of radiography.

digoxin Traditional medicine derived from the foxglove leaf; as a glycoside it slows and strengthens contraction of the cardiac muscle; *see also* INOTROPIC.

dilatation Stretching or enlargement, usually applied to a hollow organ or opening. **Gastric dilatation** is distension of the stomach with gas; a disorder usually affecting the larger breeds of dog; it arises mainly soon after feeding and can rapidly become life-threatening, as it impairs respiration; *see also* AEROPHAGIA, TYMPANY.

diluent Substance that makes a solution more dilute; in the case of a freeze-dried vaccine it is the fluid that is added to dissolve the pellet prior to injection.

dilution gene Recessive gene that reduces the pigment in hair so that black coat colour is diluted to blue and chocolate is diluted to lilac.

Dioctophyma renale Type of worm occasionally found in the kidneys of dogs and wild carnivores.

dioestrus The luteal phase of the reproductive cycle, between metoestrus and the next oestrus; *see also* METOESTRUS.

Dipetalonema reconditum A filarial worm of the dog, transmitted by fleas and lice; microfilariae may be found in the bloodstream and adult forms in connective tissue and viscera.

diphasic Having two distinct forms, characteristic feature of the temperature recording in certain viral infections.

Diphyllobothrium latum Known as the fish tapeworm, may inhabit the intestine of cats or dogs that have fed on raw fish.

diploe Folding over or overlapping of bones, as found in the skull.

diploid Having the normal number of chromosomes; all cells of the body are diploid, apart from ova and sperm, which are haploid and have only half the number of chromosomes; the diploid number is restored when an ovum is fertilized.

Dipylidium caninum The most common tapeworm of pet dogs and cats in the UK; fleas and lice are the usual intermediate hosts.

Dirofilaria immitis Heartworm of the dog, living in the heart and large blood vessels; microfilariae may be demonstrated on the blood smear; transmission is by mosquito bites, and the condition occurs in tropical and subtropical regions or in imported animals.

dirty Unclean or contaminated; *see also* WOUNDS.

Disability Discrimination Act 1995 Act of Parliament that prohibits discrimination on grounds of disability and applies to employers with 20 or more staff. Only applicable in Northern Ireland as replaced by the Equality Act 2010 in rest of UK; *see also* EQUALITY ACT.

disbud Term used for the removal of the growing horn buds in young animals such as goats.

disc Round, flattened structure such as the optic disc, where the optic nerve enters the eye, or an intervertebral disc between adjacent vertebrae.

discharge Fluid flowing from a wound or body cavity.

discharge procedures Routine that the nurse should follow whenever a patient leaves the hospital accommodation.

discoid lupus erythematosus Rare autoimmune condition, seen as small skin plaques often on the feet or around the nose; the plaques may ulcerate and the condition is often exacerbated by sunlight; biopsy confirmation is advised; *see also* LUPUS, SLE.

discospondylitis Bacterial infection of an intervertebral disc and the adjacent end plates of the vertebrae.

disease Any morbid disorder with a specific cause; signs and symptoms can be recognized. Injuries and accidents are excluded from this definition.

disinfectant Agent that destroys or removes all bacteria, viruses and fungi, includes environmental and skin disinfectants. The major types of disinfectant are alcohol, bleaches (hypochlorite), aldehydes, chlorhexidine, iodophors and quaternary ammonia compounds; *see also* ANTISEPTIC.

disinfection The process of eliminating microorganisms from contaminated instruments, surfaces, skin, etc. by the use of physical or chemical means; does not include killing spores.

dislocation Disruption of a joint so that there is loss of contact between the articular surfaces; *see also* LUXATION.

dispensing Method of legally issuing appropriate medication to animals according to their sales group as indicated in the Veterinary Medicines Regulations 2005; current groups are POM-V (prescription-only medicine – veterinarian), POM-VPS (prescription-only medicine – veterinarian, pharmacist, suitably qualified person), NFA-VPS (non-food animal – veterinarian, pharmacist, suitably qualified person), AVM-GSL (authorized veterinary medicine – general sales list). An SQP (suitably qualified person) is someone who has passed the necessary examinations and is currently on the register of approved people; *see also* PRESCRIBING, VMR.

dissect 1) To cut or separate tissue structures, usually for anatomical study. 2) In surgery, to separate different tissue structures along natural lines by dividing the connective tissue.

disseminated intravascular coagulation *See* DIC.

dissociative anaesthesia Type of general anaesthesia produced by agents such as ketamine; the agent produces good analgesia, with only superficial sleep – the patient is dissociated from its surroundings; muscle relaxation may not be sufficient for some procedures; respiratory depression is mild and blood pressure may rise with these agents.

distad Distally, towards the periphery.

distal Furthest away, distad; *see also* PROXIMAL.

distal convoluted tubule Part of the kidney where the loop of Henle runs towards the collecting duct.

distal denervating disease A syndrome in the dog characterized by progressive, severe, flaccid paralysis of all four limbs; reflexes are depressed or absent, although sensation remains intact. The aetiology remains obscure; prognosis is good, with most animals making a full recovery, although this may take several months.

distemper Specific Morbillivirus infection principally affecting the dog and ferret but now largely controlled by the use of effective vaccines; contagious and produces severe-to-fatal disease primarily in puppies; clinical signs include pyrexia, oculonasal discharge, cough and neurological signs; after recovery, dogs may develop hard pads, distemper teeth and old dog encephalitis; *see also* CHOREA, HARD PAD.

distemper teeth Adult teeth with pitted, discoloured enamel, resulting from distemper infection in puppyhood.

distichiasis Presence of a double row of eyelashes at the lid margin, which may rub against the cornea.

disuse atrophy Wasting of a limb muscle as a result of reduced use of the limb;

causes include pain, fracture, soft tissue injury, etc.

diuretic Drug that increases urine output.

diversification As a strategy to grow a business, diversification involves taking a new product or service to a new group of customers; for a veterinary practice, this might be opening an adjacent boarding facility, for example.

diverticulum Sac or pouch opening from a hollow structure such as the alimentary tract.

DM Diabetes mellitus.

DNA Deoxyribonucleic acid. The basic structure of all genes, consisting of a double helix of deoxyribose sugars, linked by the purines adenine and guanine, and the pyrimidines cytosine and thymine. Forms part of the genetic material of the cell nucleus in the chromatin fibres, which consist of long-chain molecules of DNA and associated protein.

DNA probes Laboratory technique used to identify bacteria in tissues, especially if they are slow growing or difficult to isolate.

docking Deliberately removing all or part of an animal's tail; defined as an act of veterinary surgery. There are RCVS advisory rules on who shall carry out docking and in what circumstances it should be done.

Doctor Courtesy title that can be used by veterinary surgeons registered with the RCVS, as long as they add the descriptor 'veterinary surgeon' or 'MRCVS' so they do not imply they have a human medical qualification or PhD.

doe Female rabbit.

dog Member of the Canidae, with very many varieties (breeds) of domesticated dog; wild dogs, foxes, jackals and wolves make up the rest of the group.

dog catcher Piece of equipment consisting of a pole with a distensible rope loop for securing free-running dogs.

Dog Control Notice (England & Wales) Legislation that makes it an offence to keep a dog that has attacked a person or another protected animal or to encourage a dog to be aggressive or allow a dog to be aggressive or

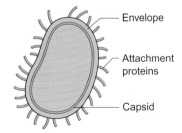

Figure 10. Distemper virus (Morbillivirus).

dangerously out of control in either a public place or a private place, Sections 55 to 67 of the Clean Neighbourhood and Environment Act 2005 apply. Other regions of the UK have similar laws.

dog erythrocyte antigen (DEA) Antigens carried on the surface of the red blood cells that determine which of the 13 different canine blood groups a dog belongs to.

dog warden Person appointed by a local authority with a statutory function to control the stray dog population and educate the public on the need for dog controls.

Döhle bodies Structures that may be identified in toxic neutrophils; see also BASOPHILIA.

dolichocephalic Dogs with long, pointed skulls, such as the Saluki; the shape of the skull will be in the breed standard.

dolor L. = 'pain'; one of the four classic signs of inflammation. See also CALOR, RUBOR, TUMOR, INFLAMMATION

dominant 1) Term used to denote a gene or trait that will always show its effect in the next generation. **2)** Behavioural characteristic where one animal ranks higher than others in its social group.

Domitor Commonly used, reversible sedative and premedicant; see also MEDETOMIDINE.

DOOP Disposal of old pharmaceuticals; most pharmaceutical waste must be placed in a disposal of old pharmaceuticals bin.

Doppler Use of ultrasound waves to assess how blood flows through a patient's vessels and heart. A regular ultrasound scan cannot demonstrate blood flow.

dorsal Towards the spine or back surface; see also VENTRAL.

dorsum The back or often the upper (top) exposed body surface, e.g. the upper surface of the paw.

dose Measured amount of drug required to obtain a therapeutic effect.

dosimeter Instrument used to measure radiation; see also FILM BADGE.

double-blind Methodology widely used in comparative clinical studies of new drugs, where neither the doctor nor the patient knows which drug is being taken.

double dentition Developmental abnormality where supernumerary permanent teeth come through the gums; should not be confused with retained deciduous teeth; common for some small breeds of dog to have extra permanent canine teeth.

doxapram A CNS stimulant often used sublingually to stimulate respiration in the newborn.

drain 1) Method of removing fluid from a cavity. **2)** Channels in buildings to remove waste water. A **Penrose drain** consists of soft rubber tubing that can be inserted into the region requiring drainage, with the lowest end protruding; it works by capillary action, drawing fluids down the inner and outer surfaces of the tube – should not be fenestrated as this reduces the surface area of the tube. A **chest drain** consists of tubing inserted into the thoracic cavity, in the lower third (to remove fluid) or the upper third (to remove free air). The external end must be carefully connected to a vacuum pump (for continuous drainage) or sealed with a tap or spigot (for intermittent drainage); a gate clamp or second seal should also be used for security; the internal end may be fenestrated to increase the number of openings that fluid can move through; see also HEIMLICH VALVE. A **sump drain** consists of outer and inner tubes; suction is applied to the inner tube while the outer is perforated to allow fluid to be drawn in.

drape Cloth or paper presterilized and used to cover the patient before and during surgery.

dressing Wound protection or material applied to the surface with or without medication to provide cover and assist in healing.

drill Apparatus used in orthopaedic surgery to make the screw holes.

drip set Apparatus for continuous injection (infusion) of fluids into a vein; colloquial term for a fluid administration set; consists of an attachment that links to the drip bag, a measuring chamber, a length of tubing and a Luer connection; sets specifically for giving blood can contain a filter to remove any small clots.

dropsy Oedema fluid in the abdomen; see also ASCITES.

drowning Death by asphyxiation if water is inhaled into the lungs; the liquid prevents the exchange of oxygen and carbon dioxide; resuscitation should always be attempted unless there has been a prolonged period of immersion.

drug Any therapeutic agent, other than food, used to prevent, diagnose or treat a disease; see also CONTROLLED DRUG.

drug eruption Hypersensitivity to a drug, characterized by acute pruritus, erythema and red weals; see also ANAPHYLAXIS.

dry–dry bandage Used on wounds discharging fluids, using a stack of gauze pads or similar absorbents with a conventional bandage over it.

dry eye Disorder resulting from inadequate tear secretion; see also KERATOCONJUNCTIVITIS SICCA.

duct Channel or passageway used for excretion and secretion.

ductus arteriosus A fetal blood vessel connecting the pulmonary artery and the aorta so that blood is diverted from the lungs; after birth, the vessel closes and becomes a fibrous remnant; see also PATENT DUCTUS ARTERIOSUS.

duodenum First part of the small intestine, running from the pylorus to the jejunum; produces many digestive juices and receives secretions from the pancreas and liver.

dura mater The outermost of the three membranes that protect the CNS (meninges); the dura is tough and blends with periosteum in the cranium; see also EPIDURAL.

durotomy Surgical incision of the dura mater, necessary for intracranial procedures and to get access to the nervous tissue of the spinal cord.

dwarfism Inability to sustain normal growth; may be hereditary or a failure of growth hormone production caused by pituitary disease. An adult animal may function normally.

dynamic compression plate (DCP) Metal plate used for internal fracture fixation; the plates are available in a variety of lengths and thicknesses; the screw holes are oval in shape, so that screws inserted eccentrically will provide compression across fracture gaps; see also ASIF.

dys- Prefix meaning difficult, abnormal or impaired.

dysautonomia Disease affecting the autonomic nervous system; see also KEY–GASKELL SYNDROME.

dyschezia Difficult or painful passage of faeces from the rectum, usually the result of a long period of voluntary suppression.

dyschondroplasia Abnormal skeletal development; see also OSTEOCHONDROSIS.

dyscoria Unequal size of the pupils or an abnormal shape of the opening.

dyscrasia Presence of abnormal cells and particles in the blood.

dysecdysis Skin moulting in reptiles; may be incomplete, especially in malnutrition or an unsuitable environment.

dysentery Term used for severe diarrhoea with blood and mucus; see also PARVOVIRUS.

dysmetria Unequal movements of the limbs as a result of damage to the cerebellum.

dysphagia Difficulty in swallowing.

dysphonia Difficulty in voice production; may be caused by a disorder of the larynx, pharynx, tongue or mouth, sometimes psychogenic.

dysplasia Abnormal development leading to disease; see also HIP DYSPLASIA, RETINAL DYSPLASIA.

dyspnoea Laboured or difficult breathing; may result from obstruction of the airway, various diseases of the bronchial tree and lung tissue or from heart disease.

dysrhythmia See ARRHYTHMIA, CARDIAC.

dystocia Difficulty giving birth; traditionally divided into fetal and maternal categories; see also PRESENTATION, POSITION.

dystrophy Condition produced by inadequate nutrition of an organ: muscular dystrophy, epithelial dystrophy of dog's retina; see also CENTRAL PROGRESSIVE RETINAL ATROPHY.

dysuria Painful passage of urine or difficult flow from the bladder.

ear The organ of hearing and balance. The **inner ear** is the deepest chamber of the ear, located within the petrous part of the temporal bone of the skull; it consists of the semicircular canals (vestibular apparatus), the coiled cochlea and the vestibule (composed of utricle and saccule); the vestibular apparatus provides positional information concerning head movements and balance, while the cochlea provides hearing; *see also* DEAFNESS, OTITIS INTERNA, SEMICIRCULAR CANAL. The **middle ear** consists of the chamber of the ear, within the tympanic part of the temporal bone, housing the auditory ossicles – the malleus, incus and stapes; it transmits sound from the external ear canal (across the tympanic membrane) to the oval and round windows of the cochlea; *see also* COCHLEA, OTITIS MEDIA. The **outer ear** includes the pinna (ear flap) and external auditory canal; *see also* OTITIS EXTERNA.

ear canal The funnel-shaped, cartilaginous canal of the outer ear, running from the ear flap to the tympanic membrane; composed of vertical and horizontal parts; external auditory canal.

ear canal ablation *See* TOTAL EAR CANAL ABLATION.

ear drum Tympanic membrane; the thin membrane dividing the external and middle ear; transmits sound waves from the external ear to the malleus, incus and stapes of the middle ear; *see also* TYMPANIC MEMBRANE.

ear mites *Otodectes cynotis*; surface-living, visible to the naked eye and can be seen on auriscopic examination; a common cause of otitis externa. All animals within the household will require treatment, as the mites are not host-specific; cats in particular can tolerate a large ear mite burden with few clinical signs; repeated treatment may be necessary to break the life cycle of the mites; *see also* OTODECTES CYNOTIS.

EBL European bat Lyssavirus; *see also* RABIES.

Ebola A virus of the Filoviridae family with infection first recorded in 1976, with a high mortality rate in humans. Fruit bats are thought to be the natural host, but the disease is spread between humans via direct contact with infected bodily secretions. Dogs have been shown

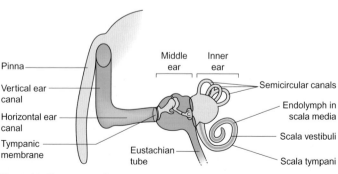

Figure 11. Ear components.

Pinna

Vertical ear canal

Horizontal ear canal

Tympanic membrane

Eustachian tube

Middle ear   Inner ear

Semicircular canals

Endolymph in scala media

Scala vestibuli

Scala tympani

to develop antibodies to the virus but are not known to be carriers of the virus.

EBP Eosinophilic bronchopneumopathy; a form of chronic inflammatory airway disease of dogs and cats.

eburnation Sclerosis of bone; usually a response to chronic injury such as degenerative joint disease; the subchondral bone plate thickens and hardens, becoming less able to absorb concussive forces during locomotion.

ecbolic A drug that stimulates smooth muscle contraction; *see also* OXYTOCIN.

ecchymosis Leakage of blood into the tissues to cause a bruise; *see also* PETECHIA.

eccrine Sweat glands, an **eccrine carcinoma of the foot** is a neoplastic condition; *see also* SWEAT GLAND.

ecdysis The shedding of an outer layer of skin as in snakes.

ECG Electrocardiography. Electrical tracing (electrocardiograph) of activity in the heart; usually obtained by attaching three recording leads to the animal placed in right lateral recumbency.

Echinococcus granulosus Small tapeworm of the dog; the larvae infect ruminants, pigs and horses and can infect humans, where they cause hydatid cysts (hydatidosis) in the liver and lungs; control measures include effective, regular worming of dogs, good hygiene and not feeding uncooked offal to dogs.

echocardiography Ultrasound scanning of the heart and major vessels; *see also* ULTRASOUND.

echogenicity The ability of an organ, substance or tissue to reflect ultrasonic waves and produce echoes (term used during ultrasound examinations).

echoic Refers to the acoustic density of tissues as seen on an ultrasonic image of bodily tissues. When an anatomical structure's acoustic density is greater than normal, it is said to be **hyperechoic**. Likewise, a structure that is lower in density than normal is said to be **hypoechoic**.

eclampsia Nervous signs resulting from low blood calcium levels; occurs shortly before parturition or 4–6 weeks after, when milk demand is at its peak and large calcium reserves have to be mobilized by the mother; signs vary but can include fits; treatment includes slow intravenous infusions of calcium borogluconate; offspring should be removed and hand-reared.

ECM Extracellular matrix; a mixture of polysaccharides and proteins that fills the spaces between cells and gives support to tissues.

ECSWT Extracorporeal shockwave therapy, also known as radial pressure wave therapy; a treatment used in horses for the management of orthopaedic problems.

-ectasis Distension of any tubular structure.

ectoderm The outer layer of cells in the embryo, giving rise to the skin and its associated structures.

-ectomy Surgical removal of a part, e.g. splenectomy – surgical removal of the spleen.

ectoparasite A parasite that lives on the outer surface of the body, e.g. mites, lice, ticks and fleas.

ectopic Aberrant, occurring in the wrong place, e.g. **ectopic ureters** enter the bladder at a site other than the trigone and may even enter the vagina or urethra; ectopic ureters are often a cause of urinary incontinence.

ectopic beats Contractions of the heart that are initiated by a region other than the S–A node.

ectopic cilia Single hairs or small hair clusters that arise from the conjunctiva and irritate the cornea; usually require surgical removal; *see also* DISTICHIASIS.

ectropion Outward drooping of the lower eyelid, usually an inherited defect; treatment is surgical.

eczema General term for any patch of inflamed skin.

EDTA *See* ETHYLENEDIAMINE-TETRAACETIC ACID.

efferent Conducting away from, e.g. an **efferent nerve** carries an impulse away from the spinal cord to a gland or muscle; **efferent blood vessels** take blood away from an organ.

effleurage A gentle form of massage that should ideally be performed first before any other physiotherapy techniques are applied. Effleurage massage is directed towards the heart, which improves circulation and promotes the drainage of lymphatic fluid.

effusion Fluid that leaks out from blood vessels or lymphatics, e.g. joint effusion collects within a traumatized joint; pericardial effusion collects within the pericardial cavity.

egg-bound Common condition of birds where an egg gets stuck in the oviduct; the egg can usually be massaged out; low calcium or stress may predispose.

egg tooth A small sharp tip on the beak of a chick inside an egg which they use to break through the membrane into the air sac and then break out of the shell. The egg tooth falls off the beak a few days after hatching as it is no longer required.

Ehlers–Danlos syndrome Rare disorder characterized by hyperelasticity of the skin and increased joint laxity.

Ehmer sling Hindleg sling used to maintain the limb in flexion and prevent weight bearing; may be used after replacement of luxated hips; requires careful padding and application to ensure that it does not rub, slip or impair circulation.

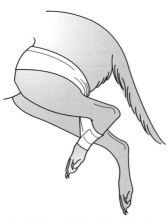

Ehmer sling applied in a figure of eight to hold the hindlimb in flexion

Figure 12. Ehmer sling.

ehrlichiosis Disease caused by *Ehrlichia canis*; the Gram-negative bacterium gives rise to neurological signs and is spread by ticks; rare in the UK but more common in the USA.

eicosanoid Compounds in cell membranes, derived from polyunsaturated fatty acids. They act as a type of hormone and play a part in inflammatory process response; *see also* ESSENTIAL FATTY ACID.

Eimeria **spp.** Coccidia; many species of protozoal parasites that cause enteritis in their host animals.

ejaculation The expulsion of prostatic fluid followed by a sperm-rich fraction through the penis; the process taking approximately 15 minutes in the dog but more rapid in the cat.

elastin Protein found in elastic fibres of loose connective tissue; *see also* CONNECTIVE TISSUE.

elbow The ginglymus (hinge) articulation between the distal humerus, radial head and proximal ulna.

elbow dysplasia Developmental disease of the elbow joint; the three forms most commonly recognized are un-united anconeal process, osteochondrosis and osteochondritis dissecans. Elbow joint incongruity also seen. Has a high genetic component, affects mainly large and giant breeds, leads to irreversible DEGENERATIVE JOINT DISEASE.

elective Proceeding from choice; includes all surgery planned in advance and performed at the best time for the patient, the owner and the veterinary surgeon.

electric burn Tissue damage from passage of a large electric current through an area.

electric shock Passage of an electric current through the body, resulting in muscle spasm (which may affect the heart muscle, leading to cardiac arrest); can occur in puppies that chew electric flex, etc. Care must be taken to ensure that the causal electrical equipment is switched off and unplugged before approaching an animal that has just had an electric shock. Use rubber gloves or a broom handle to make first contact.

electrocardiograph *See* ECG.

electrocoagulation Haemostasis using a small metal blade that is electrically heated, or by passing an electric current through the localized blood vessel; *see also* DIATHERMY.

electrodiagnostic testing (EDT) Use of fine-needle electrodes and nerve stimulators to record nerve conduction velocities and the response of muscles to nervous stimulation; *see also* ELECTROMYOGRAPH.

electroencephalograph (EEG) Trace of the electrical activity in the brain; as little is known about EEG patterns in animals, the test may provide limited information.

electrolyte A salt that can conduct electricity in solution as it breaks down into positive and negative ions, e.g. NaCl, NaHCO$_3$.

electromagnetic radiation (EMR) Waves of radiation, including radiowaves, infrared, light, ultraviolet radiation, X-rays and gamma radiation.

electromyograph (EMG) The recording of electrical activity in muscles by introducing fine-needle electrodes into the tissue; part of electrodiagnostic testing; *see also* ELECTRODIAGNOSTIC TESTING.

electron Elementary particle that carries a negative charge and circles around the nucleus of an atom; electricity results from a flow of electrons.

electrophoresis Movement of particles when an electric field is applied; negative particles will move towards the positive anode while positive charges will move towards the negative cathode.

electroretinograph (ERG) Trace of the electrical activity of the retina in response to light; may be used to test retinal function prior to cataract surgery, when the lens opacity prevents ophthalmoscopic examination of the retina.

element Simple substance that cannot be subdivided into other substances, contributes to a compound when combined with other elements (e.g. C, element; CO$_2$, compound).

elimination diet Hypoallergenic diet consisting of proteins that an animal is unlikely to have come into contact with before; once a patient is stabilized on an elimination diet, other protein sources can be added one by one so that the allergen can be identified.

Elizabethan collar 'Buster' collar; a plastic cone that fits around the neck but extends up to or beyond the end of the nose; prevents the animal from scratching or rubbing the head or chewing at the body; widely used postoperatively (e.g. after ocular surgery) to prevent wound interference, etc.

EM Electromicrograph or electron microscopy.

emaciation Extreme thinness; may result from starvation, chronic disease, etc.

emasculation *See* CASTRATION.

emasculators Surgical instrument used for castrating horses.

embolism Obstruction of a blood vessel by an embolus.

embolus, *pl.* emboli Plug of fibrin and platelets that blocks a blood vessel.

embrocation Liniment or ointment.

embryo The developing fertilized egg before it becomes a fetus.

emesis Vomiting.

emetic An agent that induces vomiting (e.g. a side effect of xylazine in the dog); may be used if the animal has eaten recently but requires emergency surgery or if it has ingested a non-corrosive poison; *see also* WASHING SODA.

emollient An agent that softens the skin.

Emotional Intelligence Quotient (EQ) A measure of a person's ability to understand other people and work effectively with them; based on five core areas of self-awareness, self-regulation, motivation, social skills and empathy.

emphysema Pathological accumulation of air in the tissues; if alveoli over-dilate, the alveolar membranes can rupture and air enters the connective tissue between alveoli; the condition leads to expiratory dyspnoea and cyanosis.

employee A person who works full- or part-time under a contract of employment; this contract may be written or implied; see CONTRACT OF EMPLOYMENT.

Employment Rights Act 1996 Act of Parliament that states that employees should have an employment contract within 2 months of starting work.

employer A legal entity (person, institution or business) that takes on a worker under a contract of employment.

empyema Pus within a body cavity; usually implies pyothorax.

emulsification Process of rendering large lipid drops into smaller and more absorbable particles in the intestine. Also refers to suspension of oils in water, as in dispensing liniments, etc.

emulsion Mixture of two liquids, one suspended as fine particles within the other.

enamel Hard substance forming the outer covering of teeth.

enamel hypoplasia Dental condition where the teeth appear mottled because of imperfect enamel formation, at one time common in puppies and adults after distemper virus infection but may be caused by any severe systemic disease in the young dog.

enarthrosis Ball-and-socket joint such as the hip.

encapsulated Enclosed within a limiting membrane.

encephalitis Inflammation of the brain tissue.

encephalitozoonis An infection caused by *Encephalitozoon cuniculi,* a parasite that affects rabbits predominantly but can affect rodents, dogs, cats and humans. It most often occurs in animals whose immunity is compromised.

encephalomeningitis Inflammation of the brain and its meninges (meningoencephalitis).

encephalomyelitis Inflammation of the brain and spinal cord.

encephalon The brain.

encephalopathy Any disease or disorder of the brain.

endarteritis Inflammation of the endothelial lining of an artery.

end artery An artery that is the sole supply to a region and has no collateral vessels, e.g. retinal vessels, coronary vessels; should the artery be occluded, the area of tissue it supplied will become devitalized.

endectoside An antiparasitic drug that is effective against both endoparasites and ectoparasites.

endemic Describes a disease that is always present within a given population.

endocardiosis Progressive degeneration of the cardiac A–V valves; a common occurrence in ageing dogs and in younger animals of breeds such as the Cavalier King Charles spaniel; may also be accompanied by degenerative changes within the chordae tendineae; leads to valvular incompetence and congestive heart failure (predominantly left-sided).

endocarditis Vegetative lesions on the A–V valves caused by seeding of bacterial infection from a remote location via the bloodstream; common septic foci include teeth and gums, bite wounds and infective arthritis; organisms involved include *Staphylococcus* spp., *Streptococcus* spp. and *Escherichia coli.*

endocardium The inner membrane lining the chambers of the heart and covering the valves.

endochondral ossification Type of ossification occurring at growth plate regions in long bones (epiphyseal plates) and beneath the articular cartilage, brings about limb lengthening and enlargement of the articular surfaces; cartilage cells proliferate and form long columns of hypertrophied cells; the cartilage matrix mineralizes and the chondrocytes are replaced by osteocytes, which remodel the matrix to form bone.

endocrine Internally secreted.

endocrine glands Ductless structures that secrete hormones directly into the bloodstream, e.g. adrenal gland, thyroid gland.

endocrinology The study of endocrine glands and the hormones they produce.

endocytosis The uptake by the cell of external material; *see also* PHAGOCYTOSIS.

endolymph The fluid contained within the scala media of the inner ear.

endometritis Inflammation of the lining of the uterus, usually caused by infection; may occur after parturition.

endometrium The lining of the uterus.

endomysium The connective tissue layer surrounding a muscle fibre.

endoneurium The innermost connective tissue layer surrounding a nerve fibre.

endoparasite Parasite living within the body of the host; including roundworms, tapeworms, protozoa, lungworm, etc.

endoplasmic reticulum Folded membranous structures within a cell, close to the nucleus; rough endoplasmic reticulum is encrusted with ribosomes and synthesizes proteins; smooth endoplasmic reticulum lacks ribosomes and produces lipid secretions.

endoscope Any instrument with a light source and viewing channel for looking inside the body; the first endoscopes were rigid structures, but the use of fibreoptics has allowed them to become flexible for internal examination of curved structures such as the stomach and colon. They can also be used for collecting tissue samples or removing foreign bodies.

endoscopy Examination of body cavities using an endoscope.

endosteal Relating to the endosteum or lying adjacent to it, e.g. **endosteal blood vessels**.

endosteum Membrane lining the medullary cavity of the long bones.

endotendineum Connective tissue sheath surrounding a strand of tendon.

endothelium Thin lining membrane of body cavities and blood vessels; derived from the embryonic endodermal layer.

endothermic Chemical reaction that takes in, or requires, heat.

endotoxic shock Caused by the release of endotoxins from bacterial infection.

endotoxin Harmful substance released by some bacteria when their cell wall ruptures; most commonly ingested in rancid food, causing abdominal discomfort, vomiting and diarrhoea. *Escherichia coli* produces an endotoxin that causes necrosis.

endotracheal tube (ET tube) Rubber or polymer tube placed into the trachea of anaesthetized or unconscious animals to maintain a patent upper airway and allow the administration of anaesthetic gases or oxygen. Available in a wide range of sizes, with and without inflatable cuffs; the cuffs should be inflated to limit the escape of anaesthetic gases into the environment and prevent aspiration of water, saliva, blood, etc.

endplate potential The electrical potential developed at the motor endplate, where a nerve axon contacts a muscle fibre.

end-to-end anastomosis Surgical technique for the repair of resected intestine, blood vessels, etc., where the open ends of two hollow structures are sutured together to make one continuous tube.

enema A liquid introduced into the rectum; may be used to encourage defaecation and evacuate the bowel, to administer a drug or as part of a radiographic contrast study of the terminal digestive tract.

enflurane (Ethrane) Volatile anaesthetic agent for induction and maintenance, sweet-smelling; provides rapid anaesthesia and recovery but is relatively expensive. It is a halogenated ether.

enophthalmos Retraction of the eyeball into the socket, e.g. after debilitating illness when the retrobulbar fat pad has reduced in size; *see also* HORNER'S SYNDROME.

enostosis A bony growth, usually inwards and likely to cause pain.

enteral Via the gut; **enteral nutrition** is the supply of nutrients into the gastrointestinal tract by routes other than the mouth, e.g. nasogastric tube, PEG tube.

enterectomy Surgical removal of a portion of small intestine.

enteric Relating to the small intestine.

enteritis Inflammation of the small intestine.

enterokinase Enzyme produced in the small intestine at the brush border; activates trypsinogen to form trypsin; *see also* TRYPSINOGEN.

enterolith Concretion of hardened material, usually faeces, that may cause intestinal obstruction.

enteropathy Any disease of the intestines, e.g. **protein-losing enteropathy, mucoid enteropathy** of rabbits.

enterotomy Surgical incision into the small intestine to remove a foreign body, for example; care must be taken to ensure that the rest of the abdomen is not contaminated with intestinal contents.

enterotoxaemia An acute diarrhoea in young rabbits caused by *Clostridium* *spiroforme*, causing death within 48 hours.

enterotoxin A toxin that has its effect on the gastrointestinal tract; *see also* ENDOTOXIN, EXOTOXIN.

enthesophytes Mineralized linear bodies seen on radiograph, may represent areas of calcified bone or tendon.

entropion Curling inward of the eyelid margin, so hairs may contact the cornea and cause irritation; hereditary in many breeds such as the Shar-Pei and Cocker spaniel; requires surgical correction.

enucleation Total removal of the eyeball.

enuresis Urinary incontinence caused by weakness of the bladder sphincter muscle.

enzootic Describes a disease occurring within a particular geographical region or area, e.g. rabies is enzootic in much of Asia.

enzyme Protein produced by a cell that catalyses a specific chemical reaction; many are routinely used as biochemical markers to locate damage to specific organs, e.g. raised serum alkaline phosphatase levels may indicate increased bone turnover.

enzyme-linked immunosorbent assay (ELISA) Rapid laboratory test where a colour change is linked to enzyme activity; used to detect feline leukaemia virus, for example.

eosin Red stain used routinely for histological examination of tissues. **Haematoxylin and eosin stain**, commonly known as H&E, is used in histology; *see also* HAEMATOXYLIN.

eosinopenia Reduced number of circulating eosinophils, most commonly a result of corticosteroid therapy.

eosinophil Granular type of white blood cell; has striking red granules within the cytoplasm; contributes to the allergic response and is important in the inactivation of histamine; produced by the bone marrow.

eosinophilia Raised number of circulating eosinophils; causes include tissue injury (with the release of histamine), parasite burden, allergic responses or oestrus.

eosinophilic Describes diseases where there are collections of eosinophils, such as in the intestine wall in a type of chronic enteritis. The non-healing **eosinophilic ulcer** of the cat's nose and upper lip, also known as rodent ulcer, is sometimes neoplastic; *see also* EBP.

eosinophilic myositis Inflammatory myopathy affecting the masticatory muscles, especially in German shepherd dogs; occurs in acute, recurring bouts and may lead to marked atrophy and fibrosis of affected muscles; often responds to steroids; the exact aetiology remains unclear.

epaxial muscles Muscles around the vertebral column along the dorsum, lying above the level of the transverse processes; comprise the iliocostalis, longissimus and transversospinalis muscle systems; act to extend the spine and produce lateral movements.

ependyma Thin membrane lining the ventricles of the brain and the central canal of the spinal cord.

EPI *See* EXOCRINE PANCREATIC INSUFFICIENCY.

epicardium Outer membrane surrounding the heart; *see also* PERICARDIUM.

epicondyle Bony prominence on a condyle; usually a site of soft tissue attachments.

epidemic Outbreak of disease above the normal expected levels.

epidemiology The study of the patterns of disease within populations.

epidermis Superficial layer of the skin.

epididymis, *pl.* epididymides Convoluted duct attached to the ventrocaudal aspect of the testis; conveys sperm from the testis to the vas deferens.

epidural Outside the dura mater; **epidural anaesthesia** is achieved by injecting local anaesthetic into the fat-containing **epidural space** outside the spinal cord.

epigastric Involving the region around the stomach.

epigenetics Functional changes to the genome that do not involve a change in the DNA base sequence (the orders of ATCG), e.g. the addition of a methyl group to cytosine may alter how genes are expressed without altering the base sequence. This may help explain how stem cells of the embryo can differentiate into the different tissues of the body whilst having the same DNA.

epiglottis Cartilage at the base of the tongue; acts as a stopper to close off the airway during swallowing.

epilepsy Abnormal patterns of activity within the brain, resulting in collapse, loss of consciousness and convulsions; *see also* GRAND MAL.

epimysium Fibrous outer connective tissue sheath surrounding a muscle.

epinephrine Alternative name for adrenaline; used in the USA and now also in the UK.

epineurium Fibrous outermost connective tissue surrounding a nerve.

epiphora Overflow of tears; chronic epiphora leads to tear-staining of the facial hair coat; commonly caused by blockage of the nasolacrimal duct.

epiphyseal Relating to the epiphysis.

epiphysis Proximal and distal extremities of a long bone; forms from a separate centre of ossification from the shaft of the bone and is separated from the shaft by growth plate regions in skeletally immature animals; *see also* ENDOCHONDRAL OSSIFICATION.

epiploic foramen Connecting opening between the abdominal cavity and the omental bursa, also known as the foramen of Winslow.

episcleral Around the margins of the sclera of the eye.

episiotomy Surgical incision into the vulva to help the delivery of offspring.

episodic weakness Periods of muscle weakness and collapse; associated with conditions such as alkalosis, hypoglycaemia and myasthenia gravis.

epispadias Congenital abnormality where the urethra opens out onto the dorsal surface of the penis.

epistaxis Nosebleed.

epithelioma Neoplasm arising from any of the elements of the epithelium.

epithelium The surface of the body, including skin, mucous membranes, cornea, serous surfaces and associated glands; types include ciliated, columnar, cuboidal, pseudostratified, stratified and squamous.

epizootic Epidemic.

epoetin Drug form of erythropoietin used in treatment of anaemia, stimulates erythropoiesis hormonally; given by injection at frequent intervals.

epulis A hard, neoplastic proliferation of the gums.

equator of the lens Peripheral region of the lens, where the supporting zonules attach.

equine Relating to the horse, e.g. equine veterinary nursing.

equine herpes virus A serious disease of horses caused by varieties of the virus family herpesviridae that can cause respiratory disease, abortion, foal mortality and neurological signs.

equine influenza A viral disease of horses that is similar to human flu, causing elevated temperature, cough, runny nose and poor appetite; a vaccine is available.

equine sarcoid A common and benign form of skin tumour in the horse caused by a papillomavirus infection. Lesions can vary in size and shape and can be single or multiple anywhere on the skin, although most commonly on limbs, abdomen and head. Treatments can include surgical excision, laser therapy or cryotherapy.

equine viral arteritis Infection with an arterivirus causing fever, cough and other respiratory signs; spread by secretions so is a notifiable disease in stallions.

equine viral infectious anaemia A notifiable viral disease of horses caused by a lentivirus from the retrovirus family. It is usually transmitted between horses by blood-feeding insects such as the horse fly, thus fly control is important to prevent spread of infection. Once a horse is infected, it is infected for life and infection can be chronic or acute. Common signs include fever and anaemia in acute cases and prolonged fever, weight loss and more severe anaemia in chronic cases. There is currently no effective treatment or vaccine available.

erection Filling of the corpus cavernosus with blood so that the penis becomes erect.

eructation Belching, regurgitation of free gas from the stomach; *see also* AEROPHAGY.

erysipelas Skin disease caused by *Erysipelothrix rhusiopathiae*; characterized by the acute appearance of inflamed, reddened patches; can also cause bacterial endocarditis.

erythema Reddening of the skin caused by dilation of capillaries.

erythroblast Immature forms of erythrocyte, e.g. normoblast, reticulocyte.

erythrocyte Mature red blood cell; the most numerous cell in the bloodstream; lacks a nucleus (except in birds) and is packed with haemoglobin, which carries oxygen to the tissues; discoid in shape and deformable, so it can pass easily through capillaries.

erythrocyte sedimentation rate *See* ESR.

erythrocytopenia Abnormally low number of circulating red blood cells; causes include haemorrhage, haemolysis, reduced production by the bone marrow and heavy parasite burdens; *see also* ANAEMIA.

erythrogenesis The formation of red blood cells; *see also* ERYTHROPOIESIS.

erythrolysis Haemolysis, the breakdown of red blood cells.

erythron Erythrocytes and all the tissues that produce red blood cells.

erythropoiesis The process of red blood cell formation; occurs within the red bone marrow; maturation time is approximately 4–7 days.

erythropoietin Kidney-secreted hormone that stimulates bone marrow to produce more oxygen-carrying red blood cells (drug: epoetin).

Escherichia coli Gram-negative, rod-shaped bacteria; widely distributed and part of the normal gut flora; pathogenic strains produce enterotoxins that cause diarrhoea. A cause of death of young puppies; *see also* FADING PUPPY/KITTEN SYNDROME.

ESF External skeletal fixation (of fractures).

Esmarch bandage Rubber bandage that can be used to exsanguinate a limb prior to surgery to control haemorrhage; the bandage is applied from distal to proximal, squeezing blood out of the limb; the distal end is then unwrapped to expose the required surgical site but a loop is left proximally to act as a tourniquet; operating time is limited as tissue hypoxia can occur; the bandage may also mask haemorrhage, blood loss only becoming apparent when the bandage is removed.

esophagus Alternative spelling (US) for oesophagus.

ESR Erythrocyte sedimentation rate. The rate at which erythrocytes settle in a standing blood sample; observed under standard conditions, it is used as a test for many chronic conditions.

essential fatty acids The essential fatty acids include linoleic acid (double bonds n = 3) and arachidonic acid (n = 4; cats only); such fatty acids form part of cell membranes and are used in the synthesis of prostaglandins; deficiency leads to reproductive failure, poor coat and skin, delayed wound healing and emaciation. Plants contain n = 6 acids and algae have n = 3 acids (so marine-feeding animals commonly have n = 3 acids in diet); *see also* EICOSANOID.

ethanol An alcohol, each molecule containing two carbon atoms.

ether One of the earliest volatile anaesthetic agents; highly inflammable and explosive; decomposes readily so has to be stored in dark glass; irritant to mucous membranes, commonly causes postoperative nausea; superseded by agents such as halothane and isoflurane; may be applied to ticks to facilitate removal.

ethics Code of practice for correct conduct of all veterinary staff.

ethmoid Like a sieve; the ethmoid bone of the cranium is perforated with many fine holes that allow the passage of fibres of the olfactory nerve as they run cranially to innervate the nasal membranes and olfactory organs.

ethmoturbinates Scrolls of bone arising from the ethmoid bone and dividing the nose into nasal chambers.

ethylenediaminetetraacetic acid (EDTA) An anticoagulant used in blood collection tubes if the sample requires haematological tests.

ethylene glycol A component of antifreeze; has a sweet taste and is a common cause of poisoning in dogs and cats, signs include vomiting, weakness, collapse, haematuria and convulsions.

ethylene oxide Vapour used to sterilize equipment; the gas is highly effective against microorganisms and spores; the process can also be carried out at room temperature, so heat-sensitive items can be sterilized; however, the procedure takes at least 24 hours (items have to be left to air) and specialist fume cabinets are required.

eukaryocyte Organism in which the chromosomes are enclosed in a nucleus.

eustachian tube A structure running from the middle ear to the nasopharynx; a route for ascending middle ear infections.

euthanasia Humane destruction of an animal; means 'good death'.

euthyroid Having normal thyroid function; *see also* THYROID.

euthyroid sick syndrome Syndrome where the thyroid secretes a normal level of triiodothyronine (T_3) and thyroxine (T_4) but circulating levels are low because of starvation, surgery, hepatic or renal disease, diabetes mellitus or other chronic illness.

EV *See* EXTERNAL VERIFIER.

evacuant A laxative enema.

eversion Turning outwards; used sometimes to describe the prolapse of the bladder or uterus; *see also* ECTROPION.

evidence-based practice The interdisciplinary use of current clinical evidence in making decisions about patient care.

evidence-based veterinary medicine (EBVM) Clinical care based on a combination of clinical expertise, critical consideration of the best available scientific evidence and patient circumstances.

evolution The process of genetic change and development.

exacerbate Make worse or more severe.

excision Surgical removal of a part.

excision arthroplasty Surgical removal of an articular surface, e.g. **femoral head excision** for Legg–Calvé–Perthes disease.

excitement, involuntary The second stage of general anaesthesia; the animal is unconscious, but there may be struggling and paddling; breath-holding is common.

excitement, voluntary The first stage of anaesthesia; the animal is conscious and may struggle to prevent induction.

excoriation A scratch.

excretion The elimination of waste materials from the body.

exercise Physical activity; a minimum level of regular activity is required to ensure that the animal maintains healthy locomotor and cardiovascular systems; activity also helps to relieve boredom.

exercise intolerance Reduced capacity to exercise; can be due to lack of fitness, anaemia, cardiac disease and many other causes.

exhale Breathe out; *see also* EXPIRATION.

exhaustion Severe tiredness and collapse after strenuous, sustained effort.

exuberant Term used to describe the proliferative healing of wounds by granulation; *see also* SECONDARY INTENTION HEALING.

exocrine Refers to secretion via a duct, e.g. the secretion of saliva from the parotid salivary gland is via the parotid duct.

exocrine pancreatic insufficiency (EPI) Reduced function of the exocrine pancreas caused by atrophy of the acinar cells or as a sequel to chronic pancreatitis; the lack of lipase, amylase and trypsin normally produced by the exocrine pancreas gives rise to the symptoms of weight loss, poor condition and fatty, odorous faeces; diagnosis may be confirmed by measuring trypsin-like immunoreactivity in a serum sample. Treatment includes supplementation with pancreatic extracts and vitamins, and feeding a low-fibre, low-fat diet; *see also* TRYPSIN-LIKE IMMUNOREACTIVITY.

exocytosis The expulsion of material by a cell; *see also* ENDOCYTOSIS.

E

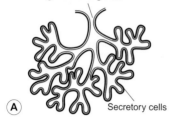

Main duct branches to
form a compound gland
e.g. duodenal glands

(A)   Secretory cells

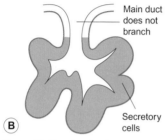

Main duct
does not
branch

(B)   Secretory cells

Figure 13. Exocrine gland.
(a) Compound tubular; (b) simple
branched acinar.

exophthalmos Protrusion of the eyeball; considered normal in some breeds such as the Pekinese; the exposed cornea may be prone to ulceration.

exostosis Proliferation of hard tissue, may be a benign neoplastic change; cartilaginous exostoses are found predominantly affecting the digits and metacarpal/tarsal regions.

exothermic Chemical reaction that gives out heat to the surroundings.

exotoxin Toxic substance produced by growing bacteria and released into the tissues.

expectorant An agent that increases the elimination of secretions from the respiratory tract by increasing the activity of cilia, stimulating cough reflexes, etc.

expiration Breathing out; a passive process brought about mainly by elastic recoil of thoracic structures.

expiratory reserve volume The difference between the amount of gas exhaled for a given level of activity and the maximum amount that could be exhaled.

expiratory valve The valve in a semiclosed, non-rebreathing anaesthetic circuit that allows exhaled gases to be removed.

expiry date The date by which a drug must be used in order for its effectiveness to be maximized. It is an offence to dispense a drug after the expiry date.

exploratory laparotomy Surgical opening of the abdomen to examine the enclosed organs visually and reach a diagnosis.

exposure Use of imaging (X-rays) to visualize an area of the body.

exposure factor Time, milliamperage and kilovolt settings; these are used in radiography to adjust the exposure (amount of radiation)

express 1) Press or squeeze out. **2)** Show physical outward signs that reflect genetic make-up, e.g. a dog with certain coat-colour genes will have a black coat.

exsanguinate To remove the blood from, until bloodless.

extensor Muscle whose action is to extend a joint.

external fixation Techniques of fracture fixation where the support is applied externally, e.g. using an external fixator or a cast.

external fixator A frame of metal pins, connecting bars and clamps that are used externally to support bone fractures; the pins are driven through the skin and into the bone fragments, the pins are then clamped onto the connecting bar that is placed close to (but not touching) the skin surface.

external respiration Occurs in lungs, the site of exchange of alveolar air with blood-carried gases.

external verifier Person appointed by the RCVS to assist in veterinary nurse training at ATACs and assess the portfolios.

extinction Death of the last remaining members of a species, so that the species no longer exists.

extinction, behavioural Process used to remove an unwanted behaviour by using the withdrawal of positive reinforcement for a previously trained or learned behaviour: the behaviour should eventually cease to be shown.

extinction burst When reinforcement in training is first stopped, the animal's behaviour may at first intensify as it tries harder to achieve a reward.

extra-articular Outside a joint.

extracapsular Outside a joint capsule.

extracellular Outside the cell; often used to describe the spaces between cells within the tissues; *see also* ECM.

extracellular fluid (ECF) Tissue fluid that bathes all the cells of the body; filters out of capillaries and is collected up into the lymphatic system, returning to the circulation via the thoracic duct.

extraction Surgical removal, e.g. extraction of teeth, lens, etc.

extradural Outside the dura mater.

extramural studies (EMS) Seeing practice; work experience; the practical veterinary experience gained outside the formal term-time teaching; applies to all veterinary surgeon undergraduates; part of veterinary training when time is spent with qualified veterinarians in general practice.

extrasystole Premature heartbeat originating in the atrium, not from the primary heart pacemaker (the S–A node); *see also* S–A NODE.

extravasation Escape of fluid (usually from a damaged blood vessel) into the tissues.

extremity The distal part of a limb.

extrinsic Implies something outside the body.

extubation Removal of the endotracheal tube during recovery from anaesthesia;

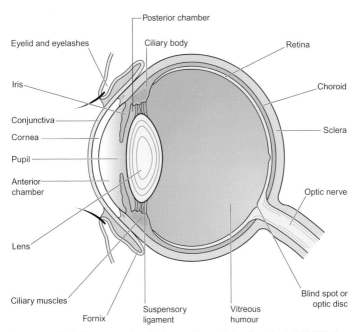

Eyelid and eyelashes
Iris
Conjunctiva
Cornea
Pupil
Anterior chamber
Lens
Ciliary muscles
Fornix
Posterior chamber
Ciliary body
Suspensory ligament
Vitreous humour
Retina
Choroid
Sclera
Optic nerve
Blind spot or optic disc

Figure 14. Eyeball: cross-section. Redrawn with permission from Aspinall V, O'Reilly M. Introduction to veterinary anatomy and physiology. Edinburgh: Butterworth-Heinemann, 2004.

this should usually be done as soon as the protective laryngeal reflexes are regained.

exuberant granulation Term used in wound healing where an open wound is allowed to repair untreated; most common in horse limb wounds, when it may be called 'proud flesh' and healing is delayed.

exudate The fluid that oozes slowly out of damaged capillaries and dries to form a scab.

eye The organ of sight; generally forward-pointing in species that hunt and more laterally located in herbivores.

eyeball The globe of the eye, sitting within the bony orbit; comprises the cornea, aqueous (anterior chamber), lens and ciliary body, vitreous (posterior chamber) and sclera.

eyelid The upper and lower folds of skin that move over the eye during the blink reaction; act to protect the eye and spread the tear film over the cornea; *see* ECTROPION, ENTROPION.

eyepiece Lens on a microscope nearest to the user's eyes; contributes to the overall magnification of the object; microscopes may have one or two (binocular) eyepieces.

F cells One of the four cell groups of the pancreas; produce the hormone pancreatic peptide.

fabella, *pl.* **fabellae** Small, paired sesamoid bones that lie just caudal to the stifle joint; they are located in the origins of the gastrocnemius muscle, within the medial and lateral heads, where they arise from the respective femoral condyles.

face mask Conical rubber mask that fits over the muzzle of an animal to allow the administration of anaesthetic gases; although available in a variety of sizes, they may not fit all animals and therefore there is increased likelihood of environmental pollution with anaesthetic agents.

facet Small, flat surface on a bone; often a region for muscle attachment or articulation with another bone.

facetectomy Surgical removal of an articular facet; removal of the articular facets of adjacent vertebrae may form part of the dorsal or lateral approach to the spine.

facial nerve Seventh cranial nerve, running from the ventral aspect of the brain through the facial canal in the petrous temporal bone and exiting the skull via the stylomastoid foramen. The facial nerve innervates the muscles of facial expression, the lacrimal glands, part of the tongue (carrying taste sensation) and some salivary glands.

facial nerve paralysis Syndrome caused by any lesion along the length of the facial nerve, resulting in paralysis of the facial muscles; more commonly unilateral, but bilateral if the lesion is central within the brain; the face and ear appears to droop on the affected side, saliva may dribble from the mouth, eyelids droop and the blink (menace) response is poor or absent.

facilitated diffusion The transfer across a cell membrane using a carrier protein to overcome the concentration gradient.

factor VIII deficiency A blood clotting disorder also known as classical haemophilia. An inherited condition present in a large number of breeds and mixed breeds. Factor VIII is a protein essential for normal secondary haemostasis (fibrin production); *see also* HAEMOPHILIA.

facultative Adjective describing bacteria that are able to adapt to and live under various conditions.

FAD Flea allergy dermatitis, the commonest cause of skin disease in cats. Caused by the sensitization effect of allergens introduced after a flea feeds from a cat. Seen as pruritus and papulocrustous skin condition; *see also* FELINE MILIARY ECZEMA.

fading puppy/kitten syndrome A perinatal condition where offspring initially feed well and appear to thrive but then lose condition, become weak and moribund and may die. It affects puppies and kittens within the first few weeks of life; generally caused by bacterial or viral infections, particularly herpes virus; non-infectious causes include hypothermia and cardiopulmonary failure. Treatment is symptomatic and supportive; the incidence of the condition can be minimized by maintaining good hygiene and ensuring that neonates receive adequate colostrum. *Escherichia coli* toxins may cause necrotizing pneumonia and renal damage.

faecalith Hard concretion of faeces; may cause tenesmus and pain on defaecation and obstruction of the rectum; faecaliths may also become tangled in the coat around the anus.

faeces Waste material excreted from the gastrointestinal tract; consists of unabsorbed food (mainly fibrous matter), digestive secretions and water.

Fahrenheit Temperature scale; converted to centigrade by applying the formula: $°C = 5/9 \times (°F - 32)$.

fainting Syncope; transient loss of consciousness resulting from insufficient oxygen reaching the brain; boxers are particularly prone to fainting attacks, possibly as a result of high vagal tone slowing the heart rate; also associated with a number of cardiac diseases.

falciform Sickle-shaped, curved.

fallopian tube Oviduct; tube arising near each ovary and running to the body of the uterus; fallopian tubes have a fimbriated end at the ovary; they collect the ova released at ovulation and convey them to the uterus; *see also* ECTOPIC.

false pregnancy Also known as pseudopregnancy, phantom pregnancy, pseudocyesis; a condition occurring to some degree in all non-pregnant bitches 6–8 weeks after a season (during metoestrus). The intensity of the signs is variable; it may be unnoticed in some bitches while others show marked signs: behavioural changes such as nest-building, excitability and protective aggression over toys, etc. are common; the mammary glands enlarge and milk may also be produced; false pregnancy had survival value for ancestral dogs living in packs as it allowed a non-pregnant bitch to provide milk for other puppies whose mother had an inadequate supply or a large litter. The condition arises because the corpora lutea that develop in the ovaries after ovulation remain for a similar length of time irrespective of whether the bitch is pregnant or not. With increasing age, false pregnancy is more likely to be complicated by pyometra; neutering during anoestrus is advisable.

falx cerebri Membrane between the two cerebral hemispheres of the forebrain; *see also* TENTORIUM CEREBELLI.

familial Occurring within close relatives or within a certain line.

Fanconi's syndrome A renal disease characterized by multiple defects in absorption from the proximal tubules of the kidney; inherited in the basenji but may also be secondary to renal injury such as heavy-metal poisoning; protein and glucose appear in the urine, and there may be other electrolyte imbalances; affected animals are polyuric/polydipsic and renal failure may occur acutely.

faradism Physiotherapy technique where specific superficial muscles are stimulated electrically, using pads placed over them; some animals may resent the skin sensation associated with the treatment.

fascia Fibrous connective tissue, also containing fat, which surrounds the body beneath the skin and ensheathes muscles and muscle groups.

fascicle Small bundle of muscle fibres.

fasciculation Twitching of muscles in groups; one of the signs of organophosphorus poisoning.

Fasciola hepatica Liver fluke; a parasitic trematode worm using a specific snail as an intermediate host and affecting ruminants, horses, humans, rats, mice and rabbits; ingested immature flukes migrate to the liver where they develop into the adult form, causing damage to hepatic and biliary tissues; can be controlled by using flukicidal wormers, by draining marshy areas where the snails live or by preventing livestock from having access to such areas.

fat A large molecule consisting of a glycerol core linked to three fatty acid side chains; in the diet it is a source of fat-soluble vitamins, essential fatty acids and energy; it also enhances the palatability of the food. Fat has a higher calorific density than either carbohydrate or protein; surplus dietary calorie intake is stored by the body as fat. Most body fat is white fat, but the 1–5% brown fat, deposited mainly around the shoulders and chest, is important for heat production. Radiographically, fat is less dense than other soft tissues, and therefore, is useful to outline organs such as the kidneys.

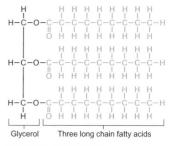

Glycerol   Three long chain fatty acids

Figure 15. Fat molecule.

fat pad Triangular area of fatty tissue within the stifle joint, just caudal to the patellar ligament; because the fat pad is less radiodense than the surrounding soft tissue, it appears radiolucent on lateral stifle radiographs and can be useful for assessing joint effusion.

fat-soluble Having an affinity for fatty substances and able to be concentrated and stored within them; a number of vitamins are fat soluble, e.g. vitamins A and D.

fatigue Tiredness; may be associated with overexertion or disease; muscle fatigue describes the physiological response of a single muscle fibre to repetitive stimulation, such that the strength of the contraction reduces as the muscle exhausts its energy supply.

fatty acid A component of fat; *see* ESSENTIAL FATTY ACIDS.

faucitis Inflammation of the mucosa caudal to the glossopalatine folds in the mouth near the tonsils.

faunivores Animals that eat other animals unlike herbivores or insectivores.

FCRD *See* FELINE CENTRAL RETINAL DEGENERATION.

FCV *See* FELINE CALICIVIRUS.

fear A response to noxious stimuli; a frightened animal may try to escape or bite at a potential danger – it is an adaptive response; aggression induced by fear can be modified by gradual exposure to the stimulus and positive reinforcement technique is used to reward for non-fearful behaviour until the stimulus predicts a pleasant rewarded outcome; *see also* PHOBIA.

feather The plumage of birds, consisting of primary (flight and tail) and secondary feathers and underlying down; each feather has a central shaft that supports many barbs; these, in turn, give rise to the smaller barbules that interlock with those on adjacent feathers to form a vane, a surface that will produce lift when swept through the air.

feather mites Chorioptes infestation in the feathers of horses, causing stamping and irritation.

feather plucking Common condition of caged birds, possibly caused by boredom or stress; may be difficult to correct as it rapidly becomes a habit; changing the environment or providing another bird nearby for company may help; birds may also peck at each other's feathers if they are kept in overcrowded conditions; faecal cortisol can be measured to assess stress in caged birds.

febrile Pyrexic; having an elevated body temperature; usually a response to infection or pain.

FCoV *See* FELINE CORONAVIRUS.

feces Alternative spelling (US) for faeces.

fecundity Fertility.

FECV *See* FELINE ENTERIC CORONAVIRUS.

feedback Part of physiological regulatory responses, where the levels of a particular substance are detected and either increase (positive feedback) or reduce (negative feedback) the production of that substance.

feeding Intake of food; feeding patterns for pets generally fall into one of three categories: free access (ad libitum, food always available), time-restricted (food is available for 5–30 minutes at intervals during the day) and meal-restricted (a set amount of food is fed); anorexic patients may be encouraged to feed by feeding a highly palatable diet, adding oil to the diet, warming the food, hand-feeding or smearing small amounts on the paws; other feeding techniques include force-feeding, intravenous alimentation, gastrotomy or PEG tube, pharyngostomy or nasogastric tube feeding; intravenous diazepam can also be used to stimulate feeding in cats. Calorie and nutrient

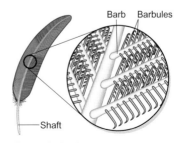

Figure 16. Feather.

requirements in the diet should match the metabolic needs of the animal, and it must be remembered that these are increased in disease states.

feeding on demand System of free access to food, discouraged as many animals are snack feeders. Weight control may be impossible; *see also* SATIETY.

Felicola subrostratus The cat louse; a macroscopic ectoparasite with six legs and sucking mouth parts; host specific, causing pruritus and alopecia.

feline calicivirus (FCV) Small, picornavirus (RNA virus) frequently found in cats in a carrier state. One of the causes of cat flu, with oculonasal discharge and oral ulceration after an incubation period of 2–5 days; recovery is usually uneventful but virulent strains may cause life-threatening pneumonia; treatment is supportive. Can also cause chronic gingivitis or sometimes lameness.

feline central retinal degeneration One of the signs of taurine deficiency. Often first recognized as dilated pupils and a cat reluctant to go out after dark.

feline coronavirus (FCoV) An RNA virus that exists as two biotypes – one of which has low virulence (FECV) while the other (FIPV) causes FIP; *see also* FELINE INFECTIOUS PERITONITIS.

feline dysautonomia *See* KEY–GASKELL SYNDROME.

feline enteric coronavirus (FECV) One of the forms of the feline coronavirus that is thought not able to progress to the illness FIP.

feline fibrosarcoma (FSA) Feline response to a vaccine, adjuvants thought to be one cause. The public will know FSA as the Financial Services Authority.

feline herpesvirus (FHV) *See* FELINE VIRAL RHINOTRACHEITIS.

feline hormonal alopecia *See* FELINE MILIARY ECZEMA.

feline immunodeficiency virus (FIV) A retrovirus that affects a cat's ability to defend itself properly against disease. Most common in feral cats and transmission is usually by a penetrating bite from another infected cat, so it is more common in biting male cats than in passive females; can cause disease in cats similar to HIV/AIDS in humans, along with FIV-associated tumours; symptomatic treatment is given. After infection, it may take months or years before immunodeficiency develops and secondary infections show up as a disease problem. Gingivitis, recurrent infections and occasional neurological signs may be found in FIV-infected cats.

feline infectious anaemia (FIA) Caused by *Haemobartonella felis*, now classified as a mycoplasma. Immunosuppressed cats are most likely to develop fever and a severe haemolytic anaemia, sometimes with jaundice; *see also* HAEMOBARTONELLOSIS.

feline infectious enteritis (FIE) Caused by a parvovirus; can be fatal in the very young; death occurs after frequent vomiting, rapid collapse from fluid losses; *see also* FPV.

feline infectious peritonitis (FIP) An infectious disease that can take different forms depending on the strain of virus and the immunity present in the cat; the wet form or effusive type is more common than the dry or non-effusive form. Caused by a coronavirus that is widely distributed in the cat community. Some cats may develop severe diarrhoea, but only 10% of cats infected with the virus go on to develop FIP. The two forms of FIP have variable rates of progression, but there is no treatment, and the condition is usually fatal.

feline leukaemia virus (FELV) One member of the retrovirus group. The disease in cats may take various forms as it is immunosuppressive; may cause lymphosarcoma or a degenerative anaemia. A large proportion of cats infected die within 3 years of first diagnosis but supportive treatment may be of value.

feline miliary eczema Flea-allergy dermatitis, feline hormonal alopecia; small crusting skin lesions develop predominantly on the dorsum but may be generalized; these can often best be detected by running a hand through the coat; affected cats spend considerable time licking at pruritic areas and may inflict serious self-trauma, with marked alopecia over the thighs and abdomen; the cause of this common condition is an allergic response to flea bites; consequently, rigorous flea control of all animals and the environment is required; corticosteroids may be used in the short term to break the itch–scratch cycle and antibiotics may also be required if the lesions are infected.

feline odontoclastic resorptive lesion disease (FORL) Also known as teeth neck lesion. The cause is uncertain; possibly diet and viral gingivitis.

feline panleukopenia *See* FELINE INFECTIOUS ENTERITIS, FELINE PARVOVIRUS, PANLEUKOPENIA.

feline parvovirus Causes an acute infection of younger cats and kittens, often called feline infectious enteritis; *see also* FELINE INFECTIOUS ENTERITIS, PANLEUKOPENIA.

feline spongiform encephalopathy (FSE) A rare disease associated with altered behaviour, aggressiveness, increase of appetite and thirst and abnormal walking; *see also* BOVINE SPONGIFORM ENCEPHALOPATHY.

feline syncytium-forming virus (FeSFV) Occurs widely in cats without symptoms but has been associated with lameness as a polyarthritis; *see also* POLYARTHRITIS.

feline torovirus A virus similar to coronavirus; has been associated with cases of diarrhoea.

feline upper respiratory tract disease Respiratory illness caused by FHV-1 and calicivirus *See also* FELINE VIRAL RHINOTRACHEITIS.

feline urological syndrome (FUS) Sandy deposits of struvite (triple phosphate) crystals that commonly block the penile urethra in male, neutered cats; possibly associated with high-magnesium dry food diets or stress; if the urethra blocks totally, the situation is an emergency; in the short term, the obstruction is cleared and the bladder catheterized; in the long term, prescription diets can be fed or urinary acidifiers used to help to dissolve crystals.

feline viral rhinotracheitis (FVR) Infectious respiratory disease caused by a herpes virus; often causes severe signs, especially in kittens and young cats; a carrier state is common after acute infection.

FELV *See* FELINE LEUKAEMIA VIRUS.

female Individuals having an XX genotype and female reproductive organs.

feminization Development of external female characteristics by a male; associated with some tumours and hormone treatments.

femoral Relating to the femur and the thigh region.

femur The thigh bone, running from hip to stifle.

fenbendazole A commonly used, broad-spectrum worming preparation effective against most nematodes and cestodes.

fenestrated drape Surgical drape with an opening or window cut out of it.

fenestration Cutting out a window or opening.

fentanyl A short-acting opioid analgesic, often combined with a neuroleptic for neuroleptanalgesia.

feral Wild, used to describe colonies of free-living cats.

Ferguson's reflex During parturition, dilation of the cervix by the fetus stimulates the release of oxytocin from the maternal posterior pituitary gland, leading to contractions of the myometrium.

ferret Popular pet, a carnivore previously semi-domesticated for hunting rabbits. Male may be twice as large as female; *see also* MUSTID.

ferrin A constituent of bile pigment containing iron.

ferritin A protein found in the liver that acts as a reserve of iron for the body.

fertile Able to reproduce.

fertilization The penetration of an ovum by a sperm, with fusion of the gametes.

FeSFV *See* FELINE SYNCYTIUM-FORMING VIRUS, POLYARTHRITIS.

fetal Relating to the fetus.

fetal membranes The two layers surrounding the unborn puppy or kitten are known as the allantoamnion and the chorioallantois. Usually only recognized when the 'water bag' appears at the vulva during the birth process.

fetid Foul-smelling.

fetlock The foreleg or hindleg joint in the horse, incorporating the distal third metacarpal/tarsal, proximal sesamoid bones and proximal phalanx (long pastern).

fetus Unborn offspring; embryo after the fetal membranes develop until birth.

fever Pyrexia; having an elevated body temperature.

FIA *See* FELINE INFECTIOUS ANAEMIA.

fibre Thread-like structure.

fibreglass Mixture of resin and fibres that hardens on contact with air; bandages impregnated with fibreglass can be used for external fracture fixation; the resulting cast is light and waterproof.

fibril Filamentous structure; often a fibre will be made up of several fibrils.

fibrillation Rapid, small contractions of muscle fibres, rather than coordinated contraction of the whole muscle.

fibrin An important clotting protein in the blood; formed by the action of thrombin on fibrinogen.

fibrinogen Precursor of fibrin; a globulin protein found in the blood.

fibrinolysis The dissolution and removal of fibrin clots.

fibrinous Made of fibrin.

fibroblast Immature fibrous connective tissue cell that can produce collagen fibres.

fibrocartilage Cartilage rich in type I collagen fibres; found where tendons and ligaments blend into bone.

fibrocyte Mature fibrous connective tissue cell, often dormant and relatively inactive.

fibroma Benign tumour of fibrous connective tissue.

fibrosarcoma Malignant tumour of fibrous connective tissue.

fibrosis Fibrous reaction to an injury.

fibrous Made of fibrous tissue.

fibula Thin bone on the lateral aspect of the hindleg; runs alongside the tibia from the stifle to the hock; distally, the fibula forms the lateral malleolus, which contributes to the stability of the tibiotarsal joint.

FIE *See* FELINE INFECTIOUS ENTERITIS.

field (of microscope) Area within which objects are visible at any particular magnification.

field of vision Area that can be seen by one eye at any one time.

fight or flight response Instinctive response to danger where an animal will either try to fight or flee, attributed to the body's physical response to stressful situations; *see also* STRESS.

fight wounds Various wounds that result from fights between animals, may be inflicted by teeth or claws; the potential for infection must always be considered; teeth puncture wounds may appear less serious but damage to deeper structures must always be borne in mind.

figure-of-eight bandage Method of applying white open-weave (nonconforming) bandage to ensure even pressure is obtained; may also be used when conforming bandage is applied to a tapering region, e.g. tail.

filamentous Made of thin threads.

filariasis The presence of filariae in the body tissues or circulation.

Filaroides osleri The most common nematode lungworm of the dog; ingested larvae travel in the lymphatics and circulation to the lungs, where they migrate to the tracheal bifurcation causing a chronic tracheobronchitis and cough; usually associated with kennelled animals. Diagnosis is best confirmed by bronchoscopy, where characteristic nodules at the tracheal bifurcation or within the bronchi are seen; treatment with suitable anthelminthics is usually effective; *see also* OSLERUS OSLERI.

film badge Personal radiation monitoring badge, worn on the trunk by staff undertaking radiographic procedures; consists of various thicknesses of metal overlying sensitive film; badges are sent for reading at statutory intervals to ensure that body radiation is below legal limits.

film focal distance (FFD) The distance between the radiographic film and the focal spot in the X-ray tube head; the distance affects the exposure according to the inverse square law – i.e. if the FFD is doubled, the exposure will have to be quadrupled; the greater the FFD, the sharper the image as there is less penumbral blurring; *see also* PENUMBRA.

filoplumes Long feathers lying close to the flight feathers that have a sensory function.

filter Sheet of aluminium or copper in the X-ray tube head that absorbs radiation of low energy that would not contribute to a diagnostic image.

filum Thread-like structure.

filum terminale Thin, fibrous continuation of the pia mater (innermost meningeal layer) from the end of the spinal cord to the coccygeal vertebrae.

fimbria, *pl.* fimbriae Fringe, e.g. at the end of the oviduct.

fin Webbing of skin stretched across supporting bones and used for locomotion by fish.

fin rot Term used to describe various conditions of the fin; may be caused by bites from other fish, *Oodinium* spp. and infections; treatment depends on the specific cause.

fine needle aspirate (FNA) Used to collect a diagnostic sample for laboratory examination.

finger sweep A method of checking the mouth in emergency airway obstruction.

Finochietto retractor Surgical instrument for retracting the chest wall to allow access to the thoracic cavity.

FIP *See* FELINE INFECTIOUS PERITONITIS.

firearms certificate Licence granted by the police that must be held by all veterinary surgeons who have dart guns or humane killers such as captive bolt pistols.

first aid Immediate life-saving aid that may be given without the need for any drugs, medication or specialist equipment.

first-intention healing How sutured surgical wounds heal – the epithelial layers are held in apposition, fibroblasts migrate across the wound and there is minimal scarring.

fissure Deep furrow.

fistula, *pl.* fistulae Abnormal tube connecting two epithelial surfaces, e.g. vaginorectal fistulae linking the vagina to the rectum may occur after whelping; if material regularly passes through the fistula, the connection develops its own epithelial lining and becomes permanently patent, e.g. teat fistulae will not heal while the animal continues to produce milk, which passes through the opening.

fit Lay term for a convulsion or seizure; *see also* EPILEPSY.

fitness to practice The responsibility of all veterinary nurses and surgeons to ensure that they are clinically competent, maintain trust from colleagues and clients and adhere to all aspects of the RCVS Code of Professional Conduct.

FIV *See* FELINE IMMUNODEFICIENCY VIRUS.

Five element theories Each element in traditional Chinese medicine represents a certain quality and stage of transformation. It is regulated by a negative feedback system and a control system. Wood, fire, Earth, metal and water are the five important elements.

fixation, external Any method of fracture fixation using apparatus applied to the outside of the limb, e.g. splinting, casting, external fixator frames.

fixation, internal Any method of fracture fixation involving the use of implants within the bone or on the bone surface, e.g. intramedullary pinning, plating, tension band wiring, rush pinning, etc.

fixative 1) A chemical that denatures protein, hardening and preserving tissue samples, e.g. formalin. **2)** In radiography, the chemical solution that dissolves and removes unexposed silver bromide crystals from the radiographic film and hardens the film, though wet processing is rarely performed nowadays.

flaccid Limp, relaxed, lacking tone.

flagellum Whip-like tail attached to many protozoa, some bacteria and cells such as sperm; used for locomotion.

flail chest Segment of the thoracic wall that becomes free moving as a result of multiple rib fractures; the free segment is sucked inwards by the negative pressure produced during inspiration and compromises respiratory function; treatment consists of stabilizing the fragment to an external frame.

flank Lateral body wall between the last rib and the hindleg.

flare, aqueous Bright reflection of light from particles within the anterior chamber of the eye.

flatulence Gas in the digestive tract.

flea Common ectoparasitic insect, living mainly in the environment but moving on to warm-blooded animals to feed on their blood; intermediate host for part of the life cycle of *Dipylidium caninum*, the common tapeworm of the dog. Flea life cycle can be as short as 3 weeks under suitable conditions or eggs can remain dormant for many months.

flea allergy dermatitis *See* FAD, FELINE MILIARY ECZEMA.

flehmen reaction Often seen in sexually aroused stallions, when they typically extend their neck and curl their upper lip. Thought to be associated with trapping pheromone smells in the nostrils so that they can be analyzed to tell if the mare is in oestrus; less noticeable reflexes are also shown by dogs and many other species; *see also* VOMERONASAL ORGAN.

flexion Movement of a joint such that the angle between the articulating bones reduces.

flexor Muscle whose action is to bring about flexion of a joint.

flexure A bend.

floaters Small bodies within the vitreous of the eye.

flocculent Tending to precipitate and form irregular, fluffy masses.

flooding The continuous exposure of the animal to a stimulus at a level that evokes a response in behaviour training until the response to the stimulus ceases.

flotation Laboratory technique where faecal samples are mixed with sugar or salt solutions of a high specific gravity; worm eggs will float in this solution and stick to a cover slip floated on the surface.

flowmeter Part of an anaesthetic circuit used to regulate the flow of gases to the patient; the scale is marked in litres/ minute and a float in the chamber is used to take the reading; most floats have a dot on them that shows that the float is rotating and gas is flowing (rotameter).

fluids Liquid substances; in nursing relates to rehydration, either oral or parenteral routes are commonly used.

fluid therapy The use of blood, plasma or synthetic fluids to replace deficits; may be administered intravenously, subcutaneously, intraperitoneally and intraosseously; fluid therapy supports the cardiovascular system and maintains renal perfusion and urine output; an important component of the treatment for many disorders, including shock.

fluke A trematode parasite (*Fasciola hepatica*) that resides in the liver of horses, sheep and cattle.

fluorescein Fluorescent dye that can be used to demonstrate corneal ulcers, check the patency of the nasolacrimal duct, etc.

fluorescent Able to absorb light of one wavelength and emit light of a longer wavelength.

fluorescent antibody testing A laboratory method of detecting antigens using a specific antibody labelled with a fluorescent marker.

fluoroquinolones Important group of antibacterial agents effective against Gram-negative organisms. Used in the treatment of otitis media caused by *Pseudomonas* species and for enteric infections such as *Salmonella*; *see also* ENFLOXIN, CIPROFLOXACIN.

fluoroscopy Radiographic technique where X-rays are generated and passed continuously through the area of interest; the image is formed on a fluorescent screen, providing a moving image; useful for guided catheterization of vessels, evaluating gut peristalsis/swallowing, etc.

Fluothane *See* HALOTHANE.

fluralaner An ectoparasiticide of the isoxazoline group, systemically active against fleas for 12 weeks and ticks for

8 weeks; in dogs it can be used as part of a treatment strategy for the control of Flea Allergy Dermatitis.

FLUTD Feline lower urinary tract disease; *see also* FELINE UROLOGICAL SYNDROME.

fly strike Infestation of flesh-eating maggots caused by the hatching of Dipteran blow-fly eggs laid on the skin or fur. Usually occurs in hot weather in animals that are debilitated and not able to groom themselves.

FNA *See* FINE NEEDLE ASPIRATE.

focal Restricted to one defined area.

focal–film distance The distance between the target in the X-ray tube and the film.

focal spot The area on the target in an X-ray tube head where the electrons strike; the region where the radiation is produced; the smaller the focal spot the sharper the resulting radiographic image as there is less blurring.

focusing cup Part of the X-ray tube head that focuses the primary beam.

fogging Radiographic term describing lack of definition in the finished radiograph; causes are overdevelopment or inadequate rinsing after fixation.

folate One of the B complex vitamins.

Foley catheter Indwelling urinary catheter with a soft bulb at one end that can be inflated with air or water to hold the catheter tip in the bladder.

follicle Collection of cells with a central hollow or cavity, e.g. **ovarian follicles** surrounding developing ova.

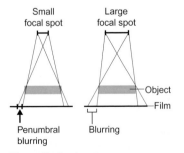

Figure 17. Focal spot.

follicle-stimulating hormone (FSH) Hormone released from the anterior pituitary; stimulates the formation and maturation of Graafian follicles within the ovary; in the male it increases spermatogenesis.

follicular stasis Disorder of tortoises and turtles, failed ovulation causing hindlimb paresis.

folliculitis Inflammation of hair follicles, with the formation of papules and pustules.

fomentation Application of heat to an area, e.g. use of a poultice.

fomite An inanimate object, such as a grooming brush or feed bowl that may transmit disease-causing organisms.

fontanelle The junction between two cranial bones in the immature animal.

food Dietary material that is consumed to meet nutritional needs.

food hypersensitivity Allergic reaction to a component of the diet; *see also* WHEAT-SENSITIVE ENTEROPATHY.

foot-and-mouth disease Highly contagious, viral, notifiable disease of cloven-hoofed animals; characterized by the appearance of vesicles around the mouth, between the digits, etc.; DEFRA must be informed if the disease is suspected, and a slaughter policy operates in the UK.

foramen Hole or aperture.

foramen magnum The opening in the occipital bone of the skull that allows the exit of the spinal cord and its enveloping meningeal membranes.

foramen ovale The hole in the septum between the atria in the fetal heart; this allows blood to bypass the lungs in the fetus; it normally closes at birth.

foraminotomy Surgical enlargement of a foramen; may be used as part of the lateral surgical approach to the spinal cord where enlargement of a spinal foramen between two adjacent vertebrae allows decompression of the exiting spinal nerve.

force feeding Providing food for a patient who refuses to eat voluntarily.

forceps Instrument for gripping and holding tissues; common types include

Allis tissue forceps, bone-holding forceps, dressing forceps and rat-toothed forceps.

forearm Region from the elbow to the carpus.

forebrain Cerebral hemispheres and thalamus.

foregut The cranial portion of the gut in the developing embryo, becoming the pharynx, oesophagus, stomach and duodenum.

foreign body Any object within the body that is not self, e.g. a piece of grit, shard of glass, barley awn, swallowed golf ball, etc.

FORL *See* FELINE ODONTOCLASTIC RESORPTIVE LESION DISEASE.

formaldehyde Formic acid; a pungent disinfectant and tissue fixative; the vapour is toxic.

formalin A 37% aqueous solution of formaldehyde, used as a tissue fixative.

formulary A collection of drug formulae and dosing information, e.g. British National Formulary (BNF).

formulation The chemical preparations of a drug, e.g. ointment, tablet, powder, liquid.

fornix Arch-shaped structure.

forte The Latin word for 'strong' used by pharmaceutical manufacturers to distinguish from a less-concentrated product.

fossa Dent or depression, usually in the surface of a bone.

fossa ovalis The point in the wall of the right atrium where the foramen ovale of the fetus allows passage of blood from the left and right atria.

fovea Cup-shaped depression or small pit; the lower part of the retina where the greatest concentration of cones occurs.

FP Feline panleukopenia or 'feline parvo'; *see also* FELINE INFECTIOUS ENTERITIS, FELINE PARVOVIRUS, PANLEUKOPENIA.

FPV *See* FELINE PARVOVIRUS.

fractionate Separate out the components of a mixture.

fracture Complete break in the integrity of a bone; usually a result of trauma but can occur with little force if the bone is diseased, e.g. fracture at the site of an osteosarcoma.

fracture disease Less than optimal return to function after bony union at a fracture site; may be caused by malunion, nerve damage, muscle contracture, fibrosis, etc.

fracture healing The physiological method by which a fracture heals; if there is a gap of more than a few millimetres between the bone ends, the initial haematoma organizes into a fibrous callus, which calcifies and finally ossifies; if the fracture is rigidly immobilized and there are no gaps or only small gaps between the fragments, direct bony union can occur; direct bony union is the more rapid process, but the repair is not as strong initially as callus.

fracture separation Type of fracture occurring in skeletally immature animals, where the fracture line is at the level of a growth plate; commonly divided into Salter–Harris types I–V.

fragmented coronoid process The most common lesion of elbow dysplasia; the medial coronoid process of the ulna fails to develop correctly and forms one or more loose fragments, which irritate the joint and cause secondary arthrosis; *see also* ELBOW DYSPLASIA.

franchise An agreement from a company for another individual or group to act as an agent and market and provide that company's product or service.

free radicals Many age-related changes are thought to result from free radicals attacking cells and allowing the contents to spill out, destroying the cell; in nutrition, as important as vitamins, minerals; some enzymes can neutralize the radicals; *see also* VITAMIN E, ANTIOXIDANT ENZYMES.

French moult Rapid shedding of flight and tail feathers, making affected birds unable to fly; exact cause is unknown.

frenulum Band of connective tissue on the ventral aspect of the tongue.

friable Brittle, crumbling.

friction Cause of skin trauma, varies in severity from that caused by collar friction to the neck to severe 'friction

burns' and granuloma caused by persistent licking.

frog A wedge-shaped area of soft, incompletely keratinized epidermis just caudal to the sole of the equine hoof; functions as a shock absorber when the hoof contacts the ground.

frontal bone Bone of the skull forming the forehead and dorsomedial aspect of the orbit.

frontal sinus Air spaces within the frontal bone that communicate with the nasal passages.

frostbite Damage to tissue caused by extreme cold; ear tips, toes and tail are most commonly affected; affected areas become erythematous initially but then slough.

fructo-oligosaccharide A compound of fructose and oligosaccharide that cannot be hydrolyzed in animals unless it is fermented in the large intestine by bacteria.

fructose Fruit sugar.

frusemide *See* FUROSEMIDE.

FSA *See* FELINE FIBROSARCOMA.

FSE *See* FELINE SPONGIFORM ENCEPHALOPATHY.

FSH *See* FOLLICLE-STIMULATING HORMONE.

FTLV Feline T-lymphotrophic lentivirus, now renamed FIV; *see also* FELINE IMMUNODEFICIENCY VIRUS.

full-pin splintage Type of external fixator frame where the pins enter the limb, penetrate both cortices of the bone and exit through the skin on the far side, thus allowing connecting bars to be placed on two sides of the limb.

fulminating Occurring suddenly and rapidly worsening.

fumigation Use of a gas or vapour to disinfect the environment.

fundus The lowest part of a hollow organ or the part furthest away from the opening; the lower part or body of the stomach adjacent to the pylorus; also used to describe the posterior surface of the eyeball as seen by the ophthalmoscope.

fungal Relating to an infection with a fungus.

fungicide Substance used extensively in horticulture to eliminate plant fungi, may be the cause of poisoning in pets; *see also* CARBAMATE, POISON.

fungus, *pl.* **fungi** Yeasts and moulds; some are commensals, some are opportunistic pathogens, while others always cause disease; *see also* CANDIDA, MALASSEZIA, MICROSPORUM CANIS, TRICHOPHYTON SPP., MYCOSIS, RINGWORM.

funicular Cord-like.

fur The hair coat of animals, characteristic of mammals.

furcation Dental disorder when the roots of molar teeth become exposed.

furosemide Commonly used diuretic (used to be called *frusemide*) promoting the excretion of potassium and loss of water via the kidneys. A loop diuretic.

fur slip Chinchillas can shed patches of fur if they are handled roughly.

furunculosis Deep pyoderma; *see also* ANAL FURUNCULOSIS.

FUO Fever of unknown origin; *see also* PYREXIA.

FUS *See* FELINE UROLOGICAL SYNDROME.

fusiform Spindle-shaped.

FVR *See* FELINE VIRAL RHINOTRACHEITIS.

gag Metal, plastic or wooden objects used to hold the mouth open, thus allowing access for dentistry, oral examination etc.; sometimes a roll of bandage between the molar teeth or a wooden block with a drilled hole is utilized to help to pass a stomach tube.

gagging Description of a choking/retching mechanism often associated with vomiting as a reflex.

gait Movement; the limbs' movement assessment, used in orthopaedic and neurological examinations to assess for defective proprioception and in joint disorders.

galactic Relating to milk.

galactose Monosaccharide derived from lactose and converted to glucose in the liver; important in kitten and puppy nutrition.

galactostasis In the bitch, excess milk in the mammary glands observed at the time of weaning or during pseudopregnancy.

gall bladder Structure in the liver for bile storage, connects to the duodenum via the bile ducts.

galliform (or gallinaceous) The group of ground-living, chicken-like birds, including poultry, turkeys, pheasants, guinea fowl and quail.

gallipot Small container used in pharmacy and surgery for ointments and lotions.

gallop rhythm Heart disorder where the beat is very rapid and similar to the beat of a horse's fastest gait.

game birds Includes pheasants and partridges; may be reared artificially or as naturally occurring animals.

gamete Mature sex cell – the sperm of the male or the ovum of the female.

Gamgee Dressing composed of a thick layer of absorbent cotton between two layers of gauze.

gamma Third letter of the Greek alphabet; often used to describe newer words for globulins and in radiation studies; *see also* GAMMA RAYS, GAMMAGLOBULIN, RADIATION.

gammaglobulin Any of a class of protein present in the bloodstream; as almost all are immunoglobulins, often used as a measure of immunity.

gamma-linoleic acid (GLA) One of the lipids responsible for mediating the anti-inflammatory reaction.

gamma rays Rays emitted by radioactive substances that have severe cytotoxic effects.

GAS *See* GENERAL ADAPTATION SYNDROME.

G cells The cells in the lower part of the stomach adjacent to the pylorus that secrete gastrin.

ganglion A group of nerve cells important in the interchange of signals, some distance away from the CNS; *see also* PARASYMPATHETIC NERVOUS SYSTEM, SYMPATHETIC.

gangrene Death and decay of part of the body caused by loss of nutrition and then invasion by anaerobic bacteria; caused by a failure of the blood supply, toxins, burns, etc.; *see also* NECROSIS.

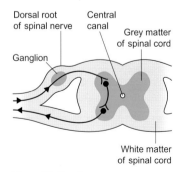

Figure 18. Ganglion.

gangrenous mastitis Toxins from infections such as *Staphylococcus* spp.; may cause necrosis of part of the mammary gland.

ganja Alternative word used for cannabis; *see also* POISONS.

gap analysis The measurement of distance between actual performance compared with desired performance.

garter snake *Thamnophis* spp., member of the Colubridae family, has only a right lung and no caecum nor pelvic spur.

gas Usually invisible vapour in which the particles are diffusely suspended, e.g. anaesthetic gas. **Alveolar gas** is the gas used in respiration that remains in the alveoli; *see also* ANATOMIC DEAD SPACE.

gaseous products of digestion (GPD) Gases that escape from the body as part of the digestive process.

gaskin Portion of the hindleg muscles proximal to the hock; term rarely used in dogs but used for horses.

gastric Relates to the stomach.

gastric dilation Distension of the stomach with gas, a disorder usually affecting the larger breeds of dog; arises mainly soon after feeding and can rapidly become life-threatening as it impairs respiration. May result from pyloric dysfunction, a foreign body, torsion, atonic muscles; *see also* AEROPHAGY, TYMPANY.

gastric dilation/volvulus (GDV) Acute illness seen in deep-chested dogs where the stomach inflates and then rotates, often involving a rotation of the spleen and then a profound vascular change affecting venous return; this is an emergency.

gastric emptying time The time it takes for food/liquid to leave the stomach and enter the duodenum. Physiologically important, can be demonstrated with contrast radiography; may be used diagnostically.

gastric haemorrhage Bleeding of the stomach lining; blood appears in the vomit; possible causes include a bleeding ulcer or a foreign body.

gastric juice Fluids of low pH secreted within the stomach, neutralizes the saliva so that pepsinogen can function; *see also* GASTRIN.

gastric lavage Used to remove toxic or excess stomach contents; a technique using two tubes: one to pump in and a wider-bore one to drain out gastric contents; can be improvised.

gastric lipase Enzyme secreted in the stomach of newborn animals to assist the digestion of milk fat; *see also* LIPASE.

gastric torsion The disease state where the stomach has rotated through 180° or 360° so that gas can no longer escape up the oesophagus.

gastric tympany A condition when the stomach is gas-filled and there has been some inability to release it.

gastric ulcer Occurs in the mucosal layer, of significance when medication has been used; *see also* NON-STEROIDAL ANTI-INFLAMMATORY DRUG.

gastrin Hormone produced by the 'G' cells of the fundus of the stomach; stimulates the production of acid secretions.

gastritis Inflammation of the lining of the stomach. Bacteria such as *Helicobacter*, food toxins in the stomach or some disease elsewhere in the body may be involved.

gastro- Relating to the stomach.

gastrocentesis Puncture of the stomach to relieve gas distension, usually an emergency procedure.

gastrocnemius Muscle of the hindleg connecting the distal femur to the os calcis of the tibia, extends the hock on contraction.

gastroenteritis Inflammation of the lining of the stomach and the intestine – usually seen as vomiting and diarrhoea or 'D & V'.

gastrointestinal tract The part of the digestive system that includes the stomach and the intestines.

gastropexy Surgical procedure to form an adhesion between the stomach and peritoneum, used to prevent the return of gastric torsion.

gastroscope Endoscope designed to examine the interior of the stomach; it is necessary that it should be flexible in order to curve to see all the surfaces of the organ.

gastrosteges The large scales on the ventral surface of a snake.

gastrotomy Surgical incision into the stomach.

gauze, absorbent Wound dressing with open-mesh weave.

GDV *See* GASTRIC DILATION/ VOLVULUS.

gecko Small reptile, sometimes kept as an exotic pet.

Geiger counter An instrument for detecting and measuring radiation, such as particles from radioactive material, consisting of a Geiger tube and associated electronic equipment. Used for measuring the exposure of personnel involved in the treatment of cats with iodine-131 for hyperthyroidism.

gel Suspension of colloid with a firm consistency. Used in laboratory tests for diffusion techniques.

gelatin Pliable substance produced by digesting collagen; used for medicinal capsules and in a modified form as a surgical dressing, often as a foam.

geld Traditional word for neutering farm animals. Castrated horses are still known as geldings.

Gelpi retractors Surgical instrument with single-point tips and ratchet for holding tissues apart.

gene The basic unit of genetic material found on the chromosome in the cell nucleus, made up of a particular sequence of base pairs (nucleotide bases pairing: adenine with cytosine, guanine with thymine) on the DNA strand. A **dominant gene** is one that produces its effect in the offspring regardless of the other allele. A **lethal gene** is one that brings about the death of the organism.

A **mutated gene** is the 'rogue' that has mutated to produce a different characteristic. A **recessive gene** is one that produces its effect in the offspring only when both alleles are the same; *see also* HOMOZYGOUS.

gene alleles Different forms of the same gene occupying the same locus on the chromosome.

gene mapping Modern technology used to study the gene locus.

general adaptation syndrome (GAS) A response to stress by the body.

general anaesthesia Method for bringing about loss of consciousness, muscle relaxation with pain removal by direct action on the CNS, produced by inhalation or injection of an anaesthetic or analgesic drug.

general anaesthetic (GA) The administration of an anaesthetic agent to bring about loss of consciousness.

General Sales List (GSL) Pharmaceutical category of medicines that may be sold to the pet owner without restriction.

generalized progressive retinal atrophy (gPRA) Degenerative condition of the retina; inherited in dogs, most commonly as an autosomal recessive trait; also occurs in Abyssinian and Siamese cats; typically, the animal develops poor night vision; *see also* CENTRAL PROGRESSIVE RETINAL ATROPHY.

generic name The chemical or compound name of a drug, for example meloxicam; *see also* TRADE NAME.

gene selection Breeding strategies; eventually could eliminate hereditary disorders.

gene therapy The introduction of genes into a cell to ameliorate a disease process.

genetics The science of studying inheritance.

genial Relating to the chin.

genicular Relating to the knee.

genital Relating to the organs of reproduction, especially the visible external organs. As an adjective, the word 'genitals' is incorrect; *see also* GENITALIA.

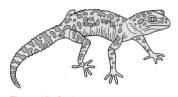

Figure 19. Gecko.

genitalia Popular term for the external parts of the reproductive organs; *see also* PENIS, VULVA.

genome The complete set of hereditary factors comprising all the genes in the chromosomes.

genotype The genetic make-up that acts together with environmental factors to give a particular individual characteristics; *see also* PHENOTYPE.

gentamicin Antibiotic effective against mainly Gram-negative bacteria but because of toxicity often used as a topical application only.

genus Group classification of organisms, higher than 'species'.

genu valgum Angulation of the femur and the tibia to produce a condition of the knee joint equivalent to 'knock knees'.

gerbil Small mammal and popular child's pet.

geriatric Relating to the state of ageing and to disease of old animals.

gestation The period of pregnancy from fertilization to birth.

GFR *See* GLOMERULAR FILTRATION RATE.

GH *See* GROWTH HORMONE.

ghost cells Pale outlines of red blood cells that may be seen microscopically in urine samples.

Giardia Genus of parasitic organisms, motile when examined in fresh faeces because they have flagella. Species cause disease in cats and dogs; often an intractable diarrhoea with the presence of mucus and blood.

Giemsa Stain used in the microscopic examination of differential blood films, protozoal parasites, bacteria, etc.

Gigli saw Fine wire chain used to saw through bone, as in the amputation of the forelimb through the humerus.

gill The external apparatus of the fish to obtain oxygen from the surrounding water, equivalent in function to the mammal's lung.

Gillies needle holder Needle holder with a short blade to cut the suture material included near the points of the forceps.

gingiva The gum.

gingivitis Inflammation of the gums, often seen as a red rim at the margin with the teeth; *see also* PERIODONTITIS.

ginglymus Joint in which movement occurs in one plane; the knee and the elbow joints are the commonest examples.

girdle An encircling structure, e.g. the **pelvic girdle**.

GIT *See* GASTROINTESTINAL TRACT.

gizzard The muscular stomach of the bird, between the proventriculus and the small intestine; the gizzard is packed with grit that is used to macerate the food.

gland A group of cells organized to produce a secretion or an excretion, traditionally divided into the two groups **endocrine glands** and **exocrine glands**.

gland of Harder Term once used for the nictitans gland on the inner surface of the third eyelid.

gland of Moll Modified sweat glands at the edge of the eyelid.

glans The tip of the penis; enlarges with altered blood flow.

glaucoma Increased intraocular pressure; pressure on the retina may result in loss of vision; a series of pathological conditions develop varying with the pressure increase and its consequences; *see also* AQUEOUS, CLOSED-ANGLE GLAUCOMA, OPEN-ANGLE GLAUCOMA, UVEITIS.

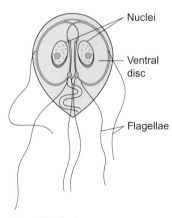

Figure 20. *Giardia* sp.

glenoid cavity Hollow depression in the ventral part of the scapula, for articulation with the head of the humerus.

glia (neuroglia) Special connective tissue of the CNS; glial cells make up about 40% of the brain.

glial cell Forms part of the neuroglia connective tissue around the neurones; *see also* NEUROGLIA.

gliosis The loss of neural elements, especially in the retina of the eye following some form of injury.

globe (eye) The optic globe is the equivalent of the eyeball.

globulin Protein substance with large molecules; immunoglobulins are produced by the plasma cells and have an important role in immunity. Serum protein electrophoresis divides globulins into five groups including alpha (α), beta (β) and gamma (γ). The gammaglobulins have the most important function in 'humoral' immunity.

glomerular filtrate The product in the kidney of diffusion from the bloodstream of an ultrafiltrate of plasma (low in proteins) into the low pressure of Bowman's capsule, ready to pass into the tubules.

glomerular filtration rate (GFR) A measure of renal blood flow.

glomerulonephritis Inflammation of the filtering glomeruli of the kidney, characterized by urine samples that are very rich in protein.

glomerulus The tuft of capillaries contained in the cup-like Bowman's capsule of a nephron. Fed by afferent arterioles and drained by efferent arterioles.

glossal Relating to the tongue.

glossopharyngeal nerve Cranial nerve IX, supplies the pharynx, tongue and salivary glands.

glossotrichia Hairs emerging from the dorsum of the tongue; a condition seen in cocker spaniels and other breeds.

glottis The vocal apparatus, consists of a space between the vocal cords and is that part of the larynx that produces sounds such as barking, mewing and purring.

glove, radiography Fine layers of lead within these gloves give some protection to the hands. The gloved hands should not be placed in the primary beam.

glove, surgical Latex rubber glove capable of being sterilized or already packed sterile. Closed- and open-gloving methods may be used in applying them to the hands.

gloving The procedure of donning sterile gloves so that there is no contamination from the hands or clothing, preserving the asepsis of the procedure. There are three methods that can be used – **1)** open, when the hand picks up the glove, only touching it on the inside; **2)** closed, the most commonly used and easiest of the three methods, when the hands are not pushed entirely through the gown cuffs so that they do not touch the gloves; **3)** plunge, when an assistant holds the gloves open and the hands are plunged into the gloves. This method is very rarely used.

glucagon Hormone produced by the pancreas that causes an increase in the blood sugar level.

glucocorticoid Any one of a group of corticosteroids that are essential for the utilization of carbohydrate, fat and protein by the body. Both natural production and synthetic hormones have powerful anti-inflammatory effects.

gluconeogenesis Formation of glucose from protein or other noncarbohydrate sources; *see also* GLYCOGENOLYSIS.

glucosamine Amino acid derivative found in many glycoproteins and polysaccharides.

glucose A simple sugar used by the body as an important energy source. Any glucose not needed for energy is stored as glycogen.

glucosuria The presence of glucose in the urine; *see also* DIABETES MELLITUS.

glutamate Involved in neurotransmission, acts at the N-methyl-D-aspartate (NMDA) receptor.

glutamic–oxaloacetic transaminase (GOT) See SGOT.

glutamic–pyruvic transaminase (GPT) See SGPT.

glutaraldehyde Compound that used to be used for the cold sterilization of instruments such as endoscopes; produces irritant vapours. Has been superceded by safer alternatives. Also used as a tissue fixative for electron microscopy.

gluteal Muscle mass of the hip, used to extend, abduct and rotate the thigh.

gluten The protein found in wheat and in other cereal grains; *see also* DIETARY HYPERSENSITIVITY, MALABSORPTION, WHEAT-SENSITIVE ENTEROPATHY.

glycaemia Implies the presence of glucose in the blood; *see also* HYPOGLYCAEMIA, HYPERGLYCAEMIA.

glycerol Clear viscous solution with a sweetish taste, used as an enema in cats and topically to moisten the skin. Also known as glycerine when used pharmaceutically.

glycine A nonessential amino acid; functions as an inhibitory neurotransmitter in the CNS.

glycogen Storage form of carbohydrate, formed and stored in the liver and muscles.

glycogenolysis The provision of energy by the conversion of glycogen to glucose; occurs in muscles as well as the liver.

glycolysis Glucose converted by enzyme activity to lactate or pyruvate, with release of energy.

glycoprotein Protein molecule combined with a protein group.

glycopyrrolate Anticholinergic compound, sometimes used in preanaesthetic medication; *see also* ATROPINE.

GME *See* GRANULOMATOUS MENINGOENCEPHALITIS.

gnatho- Relating to something involved with the jaws.

gnathotheca Keratin layer in the mandibular beak.

gnotobiotic animal An animal reared in such a way as to exclude normal bacteria – born 'germ-free' it may be infected with one organism to study the response.

goblet cell Simple glands whose function is to secrete mucus; may be found in the lining of epithelial surfaces.

goitre Condition seen as a swelling of the neck from enlargement of the thyroid gland.

golden hour The first hour immediately following trauma during which a critically ill patient can be saved (or lost); *see also* TRAUMA.

Golgi complex The organelle complex in the cell; consists of a series of tubes that store lysosomal enzymes.

gonad Male or female reproductive gland that produces the gametes and hormones; *see also* OVARY, TESTIS.

gonadotrophin Any of those hormones synthesized by the pituitary gland that have an effect on the gonads; release of gonadotropins is stimulated by gonadotrophin-releasing hormone (GnRH); *see also* FOLLICLE-STIMULATING HORMONE, LUTEINISING HORMONE.

goniometer Special lens instrument for measuring intraocular pressure by measuring iridocorneal angles; *see also* OPEN-ANGLE GLAUCOMA, CLOSED-ANGLE GLAUCOMA.

gonioscopy A procedure during which the junction between the iris and the cornea is viewed directly using a special lens.

gonitis Inflammation of the stifle (femorotibial) joint.

goodwill An intangible asset of a business, based on its reputation that is taken into account as a value asset when a business is sold.

gouge A curved chisel used in orthopaedic operations to cut and remove bone.

Graafian follicle Small follicle containing an oocyte that develops in the ovary; it matures to release an ovum and forms the corpus luteum.

gracilis muscle A fine, 'slender' muscle that connects the pelvic symphysis to the tibial crest; adducts the limb.

Graefe's knife A knife with a fine point used in cataract surgery.

graft operation Any tissue or organ that is removed from one site and located elsewhere.

gram Unit of mass equivalent to 1/1000th of a kilogram.

Gram's stain Staining of bacteria by application of dyestuffs, iodine and ethanol: bacteria that retain the crystal violet colour are **Gram-positive** and those that can be decolourized and then retain carbol fuchsin, a red dye, are **Gram-negative** organisms.

grand mal (fit) Major convulsive attack, as occurs in epileptic fits; *see also* EPILEPSY, SEIZURES.

granular casts Structures found in urine specimens that indicate protein leakage from the distal tubules of the kidney but are not specific to disease states.

granulation, healing by Process of wound healing where fibroblasts and vascular elements progressively fill up a wound defect so that eventually epithelium can grow across; *see also* SECOND-INTENTION HEALING.

granulocytes White cells of the blood that have granules in the cytoplasm and a multilobular nucleus: neutrophils, eosinophils, basophils. Also known as polymorphonuclear leukocytes.

granuloma Description of a tissue mass that has an appearance similar to granulation tissue. May appear like a tumour but is usually the result of a chronic inflammatory process.

granulomatous meningoencephalitis (GME) An inflammatory disease of the central nervous system.

grass seeds Spiky grass awns that may penetrate the skin or cause severe irritation on entering orifices such as the ears, mouth, eyelids and prepuce; *see also* OTITIS EXTERNA, INTERDIGITAL ABSCESS.

grass sickness A very serious, often fatal condition of horses and donkeys where damage to parts of the nervous system controlling involuntary functions such as digestion leads to gut paralysis; the exact cause remains unclear but it may be due to a bacterial toxin.

gravid Pregnant; *see also* PRIMIGRAVIDA, MULTIGRAVIDA.

grazed wounds Abrasions, open wounds; often the result of friction in RTA, etc.

greenstick fracture A partial bone fracture, usually occurring in young animals in which the bone is bent but only broken through one cortex.

grey matter The parts of the brain and spinal cord that contain the cell bodies of neurones.

grid Structure like a grating, used in radiography as a series of vertical lead strips that reduce or eliminate scatter from the primary beam.

griseofulvin An antibiotic administered by mouth to treat fungal infections of the skin such as ringworm; should be handled with care: teratogenic.

grit Vital part of the diet for birds, as it is stored in the gizzard where it helps physically break down food during digestion.

groin Part of the body medial to the hindleg, includes the region of the inguinal canal, a point of weakness.

growth hormone Anterior pituitary hormone (also known as somatotrophin) that regulates the rate of growth of the long bones; *see also* ACROMEGALY.

growth hormone–inhibiting hormone Hypothalamic hormone that inhibits secretion of growth hormone; *see also* DWARFISM.

growth hormone–releasing hormone Hormone secreted by the hypothalamus that increases output of growth hormone.

growth plate Also known as the epiphyseal plate; found as cartilage at the ends of most bones in young animals; *see also* PHYSIS, ENDOCHONDRAL OSSIFICATION.

gubernaculum Fibrous band that connects the testis to the scrotum, aiding the descent of the gonad from the abdomen to the normal position in the adult.

guinea pig Small mammal and a popular pet, of South American origin. Reputedly domesticated 3000 years ago; prefers a dry, cold winter because of their original habitat.

Gumboro disease Infectious bursal disease; highly infectious viral disease of chicks that affects the bursa of Fabricius with resulting profound lymphopenia; a vaccine is available.

guppy Small warm water fish, grows to 4 cm or more.

gustation Process of sampling food and odours; sensation of taste.

gut 1) Popular word for any part of the intestinal tract. **2)** Name of soluble suture material; *see also* CATGUT.

gutta-percha A rubbery substance derived from the latex of tropical trees of the genera *Palaquium* and *Payena*, used in equine dentistry as a filling substance.

guttate Resembling a drop of water in shape; speckled or spotted.

gutter splint External splint shaped to support a fractured limb.

guttural pouches Paired air-filled sacs situated between the ear and throat at the end of the eustachian tubes in the horse.

guttural pouch mycosis An equine condition caused by the presence of a fungal organism, most commonly *Aspergillus* spp. in the guttural pouches. The fungus causes plaques to form on the internal walls of the pouches, which can cause erosion of the walls of adjacent blood vessels such as the internal carotid artery. The most common clinical sign is epistaxis. Diagnosis can be confirmed via endoscopy of the guttural pouches. Treatment is usually with topical or systemic antifungal therapy. Sometimes

occlusion of the affected blood vessels is indicated to prevent a fatal haemorrhage.

gynaecomastia A condition in which the mammary glands of a male resemble those of a female about to lactate, a disease sign of some hormonal imbalance.

gyrus Convolution of the brain surface, in the cerebral cortex, between the sulci (clefts).

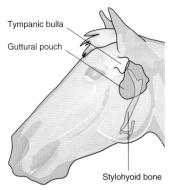

Tympanic bulla

Guttural pouch

Stylohyoid bone

Figure 21. Guttural pouch of horse. Redrawn with permission from Barakzai S. Handbook of equine respiratory endoscopy. Edinburgh: Saunders, 2007.

HAB Human–animal bond.

habit Behaviour pattern acquired by frequent repetition of some act.

HAC *See* HYPERADRENOCORTICISM; CUSHING'S DISEASE.

hachement Used in physiotherapy as a hacking action to massage muscles.

hackles Hairs at the crest of the neck, raised during anger or fright situations to protect and to threaten. Most obvious in terriers and other dog breeds.

haem- (hem- in USA) Stem word to denote blood.

haemachezia Occult blood, as in a faeces sample examination.

haemagglutination Ability of an antibody, virus, etc. to cause agglutination (clumping) of erythrocytes.

haemagglutination inhibition (HI) test Method of testing for viral antibodies in serum.

haemangiectesis Blood under the skin surface associated with dilated blood vessels.

haemangioma Benign tumour of blood vessels, found especially in the spleen and sometimes under the skin.

haemangiopericytoma Vascular tumour containing spindle cells.

haemangiosarcoma Malignant tumour most commonly found in the spleen but occurring at other vascular sites of the body.

Haemaphysalis leporispalustris One of the common rabbit ticks; also lives on other small mammals and birds.

haematemesis Vomiting of blood. May appear bright red if fresh or can have a 'coffee grounds' appearance, suggesting contact of the blood with the acid gastric juices.

haematidrosis Appearance of blood in the sweat.

haematin Chemical derived from the breakdown of blood that still contains iron.

haematinuria The presence of haematin in the urine.

haemato- (hemato- in USA) Stem word for blood.

haematocele An accumulation of blood in a cavity.

haematochezia Blood in the faeces that is obviously fresh and red; *see also* OCCULT BLOOD.

haematocrit The measurement of the percentage of erythrocytes in the whole of the blood. The term is also used for the tubes used to centrifuge heparinized blood; *see also* PACKED CELL VOLUME.

haematogenous Carried in the bloodstream.

haematological tests Relating to the examination of blood cells; does not include blood biochemistry.

haematoma Swelling caused by extravasated blood; result of an injury to the blood vessels or a clotting disorder.

haematopoiesis Formation of blood cells.

haematosalpinx An accumulation of blood in the uterine tube.

haematoscheocele Accumulation of blood in the scrotum after a castration.

haematoxylin Natural blue dyestuff used as a microscope stain, often combined with eosin to study tissues histologically. **Haematoxylin and eosin stain** is used in histology, known as H&E; *see also* EOSIN.

haematuria The presence of blood in the urine; the urine may be bright red or smoky brown in colour depending on how recently the blood was lost.

haemobartonellosis Haemolytic anaemia disease produced by a group of intracellular organisms that parasitize blood cells. *Mycoplasma haemofelis* (formerly known as *Haemobartonella*

H

felis) is the cause of feline infectious anaemia and may be associated with lowered immunity, as with feline leukaemia.

haemoconcentration Loss of the fluid components of plasma leads to an increased concentration of blood cells, used to measure conditions such as shock and dehydration.

haemocytometer Counting chamber instrument (improved Neubauer) for counting blood cells, used under the microscope; the kit includes pipettes and cover glasses.

haemodialysis Technique used to remove toxic products from the blood during renal failure, across a semipermeable membrane.

haemoglobin Protein–iron compound found within the red blood cells, transports oxygen from the lungs to the body tissues.

haemoglobinuria Coloration of the urine caused by the presence of haemoglobin; indicates severe blood haemolysis.

haemolysis Breakdown of red blood cells so that haemoglobin is released into the plasma. Occurs in samples of blood incorrectly handled and makes testing more difficult. Haemolysis will occur in the living animal in some types of anaemia, in toxic conditions and in immune reactions.

haemolytic anaemia A reduction in the number of red blood cells caused by an agent damaging the cells.

haemopericardium Accumulation of blood in the pericardial space; may result from chest injury, tumours or rupture of a blood vessel.

haemoperitoneum Blood loss into the peritoneal cavity; may be tested for by paracentesis.

haemophilia Disorder where blood clots slowly; a hereditary disorder that may be a cause of neonatal death. **Haemophilia A** is an inherited lack of clotting factor VIII; occurs in the cat, dog and horse, with females being carriers and males affected. **Haemophilia B** is an inherited lack of clotting factor IX that occurs in the dog and cat; *see also* VON WILLEBRAND'S DISEASE, VON WILLEBRAND FACTOR, FACTOR VIII DEFICIENCY.

haemopneumothorax Life-threatening condition, often the result of an RTA, when there is an accumulation of both blood and air in the pleural space.

haemopoiesis The formation of blood cells, including platelets.

haemoptysis Coughing up blood; rare in domestic animals but indicates lung trauma.

haemorrhage The loss of blood from arteries, veins or capillaries. Haemorrhage may be classified as internal or external; other descriptions describe the location or the time it occurred; *see also* EPISTAXIS, REACTIONARY, HAEMORRHAGE.

haemorrhagic gastroenteritis (HGE) An acute disease often associated with allergy or *Escherichia coli* toxin.

haemosiderin Form of iron stored by the cells; usually derived from diet or excess haemolysis.

haemostasis The arrest of haemorrhage; involves pressure applied to blood vessels, natural retraction and clot formation.

haemostat 1) Method of stopping blood loss. **2)** The name given to instruments such as artery forceps.

haemothorax Bleeding into the pleural cavity; *see also* DYSPNOEA.

hair Keratinized, thread-like structure arising from the hair bulb of the epidermis; characteristic of mammals; pigmentation and hair length differs between species and individual strains, e.g. dog and cat breeds. **Guard hairs** are stiffer hairs that form the outer protective coat. **Lanugo hair** consists of fine hairs formed during fetal development. **Wool**

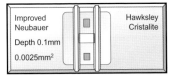

Figure 22. Haemocytometer: improved Neubauer.

hair is hair that forms the undercoat, makes up the soft 'puppy' coat and comprises the insulating layer closest to the skin of adults.

hairball Characteristic of cats that lick guard hairs, which then accumulate in the stomach; most cats vomit these as sausage-shaped pellets. If not removed they can cause an obstruction. Also a problem in rabbits.

half-life 1) The time taken for 50% of a drug to be excreted by the body. **2)** Similarly, the time of radioactive isotope decay.

halide salts Chemical group of halogen elements; includes iodine, chlorine and fluorine. Silver halide is used in X-ray film.

halitosis Breath odour that is unduly offensive; *see also* LABIAL ECZEMA.

hallucinogenic An agent that affects the brain and produces a false perception. Controlled drugs listed as Schedule 1 (S1) are not substances that veterinary surgeons in the UK may purchase.

halogen Any element of the group bromine, chlorine, fluorine, iodine.

halothane Volatile liquid anaesthetic substance, administered by inhalation. It is made from a halogenated hydrocarbon, which decomposes in ultraviolet light.

Halsted sutures Pattern of interrupted suture used in organ closure; of special value for friable tissue repair.

Halti A proprietary name for a type of head collar used in dog training.

Hammondia Species of protozoa found in the intestine of cats. Oocysts appear similar to those of *Toxoplasma*; the intermediate host is the rat.

hamster Small brown mammal frequently kept as a child's pet; includes the golden hamster, *Mesocricetus auratus* and the common (brown) hamster, *Cricetus cricetus*.

hamuli The small hooklets on a bird's feather.

hand The commonly used scale for measuring the height of horses. One hand is approximately 10 cm (4 in). The height of a horse is the distance from the ground to the top of the shoulder in hands.

hangers Metal structures used in wet radiographic processing to stretch and dry film. Channel and clip varieties are used.

haploid Condition in the gamete cells where only half the normal number of chromosomes are present; *see also* DIPLOID.

harderian gland Name formerly used for the nictitans gland, which occupies the inner surface of the third eyelid; *see also* NICTITANS GLAND.

hardpad Traditional name for the form of canine distemper where hyperkeratosis of the nose and foot pads was seen. The word was associated in many dog breeders' minds with severe or fatal viral infections.

hard palate Structure that forms the roof of the mouth, made up of the three bones: maxilla, premaxilla and palatine, covered with tough mucous membrane.

hare lip Failure of the upper lips to fuse during embryonic development; a congenital disease, may be inherited as a recessive gene; *see also* CLEFT PALATE.

Hartmann's solution Solution used for fluid therapy: isotonic, containing balanced sodium, potassium and calcium chlorides, phosphates and lactates.

harvest mites Surface mites that cause intense pruritus of dog's feet; scabs and crusts may be present; most often seen in the autumn after walking in fields, etc.; caused by larval forms of *Trombicula* sp. or *Neotrombicula autumnalis*.

haustra (*sing.* haustrum) The dilated areas of the wall of the colon that allow further digestion and compacting of faecal volume after water absorption.

haversian system Bone structure of microscopic concentric lamellae with a central canal for nutrition of compact bone; carries blood vessels, nerves and lymphatics.

haws Protrusion of the third eyelid, a term used by cat owners for the third eyelid syndrome. Dog owners use the term to refer to exposure of the lower lid also.

hay Dry grass fed to horses and rabbits, or if used as bedding, forms a diet supplement. Good quality hay has

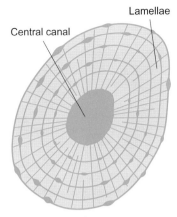

Central canal

Lamellae

Figure 23. Haversian system.

8–12% protein, 30–35% fibre and is a good source of carotene.

Hayem's solution Laboratory solution used for diluting blood for red cell counts.

Hazardous Waste Regulations 2005 In England and Wales, any business generating more than 200 kg of hazardous waste has to register with the Environment Agency.

HCM Hereditary cardiomyopathy.

HD Hip dysplasia.

HE Hepatic encephalopathy.

head The anterior part of a bone, or more specifically, the front of the animal that contains the brain and the organs of special sense.

'head gland' disease Disorder of puppies characterized by an oedematous nose and the face below the eyes; may become pus-filled and local lymph nodes then discharge purulent material.

headshaker A horse that suddenly and involuntarily shakes its head violently when being ridden.

Health & Safety at Work Act 1974 The legal act of Parliament giving employees safety protection in the workplace; employers have to comply with the Act, and employees also have responsibilities under the Act.

heart Hollow organ responsible for the blood circulation by the muscular contraction of the four chambers. Divided by a septum, the left and right chambers contract synchronously, controlled by the electrical impulses from the S–A (sino-atrial) node.

heart block Term used to describe an interruption in the heart rhythm as the conduction of the electrical impulses from the S–A node is impaired.

heart bypass Diversion of the flow of blood from the heart to a bypass machine to allow access to the heart for surgical intervention.

heart failure Condition in which the pumping action of the ventricles is inadequate; *see also* MYOCARDIAL DEGENERATION.

heart valve One of four structures inside the heart that allow for the forward propulsion of blood when the heart muscles contract, squeezing the blood inside the heart, but preventing backflow. Variously known as mitral (left A–V), aortic, tricuspid (right A–V) and pulmonary valves.

heartworm Parasitic condition in dogs, with blocking of the pulmonary artery by numerous *Dirofilaria immitis* worms. Confined mainly to southern areas of the UK but widespread in the USA.

heat In addition to the usual meaning of a rise in temperature, popularly used to describe the onset of oestrus in dogs and cats.

heat of nutrient metabolism (HNM) Produced by the intermediary metabolism of absorbed nutrients.

heat stroke Condition of collapse associated with an elevated body temperature, haemoconcentration and failure of body enzyme systems; *see also* HYPERTHERMIA.

hedgehog Small mammal with spiny exterior, species of *Erinaceus*.

Heimlich manoeuvre Technique using rapid abdominal compression caudal to the xiphisternum to dislodge a foreign body stuck in the trachea or the back of the throat; may be attempted with care in dogs.

Heimlich valve One-way valve put into a chest drainage system to prevent influx of air.

H

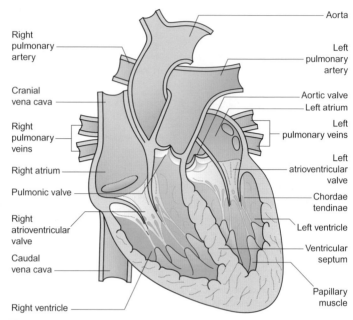

Figure 24. Heart: cross-section. Adapted with permission from Aspinall V, O'Reilly M. Introduction to veterinary anatomy and physiology. Edinburgh: Butterworth-Heinemann, 2004.

Heinz bodies Found on examining blood smears as dark stains in the erythrocytes, in cases of haemolytic regenerating anaemia.

Helicobacter Bacterium found in the intestinal tract of domestic species, specially adapted to resist the acid of the stomach wall; has been associated with gastritis, especially in cats, which have their own subspecies, *H. felis*.

helminth Description for parasitic worms which include cestodes, nematodes and trematodes.

heme- US form of prefix haem-.

hemeralopia Defective vision in bright light, also known as day blindness; *see also* CENTRAL PROGRESSIVE RETINAL ATROPHY.

hemi- Prefix used in words where 'half' is the important feature.

hemianopia Blindness of one half of the visual field, as in unilateral injury to the optic nerve tracts.

hemilaminectomy Surgical procedure to remove the vertebral lamina on one side of the spine only in order to reduce pressure on the spinal cord.

hemimandibulectomy Removal of one half of the lower jaw. Procedure used in the treatment of jaw neoplasia.

hemimelia Congenital absence of all or the distal part of the limb, seen rarely in newborn puppies and kittens.

hemipenis The rudimentary penis-like structure that functions in snakes and lizards but does not contain the urethra; may be subject to prolapse.

hemiplegia Paralysis of one side of the body only; indicates a brain lesion or high cervical injury; *see also* PARAPLEGIA.

hemisphere, cerebral Half of the forebrain, includes cortex, lateral ventricle and basal ganglia.

hemithyroidectomy Operation to remove one of the two lobes of the thyroid gland.

Hendra virus A paramyxovirus and the cause of respiratory/neurological disease in horses in Australia. Most horses die or are euthanized in 48 hours and the disease is zoonotic.

Henle, loop of Part of the kidney drainage system, the first U-loop after the nephron.

heparin Anticoagulant of natural origin from animal tissue. May be used to obtain plasma.

hepatic Relating to the liver.

hepatic encephalopathy Neurological syndrome where hepatic dysfunction allows toxic substances such as ammonia to build up to levels that affect the central nervous system.

hepatitis Inflammation of the liver, more specifically a viral infection or sometimes the result of toxicity.

hepatobiliary Refers to the liver substance and the bile duct system.

hepatoid cells Cells with microscopic appearance of liver cells, typically reported when anal adenoma tissue is biopsied.

hepatoma Tumour of the liver; may be confused with a benign enlargement of the liver.

hepatomegaly Enlargement of the liver, to the extent that it can be felt beyond the rib cage (on the right). More common in the cat, as the liver in the dog tends to reduce in size if diseased.

hepatoportal Involving the conduction system of fluids, the hepatic portal system; when bypassed as a congenital disorder, it is known as a shunt; *see also* PORTOCAVAL.

hepatosis Non-specific term for some dysfunction of the liver.

herbage One of the most common constituents of commercial feeds for smaller pets such as hamsters and guinea pigs is alfalfa (lucerne). It can be supplied as pellets or in dried chopped form. It has a modest protein content and is rich in fibre and minerals such as calcium but low in phosphorus.

herbicide Agricultural product that may be toxic to pets, particularly in a concentrated form. Sometimes selective weed killers may be licked off the coat or the feet in kittens, etc.

hereditary Characteristic that can be transmitted by one or more parent to their offspring.

Herman's tortoise One of three species of tortoise found in the UK.

hermaphrodite Animal that contains both female and male reproductive organs.

hernia Defect or weakness of the body wall allowing the protrusion of viscera to occur through one of the body's normal openings.

herniorrhaphy Operation to incise the hernial sac and repair the defect.

herpesvirus An important group of viruses for animals, causing diseases such as cat flu, abortion and fading puppies.

Hering–Breuer reflex Regulates the filling and emptying of the lungs. Stretch receptors on the walls of the bronchi and bronchioles transmit impulses to the respiratory centre of the brain, allowing for rhythmic breathing movements.

hetero- Stem word used to describe the opposite or dissimilar.

heterochromia Difference in colour, usually used to describe the irises of cats that have two different colours.

heterograft Tissue or organ grafting where material from one species is donated to another species; *see also* XENOGRAFT.

heterophil The main leukocyte of bird and reptile blood; similar to the mammalian neutrophil.

HG *See* HAEMORRHAGIC GASTROENTERITIS.

hiatus Opening or aperture; used anatomically for the apertures in the diaphragm for the passage of the oesophagus, blood vessels, etc.

hibernation The winter period of dormancy used by many cold-blooded animals to conserve energy. Nursing of hedgehogs and tortoises in the post-hibernation period is critical for anorexic animals.

hilus Anatomical term for a sunken pit – the hilus of the kidney, etc.

hindbrain That portion of the brain that includes the pons, the medulla oblongata and the cerebellum.

hip The part of the body around the articulation of the femur with the pelvis, or more specifically, the hip joint itself (coxofemoral articulation).

hip dysplasia Hereditary disease characterized by loose-fitting hip joints; has an environmental component in the development of the disorder; usually diagnosed on radiographs; a control scheme exists that is administered in the UK by the BVA and the Kennel Club.

hippocampus Part of the brain that forms the floor of the ventricles of the cerebral hemispheres. It is important to identify the area when diagnosing death from rabies.

histamine Protein found in all body tissues but particularly associated with allergic responses; *see also* ANTIHISTAMINE.

histiocyte Cell with phagocytic ability found in organs and in tissues, a fixed macrophage.

histogram Method of showing information as vertical blocks or similar portrayal of statistical information.

histology The study of tissue structure, usually by the microscopic examination of stained cells.

hive A raised skin plaque; *see also* URTICARIA.

hob A male ferret.

hobble A castrated ferret; also a method of securing a horses legs together as a form of restraint and for casting.

hoblet A vasectomized ferret.

Hobday procedure Surgical procedure to strip the mucous membrane from the inside of the vocal cords in horses to relieve roaring due to paralyzed vocal muscles of the larynx.

hock The joint between the gaskin (tibia) and cannon bone in the horse; also known as the tibiotarsal joint; has the greatest flexion angulation; *see also* OSTEOCHONDROSIS.

Hodgkin's disease A human disease of malignant lymphoma; does not occur in dogs but the name pseudo-Hodgkin's disease is often given to enlarged lymph node neoplasia in dogs.

Hohmann retractor A hand-held surgical instrument used to retract tissue to allow surgical access; usually used in orthopaedic procedures.

hole in the head disease Deep ulcers that can develop around the head of fish; freshwater head and lateral line erosion; exact cause unknown.

holistic Total care involving physiological, psychological and sociological factors in nursing.

holistic dog training Method of bringing up dogs from puppyhood where there is continual training using sympathetic methods.

holistic medicine An approach to health that considers 'wellness' of the whole animal, not just the disease or symptoms it may present with.

homatropine Medication used to dilate the pupil for a shorter time than is obtained with atropine; a synthetic compound that acts by blocking the parasympathetic nervous system.

homeo- Stem word used to denote 'the same' or 'like'.

homeopathy Method of treatment involving the use of minute doses of a substance that could produce similar symptoms to the illness if overdosed. Based on the theory that 'like cures like'.

homeostasis The ability to maintain the body to as close to the 'normal' state as possible. Internal control of the body symptoms in an attempt to overcome outside influences.

homo- Stem word used to denote 'the same', e.g. homosexual behaviour.

homozygous Having the same genetic make-up; with identical alleles.

hoof The hard, horny casing of the foot of the horse.

hookworm Nematode worms that were thought to attach themselves to the intestinal wall by their 'hooks'; the dog species are *Ancylostoma caninum* and *Uncinaria stenocephala*.

hordoleum Localized purulent infection of the eyelid, commonly known as a stye.

horizontal transmission Spread of infection or disease from one living in a group to another; *see also* VERTICAL TRANSMISSION.

hormonal Caused by some imbalance of hormone output by endocrine glands.

hormones Chemical transmitters secreted into the bloodstream by endocrine glands, used to stimulate processes or sometimes to slow them down.

Horner's syndrome Group of signs affecting the eye caused by a dysfunction of the sympathetic nerve supply; classic signs are ptosis, miotic pupil, sunken eyeball and prominent third eyelid.

host Name for an animal that carries a parasite that may serve as a source of infection to others.

hot spots Popular term used in dermatology to describe acute, weeping areas of skin; may start as an allergic response, but the animal biting or licking the area makes the skin look worse.

house dust mite Important in veterinary dermatology as the most frequent cause of allergic responses; mites belong to *Dermatophagoides* spp., *D. pharinae* and *D. pteronyssinus* being common house dust mites, faeces of these are allergenic.

house soiling Deposition of urine or faeces within the home, the first assessment has to be to decide whether it is an elimination problem or a territorial marking response.

Howell–Jolly bodies Remains of nuclei seen microscopically as opaque bodies in erythrocytes, found in some anaemias or conditions of the spleen.

HSE The Health and Safety Executive. Responsible for health and safety regulations in the UK.

human–animal bond Term used to denote a close relationship of an animal with its owner or keeper.

humane destruction Euthanasia performed in an acceptable manner.

human immunodeficiency virus (HIV) Virus causing AIDS in humans.

human resource management (HRM or HR) The function that looks after employees within a company; responsible for activities such as recruitment, training, appraisals, employment contracts and industrial relations.

humerus Bone of the foreleg loosely connected to the scapula and closely connected in the elbow joint to the radius and ulna; *see also* TROCHLEA, TUBERCLE.

humoral Relating to the body fluids, e.g. **humoral immunity**.

humour A body fluid. **Aqueous humour** is the fluid of the anterior chamber of the eye. **Vitreous humour** is a jelly-like fluid that keeps the retina in place through its 'filling' of the posterior chamber.

Humphrey ADE circuit A non-rebreathing anaesthetic circuit that can change a Mapleson A system to a Mapleson D system by moving a lever that connects the circuit to the fresh gas outlet on the anaesthetic machine.

hyaline cartilage The type of cartilage found in articular surfaces of the joints and the rings of the tracheal cartilage.

hyaline membrane Deposit found in the alveoli of the lungs; composed of cell debris and fibrin; *see also* PNEUMONIA.

hyalitis asteroid Partial opacity of the vitreous humour caused by minute calcified bodies fixed to the collagen framework (distinguishable by wobbling of the small particles when the head moves); *see also* SYNCHESIS SCINTILLANS.

hyaluronate Synthetic form of hyaluronic acid injected into osteoarthritic joints for its anti-inflammatory and lubricant effects.

hyaluronidase Enzyme that dissolves hyaluronic acid in connective tissue. An important virulence factor for pathogenic organisms such as streptococci and staphylococci.

hybrid 1) Name for a cross-bred animal; increases vigour when the parents come from different strains or species.
2) Cross-bred chicken developed to lay a high number of eggs.

hydatid A bladder-like cyst found in tissues, usually associated with *Echinococcus granulosus*.

hydration Relates to the fluid-electrolyte balance of the body and its water content.

hydrocele Fluid-filled swelling sometimes found in the enlarged scrotum when fluid accumulates around the testes.

hydrocephalus Accumulation of fluid in the brain ventricles when drainage of the CSF fails.

hydrocolloid Found in wound dressings, consisting of a microgranular suspension of natural or synthetic polymers such as gelatin, pectin and carbomethylcellulose.

hydrocortisone Glucocorticoid; pharmaceutical name used for cortisol, the hormone secreted by the adrenal cortex.

hydrogen Gaseous element with the atomic number 1, used as a measurement in a breath test for some intestinal absorption investigations; often referred to as a proton.

hydrogen bonding Weak bonds between water molecules.

hydrogen ion concentration Known by the symbol pH, a measure of hydrogen ions denoting acidity or alkalinity.

hydrogen peroxide Solution used in first aid treatment that releases free oxygen when it comes in contact with organic matter. Its mechanical cleansing effect is of special value in contaminated wounds, but it is toxic to tissues.

hydrolysis Any chemical reaction when a compound reacts with water to produce another end product.

hydrometer Instrument to measure the specific gravity of fluids.

hydronephrosis The abnormal filling of the kidney with urine; may be the result of reduced drainage through the ureter.

hydrophilic Having an affinity for water; reacting easily with water if present.

hydrophobia Literally 'fear of water'; popular term for rabies, one of the symptoms of which is painful spasms of the throat muscles that are induced by swallowing; *see also* **RABIES**.

hydropropulsion Technique of forcing water under slight pressure into a closed space to move an object, commonly applied to urethral calculi.

hydrops Watery accumulation in body tissue; when in the fetus, it is called hydrops amnii.

hydrotherapy Use of a specially designed swimming pool to exercise patients in warm water. The water gives a weightless environment to allow muscles and limbs to be exercised. Useful for patients with musculoskeletal problems to increase fitness levels and reduce obesity.

hydrothorax Fluid in the pleural space, usually serous in nature and not the result of infection; *see also* **PYOTHORAX**.

17-hydroxycorticosteroids Adrenocorticosteroid hormones with a C-17 hydroxyl group; includes cortisol, cortisone and others.

hygienist (dental) Person trained to practise certain preventive and curative treatments. For animals, the treatment must be prescribed by the veterinary surgeon and carried out under his/her supervision.

hygroma Fluid-filled cavity, usually over a joint such as the elbow, the point of the hock or the carpus.

hyoid U-shaped structure, usually refers to the apparatus that suspends the larynx behind the tongue.

hyoscine Pharmaceutical compound used as a long-acting gastrointestinal antispasmodic; known also as scopolamine. Also used occasionally as an anaesthetic agent, but is associated with delirium.

hypaxial Ventral to the vertical column; muscles that flex the lumbar spine or lower the neck; *see also* **EPAXIAL**.

hyper- A prefix that denotes 'increased' or 'abnormally raised'.

hyperactivity A state of restless movement often associated with pacing and crying; may be the sign of toxicity or encephalitis.

hyperadiposis Excessive fat; *see also* **OBESITY**.

hyperadrenocorticism Production of excessive hormone by the adrenal cortex, especially cortisol; also known as Cushing's disease.

hyperaemia Increased blood supply; may be an active response when the organ is redder and warmer than normal or passive owing to some obstruction in the venous return.

hyperaesthesia State of increased sensitivity to normal stimuli.

hyperaggression Increased response to perceived threat, often furious in nature. Rabies should be considered if the history is not known or there has been a recent sudden change in aggressiveness.

hyperbaric Greater than normal pressure (barometer measures); when applied to oxygenation, it may be used during the treatment of disease or inadvertently during anaesthesia.

hypercalcaemia Excess of calcium in the blood; may be one of the signs of overdosing with vitamin D.

hypercapnia Excess of carbon dioxide in the blood; also known as hypercarbia.

hyperchromasia Increased intensity of staining of red blood cells due to an increased haemoglobin content; see also HYPOCHROMASIA.

hypercortisolism The condition of excess production of cortisol; see also HYPERADRENOCORTICISM.

hyperechoic Abnormal increase in echogenicity due to changes in density of a structure.

hyperextension Extension of a limb beyond its normal range; a sinking carpus is an example; see also PLANTIGRADE.

hypergalactia Overproduction of milk; may be found in the first few days after birth of puppies or kittens, when the mammary glands become overdistended.

hyperglobulinaemia Increased globulins in the blood from antigenic stimulation or autoantibodies; may be an acute-phase response to infection.

hyperglycaemia Raised blood sugar level; one possible sign of diabetes mellitus.

hypericum Homeopathic remedy from the herb known as St. John's wort. Used for nerve injuries and first aid treatment of puncture wounds and crush injuries.

hyperkalaemia Elevated levels of potassium in the blood, associated with renal failure, etc. Cats have a characteristic low head carriage if affected.

hyperkeratosis Increased thickness of the stratum corneum, with crusting of the nose and foot pads being one of the most obvious signs of zinc deficiency.

hypermastia Excessive size of the mammary glands.

hypermetria A high-stepping gait; clumsy limb movements, often seen as a sign of cerebellar disease.

hypermobility A loose-fitting joint or unusual mobility when joints are manipulated.

hypermotility, intestinal Increased rate of peristalsis, often with fluid and gas sounds; see also BORBORYGMUS.

hyperonychia Increased growth of nails, often with twisting of the claws.

hyperparathyroidism Oversecretion of parathormone; see also RICKETS, RENAL.

hyperphagia Abnormal appetite or excessive food ingestion.

hyperplasia Increase in the mass of a tissue or organ (but not a cell increase, as in neoplasia).

hyperpnoea More rapid breathing with an increase in the depth of each breath taken as well as an increased rate; see also TACHYPNOEA.

hyperpolarization Part of the nerve conduction process; a fall in potential just before the resting potential returns.

hyperproteinaemia Increase in the serum protein content of the blood.

hyperptyalism Increased production of saliva; may be swallowed or may drool from the mouth.

hypersecretion Overproduction of some gland secretion.

hypersensitivity Altered state in which the animal's body reacts in an excessive way to an immune challenge. **Contact hypersensitivity** is a response of the skin to direct contact with an antigen in a previously sensitized animal. **Delayed hypersensitivity** is the type of response after 24 hours or more caused by T cells reacting with cell-bound antigen (known as type IV). **Flea bite hypersensitivity** is an excessive reaction to the protein in the flea's saliva, known also as flea allergy dermatitis or FAD; *see also* ANAPHYLACTIC SHOCK, ATOPY.

hypertension High blood pressure in the arteries. Animals with renal disease may have elevated systemic arterial pressure; cats are three times more likely to suffer from hypertension than dogs; *see also* RETINAL HAEMORRHAGE.

hyperthermia An increase in body temperature to a high level; results in collapse, haemoconcentration and failure of body enzyme systems; fatal unless rapid cooling measures can be introduced. Treatment may include immersion in cold water, spirit poured on to the feet or the skin for evaporation, application of wet towels and a fan directed to increase heat loss by evaporation, ice-cold intravenous fluids, cold-water enemas, etc.; *see also* HEAT STROKE.

hyperthyroidism Overactivity of the thyroid gland. Common in cats; signs include weight loss, aggression, excitement, tachycardia and poor coat.

hypertonic Osmotic pressure greater than another solution; in fluid therapy, usually refers to a fluid with a greater 'tension' than blood or tissue fluids.

hypertrophic cardiomyopathy Enlargement of the heart by thickening of the cardiac muscle mass as a response to an increased load; unless treated, it is usually followed by dilation and muscle weakening.

hypertrophic pulmonary osteoarthropathy Thickening of limb bones caused by some pulmonary disorder; *see also* MARIE'S DISEASE.

hypertrophy Increase in the size of an organ or tissue brought about by an enlargement of cells rather than by the increase in cell number found in neoplasia.

hyperventilation Increased depth of respiratory rate; drives off carbon dioxide and can lead to hypocapnia and respiratory alkalosis.

hypervitaminosis Signs of disease produced by injection or overfeeding with vitamins.

hypervitaminosis A Disease that may be caused in cats by being extensively fed liver obtained from animals living in sun-rich countries. Seen as spinal disease and stiffness in diseased felines; inability to groom may be one of the first symptoms.

hypervolaemia An increase in the volume of fluid in the circulation; may be produced by overenthusiastic fluid therapy.

hypha Filament of a fungus, used to help to diagnose mycotic infections under the microscope.

hyphaema Blood deposit in the anterior chamber of the eye.

hypnotic A sleep-inducing substance; thiopental used as an anaesthetic agent is one example.

hypo- A prefix that denotes 'less than' or 'below'.

hypoadrenocorticism Underproduction of adrenal cortex hormones; *see also* ADDISON'S DISEASE.

hypoallergenic Used to describe a diet with an unusual protein source for the management of dietary hypersensitivity and food intolerance.

hypoandrogenism Deficiency of male hormone production by the body, leading to infertility and feminization.

hypocalcaemia Low level of blood calcium, most likely to occur in the nursing animal; *see also* ECLAMPSIA, LACTATION TETANY.

hypocapnia Reduced level of carbon dioxide in the blood; also known as hypocarbia.

hypochloraemia Lower than normal chloride level in the blood, may be the result of repeated vomiting and loss of hydrochloric acid; *see also* ALKALOSIS.

hypochromasia Blood cells that stain less intensely; interpreted as a low haemoglobin content of the erythrocytes.

hypodermic Below the skin; usually used to describe the subcutaneous injection site, and for this reason, sometimes used to describe the syringe employed for this purpose.

hypoechoic Abnormal decrease in echogenicity.

hypogammaglobulinaemia A condition of the newborn animal where maternal immunity has failed to provide the right quantity of protective antibodies.

hypogastric Relating to the area of the abdomen below the stomach; in human anatomy, the term describes the area of the upper mid-abdomen, similar to 'cranial abdominal'.

hypoglobulinaemia Shortage of globulins in the blood; denotes low immunity status.

hypoglossal Situated below the tongue, most often used as the name of the XIIth cranial nerve, which innervates the tongue muscle.

hypoglycaemia Low blood sugar level; may be expected after insulin overdosage.

hypokalaemia Abnormally low levels of potassium in the blood, often associated with renal disease and polyuria.

hypomagnesaemia Low magnesium levels in the blood, causes muscle twitching and tetany.

hypomastia Unusually small mammary glands or a failure of the glands to develop.

hypomelanosis Underdeveloped pigmentation, usually a lack of melanin; *see also* VITILIGO.

hypometria Movement where the foot placement does not reach the intended spot, a form of ataxia.

hypo-oestrogenism Failure of oestrogen secretion or an inability to secrete, as is found in the spayed animal.

hypoparathyroidism Disorder produced by the dysfunction of the parathyroid glands or their surgical excision, characterized by a fall in blood calcium, a rise in blood phosphate and eventual tetany.

hypophyseal system Vascular conduction system connecting the pituitary gland with the hypothalamus at the base of the cerebrum.

hypophysis The pituitary gland, so-called from its position on the ventral midline of the cerebral hemispheres and the midbrain: means an outgrowth (or physis) at the undersurface (base) of the brain.

hypopigmentation Less than normal pigmentation; *see also* VITILIGO.

hypopituitarism Reduced secretion of hormones by the pituitary gland; examples are pituitary dwarves and diabetes insipidus.

hypoplasia Underdevelopment of an organ or tissue.

hypoplastic anaemia Underdeveloped red cells, usually associated with some bone marrow disease.

hypoproteinaemia Lower than normal serum protein level.

hypopyon Deposits of white cells in the anterior chamber of the eye.

hyposensitization treatment A course of injections of a specific allergen to desensitize a patient to that allergen.

hyposensitivity Reduced sensitivity to allergens; usually the aim when using a course of specific vaccines to desensitize a patient.

hypostatic Accumulation of fluid or blood in a dependent part, as in stagnant circulation of the lungs; *see also* PNEUMONIA.

hypotension Abnormally low blood pressure; may be the result of fluid or blood loss, or more frequently, caused by medication.

hypothalamus Part of the forebrain that lies below the thalamus; it has an important function in the control of the autonomic nervous system and the regulation of the pituitary gland; lower than normal body temperature.

hypothesis A theory used to explain a group of events; an explanatory argument.

hypothyroidism Underactive thyroid secretion, may be the result of drug administration or a lack of pituitary stimulation.

hypotonic Lower osmotic pressure than another fluid such as blood.

hypotrichosis Lack of hair cover or failure of growth from the hair follicles.

hypouresis See OLIGURIA.

hypovolaemia Fall in the volume of blood in circulation; *see also* SHOCK.

H

hypovolaemic shock Low volume of circulating fluid causing shock.

hypoxaemia Lower than normal oxygen tension in the circulating blood.

hypoxia Diminished blood oxygen; leads to reduced availability of oxygen to the tissues, a state that must be guarded against during and after general anaesthesia.

hypsodont Type of tooth with a long crown and a comparatively short root; may be more liable to fracture.

hysterectomy Surgical excision of the uterus. **Caesarean hysterectomy** is removal of the uterus immediately following hysterotomy to obtain puppies at full term. **Subtotal hysterectomy** is excision of the major part of the uterus but leaving the cervix in place. **Total hysterectomy** is removal of the uterus including the cervix by cutting through the anterior vagina.

hysteria A state of excitability where there is a temporary loss of control of movement and normal behaviour.

hystero- Relating to the uterus.

hysterotomy Surgical incision into the uterus.

hystricomorpha Suborder of rodents such as guinea pigs and chinchilla.

IAHO International Association of Human Animal Interaction Organizations, an association founded in 1990 to advance the understanding and appreciation of the link between animals and humans; see also DELTA.

IATA International Air Transport Association, the body that enforces the strict regulations on the carriage of animals and people by air; *see also* QUARANTINE.

iatro- Prefix denoting 'medicine', 'physician'.

iatrogenic Describes something that results from a medical treatment or surgical technique, usually an adverse reaction through inappropriate medication or an unexpected response.

ichthyosis Skin disease characterized by excessive scaling.

ictal Describing an acute epileptic convulsion; *see also* PRODROMAL.

icteric Referring to jaundice or the yellow staining of the tissues.

identification Some method of permanent marking or description; *see also* MICROCHIP, TATTOOING.

idio- Prefix used to describe something peculiar to that animal.

idiopathic Disease or condition, the cause of which is not known, or that arises spontaneously.

idiopathic inflammatory bowel disease (IIBD) One of the most common causes of enteritis in the dog and cat.

idiopathic pericarditis (IP) Pericarditis of unknown aetiology.

idiosyncrasy A reaction that is peculiar to that animal or may be an abnormal susceptibility of that animal to a drug used.

Ig Immunoglobulin; various types: IgA, IgD, IgE, IgG and IgM.

iguana Medium-sized reptile sometimes kept as a pet. Known to suffer from herpesvirus infections.

IIBD *See* IDIOPATHIC INFLAMMATORY BOWEL DISEASE.

ile(o)- Prefix indicating the ileum (intestines).

ileal Relating to the ileum.

ileocaecal Relating to the ileum and the caecum as one area.

ileocolic Relating to the ileum and colon as one area.

ileotomy Surgical procedure to incise into the ileum.

ileum The part of the small intestine distal to the jejunum.

ileus Intestinal obstruction caused by atony (loss of muscle activity); usually affects the small intestine with a loss of normal peristalsis. Fluid therapy and metoclopramide may be used for treatment; *see also* PARALYTIC ILEUS.

iliac Relating to the ilium bone that forms part of the pelvis.

iliolumbar Relating to the region of the lumbar spine and the wing of the ilium.

ilium One of the three bones that make up each half of the pelvis.

illness A disorder where there is variation from the state known as 'good health'.

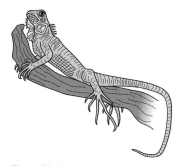

Figure 25. Iguana.

illumination, dark-ground Method of lighting a microscopic preparation from one side so that the object appears bright against a dark background.

image, X-ray The photo picture (radiograph) produced on X-ray-sensitive film. The image is essentially a shadow picture caused by different degrees of absorption of the beam by the body tissues interposed between the tube head and the film.

imaging All methods of viewing areas of the body and internal structures, such as computed tomography, magnetic resonance imaging and ultrasonography, as well as X-rays.

imbalance Unevenness in response, e.g. a hormonal imbalance.

imbibition Soaking-up of a liquid, a method of absorption.

imbrication Method used in surgery to take up excess tissue by folding or pleating it.

immature Not fully developed, yet to advance.

immature cataract Lens opacity where up to 99% of the lens is affected but the cataract is not 'total' so a tapetal reflex is still present.

immersion The submersion of an object in fluid; in microscopy, the high-power lens is immersed in oil to increase the resolution and magnification (100 times) of bacteria, etc.

immobilization The process of making a normally moving part of the body, such as a joint, unable to move. Important in fracture repair.

immobilizing drug Medication used to restrain animals without full anaesthesia, e.g. medetomidine, large animal Immobilon.

immobility Lack of or minimal movement.

immune Protection against infection, usually by specific antibodies. There are various forms of resistance to disease, usually associated with some form of immunity.

immune-mediated polyarthritis (IMPA) Disorder of the joints often associated with fever.

immune-mediated thrombocytopenia (IMT) One form of low platelet count caused by antiplatelet antibodies.

immune reaction The response of the body to the presence of antigens.

immune response Specific reaction to antigens, resulting in cellular or humoral immunity.

immune system Components of the body responsible for immunity, including the thymus, bone marrow, lymph nodes, spleen and tonsils, and blood components; *see also* LYMPHOID TISSUE.

immunization The process of stimulating immunity; may be by injection, by the intranasal route, by the oral route or any other method of administering a vaccine.

immunity The animal's ability to resist infection and foreign substances, which are usually protein in nature. **Acquired immunity** is protection that develops during life following exposure to an antigen; the term also includes the passive transfer of antibody; *see also* SERUM. **Active immunity** is protection that develops directly as a response to an antigen, produced by the body's own cells, which remain able to produce more antibody in the future if required. **Cellular immunity** is immunity resulting from antibodies on cell surfaces. It relies on T lymphocytes, which are first sensitized by exposure to an antigen. **Humoral immunity** is protection by circulating antibodies formed by specific B lymphocytes. **Maternal immunity** is protection acquired before birth or just after birth by the transfer of immunoglobulins; *see also* COLOSTRUM. **Passive immunity** is temporary protection that may be provided by the injection of antibodies as serum or immunity of the newborn through the mother's blood or colostrum.

immunoassay Laboratory method of measuring the level of substances using an antibody–antigen reaction.

immunocompetence Ability to provide protection by mounting an immune response.

immunocompromised The inability to produce a strong level of protection;

may be the result of a viral infection, an inherited defect or immunosuppressive drugs used therapeutically.

immunocyte A cell in lymphoid tissue involved in the process of developing immunity.

immunocytoma A neoplasm that may occur anywhere in the body, usually slow-growing; *see also* IMMUNOCYTE.

immunodeficiency Failure or deficiency of the immune response, may involve nonspecific factors that cause a failure of immune response or defects in specific factors such as antibodies or lymphocytes. It may be inherited or acquired during life, e.g. viral infection or toxicity.

immunodepression Lower than normal response to infection; lacking circulating antibody and/or cellular immunity.

immunofluorescence Diagnostic test applied to sections of a tissue where fluorescent antibodies attach themselves to an antigen in the tissue for which they have been specifically prepared.

immunogenic Able to stimulate an immune response.

immunoglobulin Special group of serum proteins; the globulin fraction responsible for immunity, equivalent to 'antibody'. Divided into IgA, IgD, IgE, IgG and IgM according to their origin and site of action. **Colostral immunoglobulin** is the antibody found in the first milk that is ingested by the newborn; IgG can be absorbed unchanged through the gut wall in the first few days.

immunosuppression Inability to mount a normal immune response; may result from infection or a deliberate attempt to modify a disease by using medication.

immunotherapy Method of preventing or treating disease by using an agent to modify the immune response.

impacted An object that cannot be moved; may refer to a kitten or puppy during dystocia, to the contents of the anal sacs, etc.

impacted crop Commonly due to impaction with long, spiky grass that cannot pass on through the digestive tract; impaction may be massaged out through the mouth or surgically removed; see CROP.

impacted gizzard May result from a lack of grit or eating inappropriate food, e.g. shavings or lead poisoning; affected birds appear hunched up and produce scant faeces; liquid paraffin can be tried.

imperforate Lacking an opening; most commonly applied to the newborn animal with a nonfunctioning anus.

impetigo Superficial bacterial skin infection that usually responds to antibiotics.

implantation (or nidation) The time when the fertilized ovum, having developed into an embryo, becomes attached to the wall of the uterus.

implanting Substance or object inserted into the tissues.

implied (contract) Legal situation; includes when a verbal message or phone call is received to request veterinary attention – in spite of no written agreement or no verbal negotiation over the likely fee that will be charged to attend to a request; any notes taken at the time may be valuable later.

Importation of Cats, Dogs and Other Mammals Order 1974 (amended 2000) Act of Parliament controlling the importation of mammals into the UK, setting down standard periods of quarantine.

impotence Inability to penetrate the female while the animal is in heat; may be an anatomical or hormonal defect of the opposite sex. Another form, in which there is no discharge of the fluid containing spermatozoa after penetration at mating, has been seen.

impregnation Male activity; usually refers to the act of fertilization that leads to a pregnancy.

impression smear A preparation of cells or bacteria that can be stained as a way of microscope examination and identification. Taken by pressing a clean glass microscope slide directly on the lesion.

imprinting Behavioural term for the early attachment of a newborn animal to the first available moving object, usually the mother, but other attachments are possible.

impulse An uncontrolled action; also refers to the conduction along a nerve tract.

IMT *See* IMMUNE-MEDIATED THROMBOCYTOPENIA.

inactivated Refers usually to vaccines where the organism has been treated so that it can no longer produce disease but immunity can still be stimulated.

inanimate Lifeless, breathless and almost extinct.

inanition A condition of exhaustion caused by lack of adequate nutrition.

inappetence Poor appetite, reduced food intake; often a sign of disease; *see also* ANOREXIA.

in articulo mortis (**L.**) Term used to refer to the moment at which death occurs.

inborn Condition acquired before birth; *see also* CONGENITAL.

inbred Produced as a result of mating close relatives; the risk of recessive genes coming into prominence is increased by such activity.

incarceration Confinement or constriction in a small space, sometimes used to describe a hernia.

incidence The frequency with which a certain event occurs; applied particularly to infectious disease or sometimes a genetic defect.

incineration Process of burning, recommended for clinical waste and carcasses; high-temperature incineration is essential to destroy some substances.

incipient About to come into existence; used to describe the early stage of a disease.

incipient cataract Lens opacity where only a small proportion of the lens is affected and has little or no effect on vision. Lens vacuoles may be present.

incision The act of cutting; used surgically to commence an excision or lance an abscess.

incisive Something that will cut sharply, sometimes refers to teeth.

incisive bone The bone that supports the incisor teeth, often called the premaxilla.

incisor The front teeth of the upper and lower jaws.

inclusion body Used in the diagnosis of viral infections; small particles found in the cytoplasm or nucleus of infected cells; *see also* NEGRI BODIES.

incompatibility Refers to certain medicaments that should not be used together or at the same time. There may be speedy immune responses if incompatible blood is transfused, for example.

incompetence Failure to work properly; usually applies to heart valve disease when backward leakage of blood takes place.

incongruity Used to describe unevenness in bone contact; when the radius is smaller than the ulna, the elbow joint has an incongruous surface contributing to elbow dysplasia.

incontinence Inability to control the passage of urine or faeces; commonly means urinary incontinence.

incoordination Clumsy movements, stumbling and a lack of fine control over limb placement; *see also* ATAXIA.

incubate Prepare for growth. May refer to disease, an embryo in an egg or the use of a laboratory incubator for bacterial culture.

incubation Provision for growth and development, as for tissue culture or bacteria.

incubation period The time between invasion of the body by an organism and the appearance of the first symptoms.

incubator Container with equipment to provide for optimal growth, may be a laboratory incubator for cultures or a premature baby incubator for rearing puppies or for patient care.

incurable State of chronic illness where the alleviation of the symptoms is as much as can be provided; *see also* EUTHANASIA, PALLIATIVE.

incus One of the small bones of the middle ear. (L. 'anvil'.)

index Measure or ratio; used in **therapeutic index** to show how the curative dose relates to the lethal dose.

indication Sign that suggests a certain treatment should be used or that a disease has a cause.

indigestion A failure of the normal digestive process; applies mainly to gastric digestion in humans, where it equates with abdominal discomfort; *see also HELICOBACTER*, MALABSORPTION.

individual reaction Something only a single animal reacts or responds to.

indole A breakdown product of tryptophan; occurs in urine and faeces and is responsible for foul odours.

indolent ulcer An ulcer of the skin or mucous membrane that fails to heal naturally.

induction Term applied in general anaesthesia to the first stage of rendering the animal unconscious.

induction of parturition The artificial starting of the birth process.

induction training Initial training for new staff, to familiarize them with their colleagues and the practice's ways of working.

indurated Describes abnormal hardness of the skin or an organ.

industrial tribunal An independent judicial body that hears and decides claims relating to employment, such as unfair dismissal, breach of contract, sexual discrimination, etc.

indwelling Implies an arrangement that allows a cavity to be occupied for some time, as in the use of a urinary catheter.

inert Describes a substance that does not irritate or move.

inertia Feeble or weak muscle contraction; refers to the parturition process where there is some delay before or during birth, often divided into **primary** and **secondary inertia**; *see also* DYSTOCIA.

in extremis Implies that the patient only has a short time to live.

infantilism Persistence of juvenile behaviour or psychological characteristics into adult life.

infantophagia A disturbance of behaviour where the mother eats the newborn; may be the response to a perceived threat; overattentive care by humans may precipitate this in small mammals.

infarct A small area of localized tissue necrosis produced as a result of a failure of blood supply; *see also* THROMBUS.

infarction The formation of dead tissue following a failure of oxygenated blood supply.

infection Invasion of the body by harmful microorganisms; the symptoms manifest after an incubation period when the organisms multiply.

infectious canine hepatitis (ICH) Disease caused by an adenovirus.

infectious disease Syndrome produced as a result of spreading of microorganisms causing a disease; *see also* COMMUNICABLE DISEASE.

inferior Beneath or below.

infertility Inability of the female to conceive or the male to be able to induce conception.

infestation A term restricted to established parasitic diseases, either on the surface or within the body.

infiltration Introduction of a substance into the tissues, includes cancer cells.

infiltration anaesthesia The injection of a local analgesic solution into tissues to provide anaesthesia.

inflame To light up or redden as if in a fire; a situation such as a staff/client dispute may become **inflamed**, meaning made worse.

inflammation A response by the tissues to any harmful stimulus, usually intended to limit the spread of harm to the rest of the body and to protect the vital organs. *See also* CALOR, DOLOR, RUBOR, TUMOR.

inflammatory airway disease (IAD) *See* COPD.

inflammatory response The reaction to a substance that stimulates the tissues – bacterial toxin, trauma, virus, parasite, extreme temperature, radiation may all cause such a response.

inflation Usually, distension with gas or liquid.

influenza (cat) Term used for an upper respiratory tract infection, often febrile and likely to spread. Specific viral causes; *see also* FELINE CALICIVIRUS, HERPESVIRUS.

information technology (IT) The spread of new developments and educational material by electronic communications and other modern methods.

informed consent The process of getting permission from owners before carrying out any procedures on their animals; consent should be confirmed by obtaining the owner's signature, and any consent should be based on a clear, balanced understanding of the risks and benefits of a veterinary intervention.

infra- Prefix meaning 'beneath' or 'below'.

infraorbital Below the orbit, on the floor area of the eye.

infundibulum Any structure that is funnel-shaped. The infundibulum of the brain's hypophysis and the opening of the ovarian tubes that receive the ova after ovulation are two veterinary examples.

infusion The most frequent use of this word in veterinary nursing is for fluid therapy; usually involves a slow transfer of fluid into the vein. There is also the pharmaceutical use of the word when a drug is extracted by soaking to obtain its water-soluble active part.

infusion pump A piece of equipment used for infusing fluids into patients intravenously or arterially. It can administer specific amounts of fluids very accurately over a given period of time and has a built-in alarm to indicate the end of the fluid administration or faults in the administration so that a nurse can be alerted and rectify the problem.

ingesta Food or other substances taken into the body through the mouth.

ingestion Taking in matter by mouth, involves chewing and swallowing; *see also* MASTICATION.

inguinal Relating to the area of the body between the abdomen and the hindleg, sometimes called the groin. Important as a site of weakness as the tunnel where the spermatic cord of the male and the round ligament of the female run through the inguinal canal may permit an **inguinal hernia** to develop; *see also* HERNIA.

inhalant A volatile substance that can enter the body by nose or mouth.

inhalation anaesthetic Volatile agent used in general anaesthesia; usually administered by endotracheal tube or face mask.

inhalation pneumonia Gastric contents or other semisolid substances that enter the trachea by accident and set up disease in the lungs; causes a difficult-to-treat pneumonia.

inhaled corticosteroid therapy (ICT) Used in the treatment of respiratory disorders such as asthma, chronic bronchitis and eosinophilic bronchitis.

inheritance Transmission of characteristics from parent to offspring.

inherited disease A disease that is carried on the genes, from one or both parents.

inhibin Sex hormone produced by ovary or testis that inhibits follicle-stimulating hormone production.

inhibition Prevention or reduction of activity of an organ; in psychology, a restriction on a certain activity, often controlled by behaviour training.

inhibitor Substance that slows or delays an activity.

initial First or immediate.

injected The appearance of dilated blood vessels as seen on mucous membranes. Describes an animal that has been given an injection.

injection Method of administering medication, usually requires a hypodermic syringe and a needle using gentle pressure; *see also* INFUSION.

injury Harm or hurt, usually the result of an accident.

inlet, pelvic An anatomical term for the area around the cranial rim of the pelvis; *see also* PARTURITION, PUBIS.

innate Describes a condition or a characteristic present at birth and inherited from the parents.

inner ear The deepest part of the audiovestibular system; *see also* OTITIS INTERNA, VESTIBULAR.

innervation The nerve supply of an organ or a tissue area.

innocuous Implies that something will not produce disease.

inoculation Method of administering a vaccine; a word originally used to describe a method of putting a mild form of disease into the healthy body to provide immunity; *see also* VACCINATION.

inoculum Any substance used in inoculation; originally meant smallpox scabs used for human protection against the disease.

inoperable Describes a surgical situation where further interference will not alleviate the situation.

inorganic Substance not of vegetable or animal origin; chemically, means a noncarbon compound.

inotrope Pharmaceutical agent that affects the strength of contraction of the heart muscle; drugs may be positive or negative inotropes. A **negative inotrope** is a medication that reduces the force of muscle contraction; includes beta-blockers and propranolol. A **positive inotrope** is a medication that increases the force of muscle contraction; includes drugs such as digitalis, dobutamine and enoximone.

inotropic Affecting the force of muscle contraction; usually refers to cardiac muscle.

inpatient An animal that is hospitalized to ensure nursing care with correct medication or to enforce rest.

input voltage regulator The control on the X-ray machine that ensures constant voltage supply (kilovolts) in spite of any fluctuations in the main supply.

in season Common description of oestrus in the bitch.

insect Small nonmammalian animal that has six legs and an exoskeleton and is often responsible for causing bites or stings.

insecticide Medication intended to kill insects.

insemination The introduction of live sperm into the vagina or uterus to facilitate fertilization of ova.

insensible water loss Also known as inevitable water loss, as it is the amount of fluid that leaves the body through the skin and the respiratory tract; it cannot be regulated by the body, even in times of water deprivation.

insertion The distal point of attachment of a muscle or tendon to the bone; *see also* ORIGIN.

insidious Describes a disease that develops very slowly, creeping on, and is almost imperceptible at first. Any disease is described in this way if it develops unnoticed.

insipidus Weak or watery; *see also* DIABETES INSIPIDUS.

in situ At the normal site or natural position.

insoluble A substance that will not enter into solution in a solvent; normal solvents are oils, alcohols or water.

inspirate The air inhaled at a single breath.

inspissated Refers to semidried pus as found in a long-standing abscess cavity, usually thickened or hardened by evaporation or absorption.

instar A stage in the development of an insect.

instinct Inbuilt behaviour as opposed to that learned or acquired during the lifetime.

instrument A tool, in veterinary nursing situations, usually a piece of surgical equipment.

insufficiency A lack of quantity or output, usually describing an organ that is functioning less well than normal. **Cardiac insufficiency** is the subnormal inability of the heart to pump, often a result of a valve defect or a muscle weakness. **Hepatic insufficiency**, liver disease, often precedes hepatic failure and death. **Venous insufficiency** is inadequate venous return to the heart, with tissue oedema and visible, distended surface veins.

insufflation Method of introducing a powder or vapour into a structure, used to test patency of tubes, etc.

insulation Protection or layers added for prevention of energy movement; includes loss of heat or avoiding radiant energy.

insulin Hormone produced in the pancreas by the beta cells of the islets of

Langerhans; essential for the regulation of blood glucose levels. Endogenous insulin may have to be supplemented by injections of commercially prepared insulin; *see also* DIABETES MELLITUS.

insulinoma Tumour of the beta cells of the islets of Langerhans, may first manifest itself as hypoglycaemia.

insurance, pet Method of providing for the payment of veterinary fees and other unexpected costs of animal ownership.

integer A complete number, not a part or fraction of a number.

integrins A transmembrane receptor protein that attaches the cell to its surroundings.

integument The skin; may also refer to a cover of any other organ of the body.

intelligence Intellectual ability; the ability of animals to explore, comprehend or understand, then react accordingly; *see also* COGNITION.

intensification factor Refers to X-ray screens when the exposure needs to be adjusted for the intensification of the image depending on the type of screen in use; *see also* SCREENS.

intensifying screen X-ray screen where calcium tungstate or rare earth phosphors are used to fluoresce on exposure; the image is obtained with a shorter exposure; *see also* X-RAY.

intensity The quantity of X-rays used for a radiograph; the milliamperage time, together with the distance from the tube head, controls the dose rate from the main beam of the X-ray.

intensive care Nursing care where all body functions are closely monitored; specialized nursing skills are required for critically ill and immediately postoperative patients.

intensive care unit (ICU) A dedicated facility with special equipment for monitoring and continuous attention by nursing staff.

intention, first Refers to the manner of healing; this means when a surgical incision is sutured and heals in 5 days without scarring.

intention, second Healing where there is delay caused by loss of tissue or infection; *see also* GRANULATION.

intention tremor Sign of a nervous disorder, often after a head injury, in which the limb or head trembles when the animal tries to perform a normal movement.

inter- Prefix meaning 'between'.

interbreeding Reproduction that takes place in a planned but nonpedigree manner; *see also* CROSS-BREEDING.

intercalated Inserted between, e.g. an additional degree during a veterinary degree course.

intercellular Between the cells, as for fluid that is not within the cells and is not in the circulation.

intercostal Between the ribs; a 'space' exists that is filled by muscles but provides a surgical approach to the chest.

intercourse In normal terms, refers to speech or a mutual exchange; *see also* COITUS.

interdigital Between the toes, e.g. an **interdigital abscess**.

interferons Substances that are produced by healthy cells after they become infected by a virus; inhibitory agents that can be genetically engineered.

interleukins Substances that are involved in haemopoiesis and the immune response; stimulate the T cells.

interlobar Between the lung lobes or sometimes the lobes of the liver.

intermandibular Relating to the space between the bones of the lower jaw.

intermediate host A stage in the development of some parasites' part of the life cycle which involves an invasion of an insect vector or another animal before the parasite can mature.

intermittent positive pressure ventilation (IPPV) A technique used in anaesthesia to ensure adequate ventilation of the lungs when the animal is unable to do so on its own; *see also* VENTILATOR.

internal Within the body; sometimes the word is used in anatomy for a 'medial' structure.

internal fixation Method of fracture repair using plates, pins or wires applied to the bone to minimize movement; *see also* FRACTURE, PINS.

internal respiration Diffusion of gases between blood and the interstitial tissue fluid; *see also* TISSUE RESPIRATION.

interoestrus A stage in the sexual cycle of cats; a short period of nonreceptivity.

interosseus tendon A fibrous structure between two bones.

interphalangeal Between the phalanges or the full length of the toes.

interphase The resting stage of the cell division process when the chromosomes are not individually distinguishable.

interpretation, clinical The veterinary surgeon's clinical judgement of the signs, laboratory data and other information such as that supplied by the owner or the veterinary nurse.

interpretation, radiological Reading the X-ray plates and explaining the features that are shown.

intersex An individual that shows anatomical characteristics of both sexes; *see also* HERMAPHRODITE.

interstice A small space between tissues or between two body parts.

interstitial Relating to the parts separating tissue structures.

interstitial cell-stimulating hormone (ICSH) Hormone produced by the testes; in the female, known as luteinizing hormone and produced by the anterior pituitary to stimulate the ovary; *see also* LUTEINIZING HORMONE.

interstitial cell tumour An adenoma of the testes in older dogs; often benign but may be associated with perianal adenoma.

interstitial cells of Leydig Cells in testes that secrete testosterone.

interstitial fluid Watery fluid between individual cells, forms a third of body water content when combined with plasma water within blood vessels; *see also* FLUID THERAPY.

interstitial nephritis Type of inflammation affecting the cortex and medulla of kidneys; *see also* NEPHRITIS.

intervaginal Between the sheaths, as in tendon inflammatory disorders.

interval Time or space between activity in the body. **Electrocardiograph intervals** are measurements made on a printout of the electrocardiograph to assess heart function. The **P–R interval** (PQR time) is the A–V interval in the heart contraction cycle between the beginning of atrial activity to the ventricular contraction. The **QRST (Q–T) interval** is the time of the ventricular electrical activity for contraction.

interventricular defect Congenital disease of the heart where the septum between the two ventricles is partially absent.

intervertebral disc The flexible cartilaginous plate that occupies the space between successive vertebrae.

intestinal Relating to the intestines.

intestinal atony Cessation or total paralysis of normal peristalsis.

intestinal dilation Distension of the intestine with gas or fluids; may be associated with an obstruction.

intestinal torsion Twisting of the intestine; may be associated with an old adhesion or a tear of the mesentry.

intestinal tract General term for the tube running from the pyloric sphincter to the anus; *see also* BOWEL, GUT.

intestine The longest part of the alimentary tract. The **large intestine** includes the colon, caecum and rectum. The **small intestine** includes the duodenum, jejunum and ileum.

intima The inside lining of the blood vessel.

intolerance Inability of the animal to handle a particular drug; adverse reactions develop and the medication should be stopped or an alternative found.

intoxication Physical state after absorbing poison; medical nursing measures should be applied.

intra- Prefix meaning 'inside' or 'within'.

intraarticular Within the joint cavity.

intracardiac Within the lumen of the heart.

intracellular fluid Fluid within cell walls; comprises two-thirds of the total body water content but is not readily accessible from inside cells during fluid losses, shock, etc.

intracranial Within the skull.

intradermal Within the skin thickness, as required for some injections.

intralesional Usually applies to an injection made directly into a localized lesion; *see also* ACRAL, LICK GRANULOMA.

intramammary Within the lumen of the mammary gland, usually some application of medication via the teat canal.

intramedullary Inside the bone medulla; *see also* FRACTURE, FIXATION.

intramembranous ossification Bone developed from connective tissue; does not involve conversion from cartilage, as found in the flat bones of the skull.

intramuscular (i.m.) Into the muscle; a common drug route for a slightly irritant drug injection.

intraocular Within the eye globe.

intraperitoneal Within the peritoneal cavity of the abdomen.

intravascular Inside a blood vessel.

intravascular coagulation Coagulation of the blood within the blood vessels; the end stage of shock, toxaemia, etc. Recognized when it is difficult to extract a venepuncture sample; *see also* DIC.

intravascular space The space within blood vessels to accommodate circulating blood; in fluid therapy, this important space is the first distribution point of fluids given intravenously.

intravenous (i.v.) Within the lumen of the vein; usually refers to an injection route.

intrinsic factor Widely used for an inner or inward mechanism, but one example is the glycoprotein secreted by the parietal cells of stomach to aid absorption of vitamin B_{12}.

introitus The entrance or exit of a hollow cavity or organ.

intromission The passage of one object into another.

intubation Method of providing an airway by passing an endotracheal tube into the trachea.

intussusception Invagination of a length of small intestine into itself or possibly into the large intestine.

in utero Within the lumen of the uterus.

invagination The infolding of a wall or telescoping of a structure; important activity during the development of the embryonic processes.

invasive Rapidly spreading, usually refers to a tumour or infection. In surgical procedures, means some activity that will involve entering the body; noninvasive techniques are preferred for many experimental procedures.

inventory Catalogue or list of medication, instruments, etc. made during a practice valuation. A **safety inventory** may be a management tool; *see also* CLINICAL AUDIT.

Investors in People An accreditation awarded to businesses that obtain high standards in people management and success.

inversion A turning inwards; term sometimes used for eyelids; *see also* ENTROPION.

invertebrate Animal without a bony spine, includes insects.

in vitro Done in the laboratory. (L. 'within the glass'.)

in vivo Something happening in the animal. (L. 'within the living body'.)

involuntary Describes an action that takes place without conscious will.

involuntary muscle Plain, visceral or smooth muscle; also includes cardiac muscle.

involuntary nervous system The part of the system concerned with control and homeostasis; *see also* AUTONOMIC NERVOUS SYSTEM.

involution The shrinking of the uterus to its normal size after pregnancy.

iodine Chemical element necessary for life; *see also* THYROXINE.

iodine-131 Radioisotope used in radiation therapy for the treatment of hyperthyroidism in cats.

iodophor Organic iodine compound used as a skin disinfectant.

ion An atom or group of atoms that conducts electricity.

ionic bonding Transfer of electrons from one atom to the other in forming a molecule.

ionizing radiation High-energy radiation such as is used in radiotherapy and for diagnostic radiography.

ipsi- Prefix meaning 'the same'.

iridectomy Partial removal of the iris, usually at the periphery, to promote drainage.

iridencleisis Surgical procedure to trap a sliver of iris in the limbus of the eye to control glaucoma by drainage of aqueous fluid.

iridochoroiditis Inflammation of the iris and the choroid.

iridocorneal angle Part of the anterior chamber of the eye beneath the sclera, where aqueous fluid can drain into the circulation.

iridocyclitis Inflammation of the iris and uveal tract; see also UVEITIS.

iridodonesis Trembling of the edge of the iris when the head moves; indicates a partial luxation of the lens so that the iris edge is no longer supported from behind.

iridoplegia Paralysis of the sphincter pupillae of the iris.

iris The pigmented membrane that separates the anterior chamber of the eye from the lens and controls the amount of light reaching the retina.

iris bombé An iris that bulges forward.

iris coloboma Defect with a hole in the iris.

iris cyst Small pigmented body that will sometimes become detached and float freely in the anterior chamber of the eye.

iritis Inflammation of the iris, usually a very painful condition.

iron Elemental substance, essential part of the haemoglobin molecule, and therefore, important in anaemia.

irradiate To apply ionizing radiation; see also RADIOTHERAPY.

irreducible fracture A fracture in which the bone cannot be replaced in its normal position; requires open reduction in many cases.

irreducible hernia Hernia unable to be placed in its normal position by external manipulation; requires surgery to enlarge the opening in the muscle wall.

irrigation Fluid flushing, as used in contaminated wounds, etc.

ischaemia Reduced or deficient blood supply.

ischaemic myopathy A disease of cats where aortic embolism occurs, causing sudden hindleg paralysis, often associated with advanced cardiac disease (myopathy).

ischiatic Describes the area of the body near the ischium bone.

ischiatic nerve tract Channel in birds where the ischiatic nerve passes through the kidneys in the abdomen.

ischiometer Special ruler used to calculate the degree of hip dysplasia as shown by the Norberg angle; see HIP DYSPLASIA.

ischium The area of the pelvic bone that is most caudal; exists anatomically as two separate bones.

islet of Langerhans Endocrine gland tissue situated in the pancreas; see also INSULIN.

iso- Prefix meaning 'the same' or 'equal'.

isocoria Equal size of the pupils.

isocytosis Equal-sized blood cells.

isoechoic structure During ultrasound examination any area that has the same density – a similar echogenicity level – as the surrounding structures.

isoflurane A volatile liquid anaesthetic gas administered with oxygen or a combination of oxygen and nitrous oxide for induction and maintenance of anaesthesia. It is a nonflammable halogenated ether.

isolation Separate accommodation, usually to prevent the spread of infection.

isometric contraction Contraction within muscle that increases tone and 'readiness' but does not alter the length of the muscle.

isoprenaline A drug with an action similar to that of the sympathetic nervous system: dilates the bronchioles and speeds up the heart rate.

Isospora Intracellular protozoal parasite; one of the causes of coccidiosis.

isosthenuria Urine that has the same specific gravity in spite of water deprivation or excessive drinking.

isotonic Equal osmotic strength or tonicity of fluid.

isotonic contraction Contraction of muscle that will shorten the muscle while the tone remains constant.

isotope One of many different forms of an element with the same atomic number but a different atomic weight; used in diagnostic work as a tracing device and in the radiotherapy of cancer.

isthmus of the oviduct Isthmus means any narrow bridge; specifically in birds the short segment of the oviduct where the egg shell is laid down.

itch The feeling of a need to scratch an area; *see also* PRURITUS.

-itis Word ending used when an organ or tissue is inflamed.

IU 1) Intrauterine. **2)** International unit.

IV 1) Internal verifier for the assessment of veterinary nurse training, requires an internal verification qualification. **2)** Intravenous.

ivermectin Potent anthelminthic, belongs to the avermectin group of synthetic drugs.

Ixodes Genus of ticks; *I. hexagonus* is the common hedgehog tick, which is becoming a more frequently found parasite of pets in the UK. Any tick infestation may be called ixodiasis.

Jackson cat catheter Urinary catheter designed for male cats, having a Luer fitting and a flange so that it can be sutured to the perineum.

Jackson–Rees modification Mapleson F classified. Attachment of a small reservoir bag (with an open end) to a T-piece circuit; modification allows monitoring of respiratory rate (by watching movement of the bag) and facilitates intermittent positive pressure ventilation.

Jacobson's organ Found in the nasal region to supplement olfaction in species that rely on scent detection, *see* VOMERONASAL ORGAN.

Jamshidi needle Fine biopsy needle.

jaundice Icterus; excess bile pigments in the blood, which are then deposited in the skin, conjunctiva and mucous membranes, giving a characteristic yellow colour. **Haemolytic jaundice** involves raised levels of bile pigments in the blood as a result of excessive destruction of red blood cells, e.g. following incompatible blood transfusions, AIHA, haemobartonellosis and babesiosis. **Infective jaundice** is jaundice caused by infective agents such as *Leptospira icterohaemorrhagiae*, hepatitis A, hepatitis B, etc. **Intrahepatic jaundice** is hepatogenous (hepatocellular) jaundice caused by inadequate hepatic function, e.g. viral hepatitis and liver cirrhosis. **Obstructive jaundice** is jaundice resulting from obstruction of the bile duct so that bile is reabsorbed rather than being excreted into the digestive tract; level of obstruction may be within the liver or may be extrahepatic. **Prehepatic jaundice** is haemolytic jaundice that results in elevated levels of bilirubin beyond the liver's capability to metabolize it.

jaw The bones of the face that support the teeth; the **upper jaw** consists of the paired maxillae and the **lower jaw** the paired mandibles.

jejunum Part of the small intestine from the distal duodenum to the ileum.

Jembrana disease A recently identified bovine immunodeficiency virus affecting cattle in Bali, and notifiable in Australia.

Jeyes fluid A cresol-based environmental disinfectant; toxic to cats; *see also* PHENOL.

jill Female ferret.

jird Small mammal (rat-sized) infrequently kept as a pet.

job description A written description of the work an employee is expected to undertake.

joint Articulation between two or more bones, usually to allow a degree of movement.

joint ill Infection of a joint; classically in young horses and farm animals where infection spreads haematogenously from the navel.

joint mouse A loose cartilaginous or bony fragment lying within a joint.

joule (J) The unit of work done when a point of application of a force of 1 Newton moves 1 metre in the direction of the force.

Judd tissue forceps Sometimes known as Judd–Allis forceps, used to hold tissue during surgery.

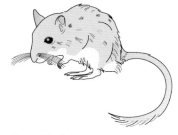

Figure 26. Jird.

jugular Relating to the throat or neck.

jugular vein Major vein on either side of the neck, draining blood from the head region.

jurisprudence The study and philosophy of law.

juvenile ataxia Incoordination that becomes apparent during puppyhood; has been reported in several breeds, including fox terriers and Jack Russell terriers; may result from changes in the brain or spinal cord, and some have a genetic component.

juxta- Prefix meaning 'in close proximity' or 'near to'.

juxtaglomerular apparatus Renin-secreting cells found close to the glomeruli in the kidney.

juxtaposition Placed next to or side by side.

kaliuresis Increased potassium excretion in the urine; occurs with the use of potassium-losing diuretics such as furosemide.

kaolin Aluminium silicate; most commonly available as a powder; when given orally acts as a demulcent and adsorbent, hence its use in diarrhoea; it is also mixed into pastes and used as a poultice.

karyoblast A form of immature red blood cell.

karyogenesis The formation of the nucleus of a cell.

karyolysis The destruction of the nucleus of a cell; a precursor of cell death.

karyon The nucleus of a cell.

karyorrhexis Fragmentation of the nucleus of a cell; this process often precedes karyolysis.

karyotype The chromosome set of an individual animal or species, particularly the number and structure of the chromosomes.

kennel cough Infectious tracheobronchitis; the most common respiratory disease of dogs; usually caused by *Bordetella bronchiseptica* and parainfluenza virus infection, although other pathogens have been reported and secondary infection can occur. Frequently arises when groups of dogs are confined together; causes a dry, hacking cough, often finishing with a retch; highly contagious; usually self-limiting but recovery from bacterial infection can be quickened by the use of antibiotics; potentially more serious in elderly or debilitated animals.

keratectomy Surgical removal of the superficial layers of the cornea; diseased tissue is removed along with a margin of healthy cornea; indications include dermoids, pannus, corneal sequestration and neoplasia.

keratin The major protein in hair, hoof and horn.

keratitis Inflammation of the cornea.

keratoconjunctivitis sicca (KCS) 'Dry eye'; inflammation of the cornea and conjunctiva as a result of insufficient tear production; particularly common in the West Highland white terrier and Cavalier King Charles spaniel; treatment includes frequent use of artificial tears, oral pilocarpine drops or parotid duct transposition. Ciclosporin ointment applied daily may be effective.

keratoconus Conical bulging of the cornea as a result of thinning of the stromal layer.

keratodermatitis Inflammation and thickening of the skin, with increased deposition of keratin within the epithelium.

keratolytic Agent that softens keratin.

keratoma Benign keratinous neoplasm.

kerion A deep pyoderma lesion; may be associated with chronic ringworm infection.

Kessler locking loop suture Suture used in the repair of severed tendons.

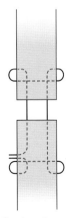

Figure 27. Kessler suture.

ketamine Anaesthetic agent that may be given intravenously or intramuscularly; causes hypertension and increased salivation and muscle relaxation is poor, hence it is most commonly used in combination with other agents to provide balanced anaesthesia. A Schedule 2 controlled drug.

ketoacidosis The metabolic acidosis arising from increased production of ketones; occurs in the later stages of diabetes mellitus and is a poor prognostic finding.

ketoconazole An antifungal medication.

ketone Organic compounds, mainly acetone, acetoacetic acid and hydroxybutyric acid, that are produced when fat is broken down, e.g. in diabetes mellitus or starvation.

key drivers The critical areas of a business that can be regularly measured and monitored to reflect progress and performance so that actions can be taken where necessary to drive the business forward.

Key–Gaskell syndrome Feline dysautonomia; characterized by dilated pupils, dry mucous membranes, constipation, mega-oesophagus and lethargy; was first reported in the early 1980s and became a well-recognized condition, but the incidence has since declined; treatment is mainly supportive (fluid therapy, nutritional support, grooming and laxatives/enemas), with recovery in more than 50%, although this may take 2–12 months.

keyhole surgery Surgery performed endoscopically, thus needing only small stab incisions.

kidneys Paired abdominal organs that form and excrete urine and also secrete renin and erythropoietic factor; lie just ventral to the spinal column, the right being slightly more cranial than the left. A filtrate is formed as blood passes through the Bowman's capsules in the renal cortex; this filtrate is then collected via ducts and concentrated as it passes through the renal pelvis into the ureter and then to the bladder.

kilocalorie (kcal) 1000 calories; a measure of energy value, commonly applied to metabolic needs and foodstuffs.

kilogram (kg) 1000 grams; a measure of weight.

kilovolt (kV) 1000 volts; a measure of electrical potential difference.

Kimsey splint Used in equine distal limb fractures.

kindling The act of giving birth – rabbits and ferrets.

kinesis Movement in response to a stimulus.

kinin Peptide that increases blood vessel permeability; *see also* SHOCK.

Kirschner–Ehmer apparatus External fixation device used for some fracture repairs; consists of metal fixation pins that pass through one (half-pin splintage) or both sides of a limb (full-pin splintage), and connecting bars with clamps; the apparatus is generally well tolerated by animals.

Kirschner wire (K wire) *See* WIRING.

kiss of life Colloquial term for mouth-to-mouth resuscitation.

kit Juvenile rabbit or ferret.

Klebsiella Genus of Gram-negative bacteria associated with respiratory infections and sometimes opportunistic pathogens in debilitated animals.

Klinefelter's syndrome Genetic abnormality where the male has an additional X chromosome (XXY); affected males are infertile and may have associated abnormalities of external and internal reproductive organs.

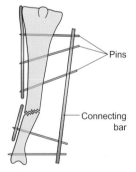

Figure 28. Kirschner–Ehmer apparatus.

knee The human equivalent of the stifle joint.

knee cap Patella, a sesamoid bone.

knocked up Suffering from luxation or subluxation of the distal interphalangeal joint; the condition is seen almost exclusively in racing greyhounds and affects the left (inside) forelimb; surgical repair offers the greatest chance of a return to racing.

knot, surgeon's Basic surgical knot consisting of three throws; for the first throw the right end of the suture material is passed over the left, the left passes over the right for the second throw and the final throw is left over right; additional throws may be used to ensure knot security when using suture materials that are liable to slip.

Knott technique Used in the diagnosis of microfilariae in blood samples.

knuckling Weight-bearing on the dorsum of the paw; knuckling denotes neurological deficits and may result from lesions of the peripheral nerve, spinal cord or higher centres; if the paw of a standing animal is placed in a knuckled-over position, the normal response of the animal should be to replace the paw correctly immediately.

Kocher forceps Ratcheted surgical forceps with serrated blades and a tooth at the end, used for haemostasis.

Krebs cycle The citric acid cycle; the final metabolic pathway for carbohydrates and fats; a complex series of enzyme-controlled biochemical reactions that occur within the mitochondria of cells, converting pyruvic acid into carbon dioxide, with the release of energy; this energy can be harnessed by using it to generate adenosine trisphosphate (ATP) molecules, which can be stored and broken down as required.

Kuhn bag An anaesthetic gas reservoir bag used as part of a T-piece circuit. It has the gas outlet on the side of the bag rather than at the end.

Kuhnt–Szymanowski operation Ophthalmological surgical technique for the correction of large ectropion defects: a skin flap is reflected below the affected portion of the eyelid, a V-shaped section is removed from the underlying conjunctiva and the defect is closed; the skin flap is then shortened and sutured back into place.

Küntscher nail Intramedullary pin that is clover-shaped in cross-section; rarely used in small animal surgery.

Kupffer cells Phagocytic cells that line the sinusoids of the liver and remove toxins, bacteria and cellular debris from blood entering the liver via the portal vein.

kyphosis Dorsal (upward) curvature of the spine; usually congenital.

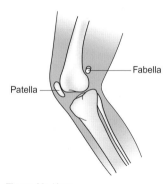

Figure 29. Knee.

labial dermatitis *See* LIP-FOLD DERMATITIS.

labial eczema Dermatosis where the lower lips in the mouth are scaly or crusty; may be associated with dental disorders.

labile Unstable, prone to change.

labium, *pl.* **labia** Lip, or lip-shaped structure.

labour The process of parturition; divided into first stage (cervical dilation), second stage (delivery of the fetus) and third stage (expulsion of afterbirth); in animals, producing more than one offspring, the second and third stages may alternate.

labyrinthitis Inflammation of the semicircular canals (vestibular apparatus) and cochlea of the inner ear; clinical signs include nystagmus, head tilt, circling and ataxia (vestibular signs) and hearing deficits (cochlear signs); often a progression of otitis media; *see also* OTITIS INTERNA.

laceration A jagged wound.

Lack Anaesthetic circuit also known as Mapleson A. A nonrebreathing system for animals over 10 kg; a coaxial circuit where fresh gas flows in the outer sleeve while exhaled gases flow down the inner tube; *see also* COAXIAL.

lacrimal canaliculus The opening of the nasolacrimal duct on the palpebral conjunctiva of the eye.

lacrimal gland The secretory glands that produce tears, which then drain via the nasolacrimal duct to the nasal chambers.

lacrimal sac The dilated proximal part of the nasolacrimal canal.

lacrimation Tear production; may be increased by any agent that irritates the eyes and is reduced in certain autoimmune conditions and by some drugs such as sulfasalazine; *see also* KERATOCONJUNCTIVITIS SICCA.

lactate dehydrogenase An enzyme released from damaged muscle and measured in serum to assess damage.

lactation Maternal production of milk to feed offspring.

lactation tetany Milk fever, hypocalcaemia causing convulsive spasms; *see also* ECLAMPSIA.

lacteal Lymphatic vessels that run within the wall of the intestine.

lactic acid A breakdown product formed during the oxidation of sugar within cells; lactic acid is then metabolized further to release energy, carbon dioxide and water; when the tissues, particularly muscle, lack sufficient oxygen (e.g. during strenuous activity), lactic acid cannot be fully metabolized and accumulates (oxygen debt arises); the lactic acid is metabolized completely when oxygen is available again, e.g. during rest.

lactophenol cotton blue Stain that may be used to demonstrate ringworm spores in a hair sample under the microscope.

lactose The main sugar in mammalian milk; a disaccharide.

lactulose A synthetic disaccharide sugar used in the treatment of hepatic encephalopathy; cannot be digested by mammals but is fermented by the gut flora; this reduces the intestinal pH and has a purgative effect.

lacuna, *pl.* **lacunae** A depression or pit, e.g. lacunae in cartilage are occupied by chondrocytes.

Lafora's disease An inherited disease of miniature wirehaired dachshunds that may not appear until 5 years of age as a progressive, myoclonic form of epilepsy.

lagophthalmus Condition where the eyelids do not close properly because of protrusion of the globe; common in breeds of dog such as the Pekinese and the pug; as the eyelids are important for distributing a tear film over the eye at each blink, the condition leads to corneal ulceration. It may be managed medically with artificial tears, though more severe cases may require surgery to narrow the palpebral fissure.

lag phase 1) Time period before colonizing bacteria start to replicate. **2)** In wound healing, the first 3–5 days after an injury where there is little or no increase in repair strength.

lag screw Orthopaedic technique where a screw is inserted across a fracture, using a large gliding hole in the near cortex and a smaller-diameter drill hole in the far cortex; this means that the screw only grips in the far cortex, and when the screw is tightened it applies compression across the fracture line.

lamella A thin layer or sheet.

lameness Gait abnormality resulting in a lack of symmetry in the stride pattern, caused by pain or mechanical restrictions.

lamina Thin layer.

lamina propria The layer of connective tissue lying beneath the surface of a mucous membrane; blood vessels, lymphatics, glands and nerve endings are located within this layer.

laminectomy Surgical removal of part of the bony neural arch of a vertebra to allow access to the spinal cord.

laminitis Inflammation of the sensitive laminae of the equine hoof.

lance To puncture or incise a swelling to allow drainage.

landmark An anatomical site that can be readily visualized or palpated and acts as a marker to locate other nearby structures.

Langenbeck retractor A hand-held surgical instrument used, usually in abdominal surgery, to move tissue away from a surgical site to allow access to other tissues.

laparoscope An endoscope inserted through the abdominal wall to examine the abdominal cavity and organs.

laparoscopy The technique of visualizing the abdomen using a laparoscope.

laparotomy Surgical opening of the abdomen, most commonly performed via the midline.

lapin Castrated male rabbit.

large intestine The distal portion of the digestive tract, comprising the caecum, colon and rectum.

larva A grub-like stage in the development of some insects and helminths.

larva migrans The developmental stage in the life cycle of some insects and helminths when larvae migrate through the host's body; **visceral larva migrans** and **ocular larva migrans** may cause clinical signs in humans and are caused by migration of *Toxocara canis* larvae through the body and eye, respectively; this is an important zoonosis, as ocular larva migrans can result in blindness.

laryngeal collapse Collapse of the larynx, leading to airway obstruction; *see also* BRACHYCEPHALIC AIRWAY OBSTRUCTION SYNDROME.

laryngeal paralysis Inability to dilate the rima glottidis due to paralysis of the laryngeal muscles. In the horse, the condition is most commonly unilateral and caused by lesions within the left recurrent laryngeal nerve; in the dog, the disease is commonly bilateral and affects older dogs of the large breeds, particularly Labradors and Irish setters. The condition is characterized by worsening stridor, which may eventually affect exercise tolerance and lead to collapse. In early stages, the condition may respond to steroids, but when more severe, surgery is required to open the airway; the preferred technique is a unilateral arytenoid lateralization or 'tie-back' procedure; *see also* STRIDOR.

laryngitis Inflammation of the larynx, often accompanied by alteration in vocalization.

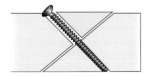

Figure 30. Lag screw.

laryngoscope Instrument with a light source and a tongue depressor, used to facilitate examination of the mouth and larynx; often used to aid intubation at induction of general anaesthesia.

laryngospasm Closure of the rima glottis caused by spasm of the laryngeal muscles; may occur during intubation or extubation of cats; prevented by the use of local anaesthetic sprays.

larynx Part of the respiratory tract between the pharynx and the trachea; used for vocalization; the larynx consists of the paired arytenoid and thyroid cartilages and the circular cricoid cartilage, suspended beneath the skull from the hyoid apparatus.

laser Light amplification by stimulated emission of radiation; a device producing monochromatic light; high-energy lasers are used in surgery for coagulation and cutting tissues; low-energy lasers are used for physiotherapy; their effects include reducing pain, reducing oedema and improving the blood supply to an area.

latent Not yet apparent, e.g. the latent image on an exposed but not developed radiograph.

lateral Towards the side, away from the midline.

lateral pterygoids Muscles in the head for mastication, responsible for side-to-side chewing movements of the lower jaw.

lateral wall resection Surgical technique used to treat chronic otitis externa; the lateral portion of the vertical canal is removed, improving aeration of the deeper structures.

latex allergy Staff who routinely wear latex gloves may become allergic to the proteins; hypoallergenic gloves may be beneficial to the wearer.

lavage Washing of a cavity or area using large volumes of sterile water, saline, etc.

laxative An agent that increases peristalsis and aids defaecation.

LDH *See* LACTATE DEHYDROGENASE.

lead poisoning Condition seen mainly in puppies; clinical signs include anorexia, vomiting and abdominal cramps, muscle spasms, convulsions and collapse; lead concentrations can be measured in the blood and treatment consists of EDTA injections to chelate the lead. May arise in parrots that have freedom in a house to chew old paintwork or in wild birds that accidentally consume lead weights left by anglers.

leads The three electrical wires used when recording an ECG.

learning theory Research shows that training by positive reinforcement using rewards produces more consistent results than punishment for incorrect behaviour.

lecithin Phospholipid necessary for the formation of cell membranes.

left displaced abomasum (LDA) Common abdominal disorder of ruminants, especially where there is increased gas production and gut hypermotility as is caused by some diets; the abomasum rotates from its usual position to the left flank and becomes distended.

Legg–Calvé–Perthes disease Aseptic necrosis of the femoral head caused by impaired vascular supply; occurs in the young of small breeds of dog, such as West Highland white and Jack Russell terriers; signs include lameness and pain on hip manipulation; the treatment of choice is femoral head excision.

leiomyoma Benign tumour of smooth muscle.

leiomyosarcoma A malignant tumour of smooth muscle.

leishmaniasis Infection with the protozoon *Leishmania* sp.; in dogs the parasite causes skin lesions, with dermatitis and alopecia around the muzzle and ears; other signs include pyrexia, lethargy, muscle wastage and hepatomegaly. The diagnosis can be confirmed by blood tests to demonstrate antibodies to *Leishmania* or by confirming the parasite in biopsies; the condition is spread by the bite of sandflies and is zoonotic.

Leishman's stain An eosin and methylene blue stain used for blood smears.

lens The transparent body between the anterior and posterior chambers of the eye; rays of light passing through the lens are bent and focused onto the retina; *see also* LENS LUXATION.

lens luxation Displacement of the lens from its normal position as a result of rupture of the suspensory fibres (*see* ZONULE OF ZINN); the condition is an emergency, as it can rapidly lead to secondary glaucoma, which destroys the retina. Primary, spontaneous lens luxation is the most common form, particularly in terrier breeds; signs include an aphakic crescent, iridodonesis and pain; surgical removal of the lens is the treatment of choice; *see also* APHAKIC CRESCENT, GLAUCOMA, IRIDODONESIS.

lentectomy Surgical removal of the lens.

lenticular Relating to the lens of the eye: **lenticular opacity** may be a false cataract.

lentigo Localized collection of melanosomes that forms a black patch on the skin.

leprosy Granulomatous skin disease of the cat, caused by *Mycobacterium lepraemurium*; possibly transmitted via the bites of infected rats.

leptocyte Form of erythrocyte seen in some cases of chronic anaemia; the cell has outer and central zones of pigment and is sometimes known as a target cell.

leptomeninx, *pl.* **leptomeninges** Two delicate, composite layers of membranes covering the nervous tissue of the brain and spinal cord; the pia mater (inner) and arachnoid mater (outer), separated by the subarachnoid space, which contains CSF.

Leptospira canicola Aerobic spirochaetal bacterium that can penetrate mucosal surfaces or areas of damaged skin; the kidney is the predilection site for the organism, where it causes an acute interstitial nephritis; clinical signs include depression, vomiting, renal pain and oliguria. The organism may be demonstrated in blood smears or urine sediment, or raised antibody levels may be detected serologically; most animals respond successfully to antibiotics and supportive fluid therapy; leptospiral antigens are now included in routine dog vaccinations and offer good protection.

Leptospira icterohaemorrhagiae Bacterium causing Weil's disease, an acute hepatitis, with pyrexia, vomiting, diarrhoea and jaundice; death can occur rapidly in peracute cases; effective vaccination is available.

leptospirosis Zoonotic disease caused by Leptospira canicola or Leptospira icterohaemorrhagiae.

lesion Any abnormality in the gross or microscopic appearance of body tissue resulting from a disease process.

lethal gene A gene that produces a fatal abnormality in the animal.

lethargy Tiredness and lack of energy; a common symptom of many diseases.

leucocyte Alternative spelling for leukocyte.

leukaemia Proliferation of abnormal white blood cells in the haematopoietic tissues and in the blood; may be subtyped according to the predominant cell type, e.g. lymphocytic leukaemia; treatment depends on the type of leukaemia and presence of secondary conditions, such as nephritis, but is generally based on the use of cytotoxic agents and prednisolone; *see also* FELINE LEUKAEMIA VIRUS.

leukocyte Any of the white cell series or their precursors; the two main divisions are the granulocytes (neutrophils, basophils, eosinophils) and the agranulocytes (lymphocytes and monocytes); granulocytes and monocytes develop from stem cells in the bone marrow, while lymphocytes are formed in the lymph nodes and spleen.

leukocytopenia Abnormally low number of circulating white blood cells; this may be a result of overwhelming infection, immunodeficiency, stress or steroid treatment; it is important that a differential cell count is performed to establish exactly which cells in the series are affected and to what degree.

leukocytosis Abnormally high total white cell count; requires a differential cell count to establish which cells in the series are affected; physiological leukocytosis occurs normally during exercise; other causes include infection and inflammation, tissue injury, parasites and neoplastic conditions.

leukodystrophy Rare, metabolic storage disease that results in accumulation of substrates within the white matter of the CNS; occurs occasionally in dogs and cats, affected animals appear normal at birth but then fail to grow and develop neurological signs; the prognosis is grave.

leukoencephalomyelopathy Rare neurological disease with degeneration of the white matter of the brain and spinal cord.

leukopoiesis The formation of leukocytes by the myeloid tissue or lymphoid centres.

luteinizing hormone (LH) In the female this hormone triggers ovulation; in the male it stimulates Leydig cells.

levator A muscle that acts to raise its insertion, e.g. **levator palpebrae superioris** raises the upper eyelid.

Leydig cells The interstitial cells located between the seminiferous tubules of the testes; secrete testosterone.

LH Luteinizing hormone.

libido Sexual desire.

lice Ectoparasites; the common biting louse is *Trichodectes canis*, the sucking louse is *Linognathus setosus*.

licensure To work in private practice in the US, a veterinarian needs to not only hold a recognized veterinary qualification but also to complete all state licensure requirements for any states they wish to work in. This includes passing the national licensure examination administered through the National Board of Veterinary Medical Examiners, as well as any state-specific examinations. Each state has different rules and prerequisites for licensure.

lichenification Hyperkeratosis of the skin, with thickening and cracking; the outer skin is leathery, folding, hairless and often darkly pigmented; a response to chronic trauma.

lick granuloma Single skin lesion, usually over the carpus or tarsus, caused by licking; may relate to boredom or stress and can rapidly become a habit; other possible causes include deep underlying infection, joint pain or other skin diseases; most animals respond to modifying the environment, antibiotics and aids such use of an Elizabethan collar.

lidocaine (lignocaine) A short-acting analgesic with rapid onset of action and duration of activity of approximately 45–60 minutes. If used with a vasoconstrictor, such as adrenaline (epinephrine), analgesia will last much longer. A local anaesthetic, available as an injection, gel or spray.

life cycle The developmental progress of many invertebrates, passing through various stages that may include intermediate hosts.

life-long learning The ongoing pursuit of knowledge throughout one's career to benefit patient welfare and for personal development.

ligament A tough, fibrous band joining two bones.

ligate Bind tightly.

ligature Suture material tied tightly around a blood vessel to prevent or control haemorrhage.

light beam diaphragm Set of four lead shutters or a cone within the tube head of the X-ray machine that are used to collimate the primary beam to include only the site of interest; collimating the beam reduces scatter.

limbic Relating to the limbus of the eye.

limbic system The part of the brain associated with emotional control and behaviour.

limbus The sclerocorneal junction in the eye.

limp 1) Flaccid. **2)** Exhibit lameness.

linea alba The fibrous band running in the midline from the xiphisternum to the pubic symphysis; the internal oblique, external oblique and transverse abdominal muscles insert on to this structure and the peritoneum also attaches in this region; midline laparotomies through the linea alba cause less soft tissue damage than incisions through the musculature itself.

linear Term used for 'straight', as in '**linear foreign body**' in the intestine or '**linear antigen syndrome**', a skin disorder of the adult dachshund.

linear accelerator Device for producing radiation used to treat some types of tumour.

line management Formal structure with a vertical chain of responsibility for other employees within a business or organization, where each employee is managed by a more senior colleague – their line manager.

lingual Relating to the tongue.

Linguatula serrata Arthropod parasite causing severe rhinitis, often with coughing and epistaxis; may require rhinotomy to confirm the diagnosis and remove the parasite, which is fortunately, very rare.

liniment Type of embrocation to rub in, usually made with oil.

Linognathus setosus The sucking louse of the dog.

lint An absorbent material used in surgical dressings.

lion jaw *See* CRANIOMANDIBULAR OSTEOPATHY.

lipaemia The presence of large amounts of lipid in the bloodstream; lipaemic blood samples can be recognized, as on standing, the plasma has a milky appearance; may follow a large, fat-rich meal or be caused by liver disease.

lipase The enzyme secreted by the exocrine pancreas for the digestion of fat.

lip-fold dermatitis Chronic inflammation of the lower lip in breeds such as spaniels; saliva collects in deep lip folds, with secondary infection and ulceration; may respond to clipping the hair, antibacterial washes and corticosteroid cream; more severe cases may require surgical ablation of the fold.

lipid Any substance that can be extracted with fat solvents.

lipofuscinosis Deposition of brown lipid pigments in internal organs.

lipoma Benign tumour of adipose tissue.

lipomatosis Presence of excessive fatty deposits in the body, often as discrete nodules.

lipoprotein Complex formed from lipid and protein molecules; in the blood most lipids are carried as lipoprotein particles of varying sizes.

liquid nitrogen Form of nitrogen stored at a very low temperature; used for cryosurgery; *see also* CRYOSURGERY.

liquid paraffin Oily liquid used as a laxative or enema. An inert mineral oil.

Listeria A genus of Gram-positive bacteria; causes listeriosis.

lithium–heparin Anticoagulant that allows biochemical tests to be performed.

litigation The practice of going to court; often includes the process of investigation before arriving at a law court action.

litmus paper A paper containing an indicator that turns red in acidic solutions and blue in alkaline solutions.

litre Measure of liquid volume; 1000 mL (2.2 pints).

Littauer Pattern of scissors used for suture removal.

litter All the offspring born to a mother in a single pregnancy.

liver The largest internal organ in the body, lying caudal to the diaphragm and close to the stomach. Functions include the secretion of bile; formation and storage of glycogen; storage and filtration of blood; metabolism of fat, protein and many drugs; and storage of vitamins A, D, B_{12} and iron.

liver enzymes Liver cells possess a wide range of enzymes undertaking many metabolic processes; several are used as laboratory markers for liver damage; enzymes that may be measured to assess liver damage include aspartate aminotransferase (AST), alanine aminotransferase (ALT) and gamma-glutamyltransferase (GGT); these enzymes do not give any indication of liver function, however, and other tests, such as bile acids, should be used to assess this aspect.

liver function tests Laboratory tests that assess liver function; the standard test was bromosulphophthalein (bromsulphalein) clearance, but this has been superseded by bile acids assays.

livid Having a purple/blue colour.

lobe Division of an organ, separated by fissures, e.g. lobes of the liver.

lobectomy Removal of a lobe of an organ.

lobule Subdivision of a lobe.

local anaesthetic A preparation that blocks the sensory conduction pathways (and motor pathways to some degree) in peripheral nerves; injectable solutions may be used to infiltrate around an area or block a specific nerve, thus desensitizing the entire area served by that nerve or in specific techniques such as epidural anaesthesia. Sprays are used to desensitize mucous membranes, e.g. for intubation. Topical gels are available but have little use in veterinary practice. Some injectable preparations also contain adrenaline (epinephrine) to prolong the duration of action; local anaesthetics without adrenaline should be available in the anaesthetic emergency drugs box and they may be given by intracardiac or intravenous injection in cases of cardiac arrest as they have antiarrhythmic effects; *see also* ANALGESIA.

local immunity Active or acquired immunity to a disease with the production of immunoglobulins at a specific site in the body, usually the site of entrance of the organism; e.g. intranasal kennel cough vaccine produces a localized immunoglobulin (IgA) response in the tissues lining the nasal cavity.

localize Pinpoint or limit to a defined area.

lochia Fluid from the uterus after parturition, often recognized as a green vaginal discharge.

lockjaw *See* TETANUS.

locomotion Movement; normal locomotion requires coordinated functioning of the CNS and locomotor systems.

locus The location on a chromosome occupied by a single gene.

loin The region along the side of the abdomen between the last rib and the pelvis.

long-acting Having an extended duration. Formulation used for antibiotics, hormones, etc., known as LA preparations.

longissimus system A group of overlapping epaxial muscles running along the dorsal and lateral aspects of the spine from the ilium to the head; action is to extend the spine and provide lateral flexion.

longitudinal In the direction of the long axis of the body.

longus system A group of overlapping hypaxial muscles located ventrally and laterally to the vertebral column; main action is to flex the spine.

loop diuretic Drug that promotes urine production by acting on the loop of Henle, e.g. furosemide; such diuretics also promote potassium loss and may cause hypokalaemia in the long term.

loop of Henle Part of the nephron – the functional unit of the kidney – extending from the proximal tubule in a loop that dips deep into the renal medulla, rising towards the cortex again and the distal tubule; this loop allows resorption of water and its integrity is important for the correct functioning of the countercurrent mechanism.

lordosis Congenital skeletal deformity with excessive downward (ventral) curving of the spine.

lore The area between the eyes and nostrils of birds, amphibians and reptiles.

louse, *pl.* **lice** Arthropod ectoparasites living on the skin surface; host-specific; they are just visible with the naked eye, have three pairs of legs and either biting (broad, e.g. *Trichodectes canis*) or sucking (narrow, e.g. *Linognathus setosus*) mouth parts; the eggs (nits) are anchored to hairs and the life cycle takes approximately 4 weeks; signs include scratching and pruritus.

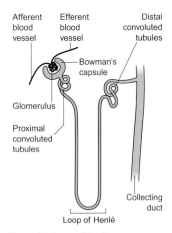

Figure 31. Loop of Henle.

lower motor neurone Ventral horn cell; the efferent nerve cell body is in the ventral horn of the grey matter of the spinal cord and its axon exits the spine and runs in a spinal nerve to innervate a specific group of muscle fibres or a gland; lesions affecting the lower motor neurone typically cause a flaccid paralysis with reduced or absent reflexes; *see also* UPPER MOTOR NEURONE.

lubricant Agents such as liquid paraffin, petroleum jelly and K-Y jelly that aid in insertion of rectal thermometers, obstetric procedures, etc.

Luer The standard fitting on the end of a syringe tube, catheter, etc; allowing a male and female connection without leaks; e.g. where a needle attaches to a syringe.

Lugol's iodine An iodine/potassium iodide aqueous solution used as part of Gram's bacterial staining method.

lumbar Relating to the region around the lumbar vertebrae.

lumbosacral disease Cauda equina syndrome; pain and neurological deficits caused by pressure on the nerve roots running in the cauda equina through the lumbosacral region of the spine; possible causes include vertebral stenosis, intervertebral disc disease, tumour, discospondylitis, etc.; decompression of the cauda equina (e.g. dorsal laminectomy) may be beneficial but the primary cause must also be addressed.

lumbosacral plexus Nerve plexus ventral to the lumbosacral spine, formed by the spinal nerves L4–S2; this plexus gives rise to the nerves of the hindlimb (sciatic and femoral nerves).

lumen The space within a hollow organ or tube.

lumpectomy Term used in surgery to indicate the removal of a mass (malignant tumour), often followed by chemotherapy or radiotherapy to prevent local recurrent disease.

lung Paired intrathoracic organs where oxygenation of the blood occurs across the walls of alveoli; *see also* ALVEOLUS, RESPIRATION.

lung lobe torsion Twisting of a lung lobe, leading to inadequate perfusion and aeration of alveoli; associated with chylothorax and other pleural effusions; may be diagnosed by radiography and bronchoscopy; requires surgical removal of the affected lobe.

lungworm Nematode parasites that live in the airways; host-specific; when larvae hatch they are coughed up, swallowed and passed in the faeces; a lungworm of donkeys, *Dictyocaulus arnfieldi* can also be transmitted to horses. *See also AELUROSTRONGYLUS ABSTRUSUS, CAPILLARIA AEROPHILA, OSLERUS OSLERI.*

lupus Immune-mediated, multisystemic disease characterized by an autoimmune haemolytic anaemia, thrombocytopenia, nephritis, erosive skin lesions, polyarthritis and other signs. Laboratory tests may confirm high levels of antinuclear antibody; the prognosis is guarded but treatment may be attempted with cytotoxic drugs and immunosuppressive doses of corticosteroid; *see also* DISCOID LUPUS ERYTHEMATOSUS, SLE.

luteinization Formation of a corpus luteum from the granulosa cells of the Graafian follicle following ovulation; *see also* CORPUS LUTEUM.

luteinizing hormone (LH) Interstitial cell-stimulating hormone; hormone produced by the anterior pituitary gland; it causes ovulation and subsequent formation of a corpus luteum in the female; in the male it promotes the secretion of testosterone by Leydig cells in the testes.

luteolysis Regression of the corpus luteum, under the influence of naturally occurring prostaglandin.

luxation Dislocation of a joint so that there is no contact between the articular surfaces; usually the result of trauma, but congenital deformities and growth plate damage may also lead to luxation.

LWR Lateral wall resection; used in the surgical treatment of otitis externa.

Lyme disease Inflammatory joint disease in humans caused by the spirochaete *Borrelia burgdorferi*; disease is transmitted via tick bites and has been reported in dogs in the UK and more commonly in the USA.

lymph Clear filtrate that bathes all cells; the fluid is collected into lymphatic vessels and flows through lymph nodes to be returned to the venous circulation via the thoracic ducts; the only cells normally found in lymph are lymphocytes.

lymphadenectasis Dilated enlargement of a lymph node.

lymphadenitis Inflammation of a lymph node.

lymphadenopathy Enlargement of lymph nodes caused by disease or as a response to infection.

lymphangiectasis Dilation of lymphatic vessels.

lymphangiogram Radiographic technique where contrast agent is introduced into lymphatic vessels.

lymphangitis Inflammation of lymphatic vessels.

lymphatic Relating to lymph nodes or vessels.

lymph node Small organs located along lymphatic vessels, e.g. submandibular, prescapular, popliteal and mediastinal; the nodes have a fibrous capsule surrounding sinuses through which the lymph filters.

lymphoblast Immature lymphocyte.

lymphocyte Small cell in the white cell series, formed mainly in the spleen, thymus and bone marrow; the cells have intensely staining nuclei, with little cytoplasm. Lymphocytes are divided into two types: **B lymphocytes** are short-lived and involved in antibody responses to infectious agents; **T lymphocytes** are long-lived and are responsible for cell-mediated immunity.

lymphoid tissue Any tissue resembling lymph node or lymphatic tissue.

lymphoma Neoplastic disease characterized by proliferation of lymphoid tissue; clinical signs associated with solid tumour masses depend on the site – if lymphoid tissue is developing at several sites it is termed multicentric; systemic effects of lymphoma cells include anaemia, thrombocytopenia, hypercalcaemia and DIC.

lymphoproliferative disease *See* LEUKAEMIA, LYMPHOMA, MYELOMA.

lymphosarcoma Malignant invasion of other tissues, e.g. intestinal wall, by lymphoid tissue.

lyophilization Freeze-drying; a common process in vaccine production.

lysis Breakdown of cells.

lysosomal storage disease Disease arising through lack of a specific lysosomal enzyme; that enzyme's substrate accumulates within cells, eventually disrupting cell function; storage diseases are rare, but the majority affect the CNS; the prognosis is grave; specific diseases include gangliosidosis, globoid cell leukodystrophy, mucopolysaccharidosis and ceroid lipofuscinosis; *see also* LYSOSOME.

lysosome Intracytoplasmic membrane-bound vesicle containing hydrolytic enzymes that are secreted by the cell.

lysozyme An enzyme that helps to destroy bacteria.

Lyssa virus The cause of rabies infection; the virus attacks the CNS; *see also* RABIES.

MAC Mean alveolar concentration (of anaesthetic gases in the lungs).

macaque Member of an Old World monkey group. The genus is *Macaca*.

macaw One of the larger parrots, usually with bright plumage and bare face patches.

MacConkey's agar An agar jelly used in bacteriology cultures for distinguishing between lactose-fermenting bacteria (such as *Escherichia coli*), seen as red colonies, and the other enteric bacteria, which produce pale colonies.

McMaster technique Method of measuring the number of parasitic eggs in a faeces sample using a special counting chamber. The eggs counted in a gram of faeces can be estimated using the 10 times objective of the microscope.

maceration Method of breaking down tissues by soaking. In obstetrics, the word is used for the breakdown of a dead fetus in the uterus.

machinery murmur Loud continuous heart noise associated with a patent ductus arteriosus; *see also* WASHING MACHINE MURMUR.

macroaleuriospores One of the positive microscopic signs of ringworm.

macroblast An abnormally large erythrocyte with the nucleus still present.

macroconidia Structures found in mycotic culture smears.

macrocyte An abnormally large erythrocyte, seen in macrocytic anaemia.

macrognathia Abnormal growth of the jaw, leads to overshot or undershot condition.

macrolide An antibiotic group that includes tylosin and erythromycin.

macromastia Abnormal development and size of the mammary glands.

macrophage A single nucleus phagocytic cell, part of the reticuloendothelial system of the tissues; *see also* MAST CELL.

macroscopic Relating to the overall appearance as seen with the naked eye.

macula The most sensitive part of the human retina, rich in cones; it does not have an equivalent in animals. The word is sometimes used for a grey spot on the cornea; often after a scar forms following injury.

macule A flat, circumscribed area of skin. May take one of four forms: erythematous, haemorrhagic, hyperpigmented or hypopigmented.

mad cow disease Popular name for bovine spongiform encephalopathy (BSE); the disease is of interest as it has been linked with spongiform encephalopathies in other animals including the domestic cat.

mad itch Condition where the animal chews at itself to relieve an irritation; in farm animals is associated with the virus causing Aujeszky's disease.

Magendie's foramen An opening in the roof of the fourth ventricle of the brain that allows the passage of CSF.

maggots The larvae of dipteran flies; can cause the death of rabbits and other animals when they invade areas of soiled skin, eating down into the flesh.

Magill circuit Anaesthetic delivery system consisting of a corrugated hose and reservoir bag; an expiratory valve at the end of the tube nearest the patient allows for the expulsion of waste gases as the animal breathes out. Used in animals over 7 kg.

magnesium Mineral element required both for bone structure and for metabolic controls (phosphokinases, acetyl-CoA). The salts, such as magnesium sulphate, are used for poulticing or as a saline laxative; struvite calculi have a complex structure that includes magnesium; *see also* CALCULI.

magnetic resonance imaging (MRI) A diagnostic imaging technique that uses strong magnetic fields to produce an image of internal structures.

magnification Any apparent increase in size, as by using a microscope or as in radiography where the image increases depending on the distance of the object from the cathode.

magnum Part of the bird's oviduct responsible for the secreting the albumen (white) of the egg.

Maine Coon cat Breed of cat noticeably larger and longer haired than other domestic varieties; colours vary.

mal French word for 'illness' or 'disease'. **Grand mal** is a form of epileptiform convulsion where there is loss of consciousness and major limb and jaw movements occur. **Petit mal** is a mild seizure that may be no more than a vacant stare and a reluctance to move. The term is borrowed from human epilepsy, when there are brief spells of dissociation and both posture and balance are maintained.

malabsorption Reduced rate of absorption of the contents of the small intestine. The malabsorption syndrome also presents as semiformed faeces, loss of fluids and electrolytes and a degree of weight loss.

malacia Abnormal softening of tissues; *see also* OSTEOMALACIA.

maladjustment syndrome Disease of newborn foals, which are sometimes described at birth as 'dummy foals'.

malar Relating to the cheek area; commonly a **malar abscess** denotes an upper molar tooth root infection; *see also* ZYGOMATIC BONE.

Malassezia Parasitic microorganism, previously known as *Pityrosporon*; a yeast found in moist skin areas often causing pruritus and hair loss.

male Denotes the masculine sex. Characterized by spermatozoa production for mating.

male sex hormones Those produced by the gonads, testosterone being produced by the interstitial (Leydig) cells.

malformation Any variation from normal anatomical structure, often congenital or acquired during early growth.

malignancy Indicates a neoplastic tumour; multiplying cells invade and destroy the tissues from which they originate and may also spread (metastasize) to other sites of the body.

mallenders Cracks in the skin behind the knee of a horse, more common in heavily feathered breeds.

malleable retractor Hand-held surgical instrument made of malleable metal used for holding tissue out of the way during surgery.

malleolus Anatomical structure in one of the bones that form the hock; if ossification is delayed in the puppy, it can lead to osteochondrosis of the hock joint. In traffic accidents, the medial malleolus usually suffers the severest injury, *see* TARSUS.

malleus Small bone of the ear, known as the 'hammer' ossicle.

malnutrition State of undernourishment as seen in starvation cases but also in patients suffering from malabsorption syndrome.

malocclusion Describes the condition of the teeth where one tooth does not meet

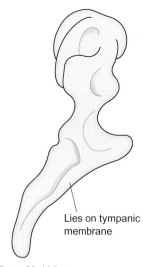

Lies on tympanic membrane

Figure 32. Malleus.

the tooth of the opposite one in the jaw. A common defect in dwarf rabbits; it may have a genetic or a nutritional cause.

malpighian Describes structures in the kidney capsule and the skin layers; named after an Italian anatomist who first described them.

malpractice Improper treatment or culpable neglect of a patient, may result in a claim for negligence or worse.

malpresentation Abnormal position of the fetus before birth, *see* DYSTOCIA.

malunion Lack of healing after a bone fracture, often a result of excessive movement, infection or nonalignment of fractured pieces of the bone.

mamma General term for the milk-secreting mammary glands characteristic of the mammalian species for nutrition of the newborn.

mammal One of the vertebrates belonging to the class Mammalia; another characteristic in addition to milk production is the growth of body hair.

mammary Adjective relating to the milk-producing gland of the female.

mammary abscess Usually, an abscess is only found in the early stages of lactation in the bitch; if it bursts, a large amount of necrotic matter comes out in the form of pus; resolution occurs in a matter of days after drainage and treatment.

mammary gland The milk-producing gland, usually described as a modified sweat gland. Most bitches have five pairs and queens four pairs. The glands are not always arranged in pairs.

mammary tumour Neoplasm, invariably malignant in the cat; common in the unspayed bitch where a large proportion are not malignant if removed in their early stages.

mammillary body Structure in the hypothalamus, thought to be part of the limbic system associated with behaviour.

mammillated Constructed like a mammary gland; the term is used for any nipple-like protrusion of the body.

mandible The bone that forms the lower jaw; the left and right sides are fused at the symphysis; *see also* RAMUS.

mandibular symphysis The semifibrous junction between the two halves of the lower jaw mandibles – a weak point: fractures are quite common in cats after head trauma.

mange A traditional word used to describe parasitic skin disease caused by mites; multiple infectious causes, each parasite needing a different treatment according to its life cycles. **Chorioptic mange** is due to *Chorioptes* sp. and affects the lower limbs of horses. **Demodectic mange** is a chronic skin infection caused by *Demodex* sp. **Ear mange** is a parasitic infection of the ear, mainly found in cats, caused by *Otodectes* sp. **Notoedric mange** occurs in cats but is rare in the UK; it is caused by *Notoedres cati*. **Sarcoptic mange** is a very pruritic or sometimes chronic scaly infection caused by *Sarcoptes* sp.

manipulation Method of moving joints to relieve stiffness; involves the forceful but passive movement of a joint beyond its normal angle of movement.

mannitol Sugar of high molecular weight, extremely effective as an osmotic diuretic but lasts only 3 hours. Used intravenously in the treatment of brain swelling.

manubrium Part of the sternal cartilages: the most cranial (first part); it is adjacent to the clavicles of the cat; *see also* CLAVICLE.

Mapleson Classification of semiclosed anaesthetic circuits made in 1954; six categories A–F, depending on the arrangement of the five key components – the fresh gas inflow, reservoir bag, breathing tube, expiratory valve and mask/endotracheal tube to patient.

Marburg disease Severe haemorrhagic fever caused by the Marburg virus; often fatal and zoonotic.

Marek's disease Neurological disease of birds caused by a herpesvirus that commonly manifests as a progressive spastic paralysis of the legs and wings; it can also cause sudden death; affected birds should be culled; a vaccine is available.

Marie's disease A disease of dogs and horses seen as a thickening of certain bones of the skeleton, often

M

as the result of some intrathoracic or intraabdominal mass; *see also* CHRONIC PULMONARY OSTEOARTHROPATHY.

marijuana Controlled substance sometimes a cause of poisoning in dog or cat through accidental ingestion or inhalation.

marketing Activities designed to communicate the value of a product or service to current or prospective customers in order to maintain or increase business growth.

mask In veterinary anaesthesia, usually a soft rubber cone that can be applied to the face of a dog or cat to provide a near-gas-tight seal to facilitate the induction of gaseous anaesthesia. Masks may also be used to filter the human's expired air during a surgical procedure or to remove harmful bacteria from the inhaled air of persons involved in such tasks as dental hygiene or carrying out some laboratory procedures.

masking down Considered a less than satisfactory method of inducing anaesthesia using a volatile agent; it involves applying a mask to the face of a preferably premedicated animal until enough anaesthetic gases reach the lungs to induce anaesthesia. This technique can be stressful for the patient and increases atmospheric pollution of the area with anaesthetic agents that can be harmful to personnel.

massage Method of manipulation of body tissues to restore function, mobilise tissues and provide pain relief. Now used quite a lot by veterinary physiotherapists and nurses. **Cardiac massage** is a specific treatment used in cardiac arrest where blood is propelled by the hand of the operator from the atria to the ventricles; pressure may be applied to the heart through the rib cage or by direct heart compression after opening the thoracic cavity; *see also* RESUSCITATION.

mass number Mass of the nucleus in an atom; equals the number of protons and neutrons.

mast cell Specialized cell most often recognized in subcutaneous tissues, facilitator of many allergic reactions. On degradation, the cells release histamine as well as heparin and other inflammatory agents. **Mast cell tumours** occur most often in the younger dog's skin, growing quite rapidly, and must be identified histologically to confirm that the growth is benign.

mastectomy Surgical removal of one or more mammary glands.

mastication Chewing process used in digestion to reduce food particles to a size where the digestive juices can act more quickly; involves mainly the molar teeth, which have a grinding action to pulverize the food.

mastitis Inflammation of the mammary tissue, most frequently the result of bacterial infection of the overfull gland or when there has been stagnation of the milk secreted.

mastoid bone One of the bones in the skull that forms part of the middle ear.

materia medica Implies the study of the drugs in use for pharmacy, their actions and effects on the body.

mattress suture Method of surgical repair where additional strength or compression of tissue may be needed.

maturation Development to a point where it is complete, especially used in physiology for the follicle in the ovary or in cell division when the number of chromosomes may be halved; *see also* MEIOSIS.

mature cataract Lens opacity that affects all of the lens; the tapetal reflex is absent and the animal is in effect blind in that eye.

maxilla The bone of the upper jaw area.

maximum permissible dose (MPD) Legal amount of radiation to which personnel may be exposed.

Mayo scissors Surgical instrument for cutting tissues; designed with narrow but rounded blunt points to allow for safe use, may be straight or half-curved in shape.

maze test An obstacle course designed to see if an animal is blind; can be made simply by placing some chairs and calling the animal through them; also used in laboratory investigation of rodent behaviours.

MCHC Mean corpuscular haemoglobin concentration.

MCV Mean corpuscular volume.

meatus A passageway or opening, as in external auditory meatus; the urethral meatus is the external opening of the urethra.

mebendazole Therapeutic drug group with low toxicity, principally in use for the broad-spectrum anthelminthic effect.

mechanism of action The way a drug works and brings about its therapeutic effect.

mechanism of labour Process leading to the normal birth of the offspring; three stages are usually described; *see also* PARTURITION.

mechanoreceptors Nerve receptors that respond to touch or any other mechanical pressure.

meconium The bowel contents of the fetus; may cause signs of colic in foals unless expelled soon after birth.

medetomidine Potent sedative, widely used for sedation, premedication and analgesia; useful when facilities for full anaesthesia are limited by time or staffing. An alpha-2-agonist licensed for companion animal use; may be used with propofol to reduce the total dose used. After an intravenous dose, 5 minutes' delay is essential before giving the propofol.

medial Towards the midline; opposite to lateral.

medial canthus The inner corner of the eyelid – the angle at which the upper and lower eyelids meet.

medial pterygoids Muscles in the head for mastication; the name comes from the Greek for 'little wing'.

median nerve One of the forelimb nerves supplying the caudal aspect of the foot.

median plane The longitudinal division of the body into two equal halves.

mediastinum The connective tissue partition or septum separating the two sides in the thorax. The structure ensheathes the heart, trachea, aorta, oesophagus and thymus gland.

medical records Essential documents; may be handwritten or kept on a computer. Records may be asked for in legal cases and must be retained for at least 7 years, preferably longer.

medication Substances administered by mouth, applied to the body or introduced into the body for the purpose of treating a disorder.

medicine 1) Any substance used as a remedy for disease. **2)** A general word used for the nonsurgical treatment of animals, as in 'the Department of Medicine and Surgery' or 'veterinary medicine'.

medium 1) A substance such as broth or agar used to culture living organisms. **2)** In radiography, a contrast substance – a contrast medium – used to outline hollow organs.

medroxyprogesterone Long-acting form of progesterone, not a corticosteroid; sometimes called MPA if acetate is included in the name.

medulla The innermost portion of an organ, often surrounded by the cortex.

medulla oblongata The part of the hindbrain above the spinal cord, contains the centres for the control of respiration and cardiac function.

medullated (myelinated) nerve fibre A nerve fibre surrounded by a myelin sheath.

mega- 1) Implies large size or giant proportions. **2)** Denotes a million.

megacolon Medical disorder of a dilated large intestine, most commonly seen in older cats; may be a sequel to pelvic fracture. Lack of exercise and house training leads to older animals retaining faeces and eventual loss of the defecation reflexes. Surgical treatment to reduce the size of the colon may be necessary.

megakaryocyte A giant cell in the bone marrow, creates the blood platelets.

megaoesophagus Disorder of the proximal alimentary canal with atonic muscle, recognized on radiograph by a dilated oesophageal tube. It may be first reported as the regurgitation of food; sometimes signs of inhalation pneumonia will also be present.

meibomian cyst A retention cyst, often seen as a rounded prominence near the edge of the eyelid; *see also* CHALAZION.

M

meibomian glands Sebaceous glands in the eyelid responsible for producing the lipid component of the tears that protect the cornea.

meiosis Cell division when the number of chromosomes in the nucleus is halved. The process is necessary in the production of ova and spermatozoa.

melaena Blood in the faeces; recognized as blackish faeces, often with a red tinge on the edges; the consistency may be softer and slimier than normal.

melanin Normal pigment of the body that accounts for the dark colour of the skin, the iris and the coat of the animal.

melano- Prefix implying black pigmentation or the deposition of melanin.

melanocytes Skin cells that produce melanin pigment.

melanocyte-stimulating hormone Product of the pituitary gland to stimulate darkening of the skin by melanocyte activity.

melanoma Tumour that has a high proportion of melanin deposited in it; despite the '-oma' name, some may be aggressively malignant, so all such tumours should not be ignored but require veterinary examination. May be found anywhere on the skin, in the eye, the mouth or the perineum.

melanosis Condition of 'blackening'; may be called melanoderma as the end stage of chronic inflammation of the skin. A specific problem is corneal melanosis, when blindness may result from a series of slow-to-heal eye ulcers.

melanosomes Packets of melanin pigment.

melatonin A hormone derivative of serotonin produced in the brain; in humans may be associated with sleep and certain depressive states, although its role in animals is not clear.

mellitus Latin word for honey, used to describe diabetes because the urine of diabetics was noticed to be attractive to insects. *See also* DM.

membrana nictitans The nictitating membrane, commonly known as the 'third' eyelid; has the function of lubricating and clearing the corneal surface of the eye; *see also* HORNER'S SYNDROME.

membrane A thin layer of tissue that covers a body surface; *see also* FETAL MEMBRANES.

menace reflex An eyelid response when a hand is used to threaten the dog or cat's eyes, used to look for cerebral injury or the ability of the retina responding as a protective reflex.

menadione The synthetic form of vitamin K; used most commonly for the treatment of poisoning by an anticoagulant such as warfarin.

mendelian inheritance Normal method by which hereditary characteristics are passed from generation to generation.

mening- Relating to the meninges, the membranes covering the brain and spinal cord.

meninges The three protective layers that cover the brain and spinal cord surface, the dura, pia and arachnoid mater.

meningioma A neoplasm affecting the brain or spinal cord: a benign growth places pressure on the nervous tissue, often causing unusual neurological signs.

meningitis An inflammatory condition of the meninges, often the result of bacterial infection; CSF may have to be collected to find out the cause of the illness.

meniscus 1) A disc-like structure, especially relevant to injury to the stifle joint, where tearing of the attachment of the menisci will add to joint instability. 2) Refers to the concave surface of a column of liquid in a glass tube, as when laboratory fluid measurements are needed.

mentation Any mental activity attributed to the agency in the brain. Used to assess head trauma: alert/depressed, delirium, stupor or coma.

mentoring A personal development tool where one person (mentor) works in partnership with another person (mentee) to guide and support them to help them maximize their career potential.

mepivacaine Local anaesthetic with rapid onset of action.

merchandizing The introduction of marketing into the veterinary scene; usually includes all those nonmedicinal products that are retailed or otherwise promoted by the veterinary practice.

mercury poisoning Toxic state caused by the unintentional absorption of mercury compounds; results in gastric irritation and fatal damage to kidney and liver.

Merkel cells Touch receptors in the skin.

meridians Acupuncture points are located along the meridians and serve in locating booster points, the network that connects the internal organs to the exterior of the body.

merle Pale coat and pale pigmentation of iris, associated with other ocular abnormalities.

merocrine Used to describe a sweat gland, from the Greek word for 'part' or 'fraction'.

merozoite Development stage of protozoal parasites such as *Coccidia*.

mésalliance Polite description for the unintentional mating of a female with an undesirable male. Frequently the cause of a request to prevent pregnancy developing; *see also* MISMATING.

mesencephalon The midbrain area; fluid flows through the **mesencephalic aqueduct** from the forebrain to reach the fourth ventricle; *see also* CSF.

mesenteric Relating to the suspensory ligaments of the abdominal viscera known as the **mesentery**.

mesh graft Pattern of skin grafting. *See also* PINCH GRAFT.

mesh, surgical Net substances or mesh grafts used in surgical repair when there has been tissue loss or weakness; *see also* HERNIA.

mesial Another word for midline or medial. Also used in dental terminology to describe the inner surface of the tooth.

mesocephalic Describes the heads of the breeds of dog and cat that have the most 'normal' skull shape; *see also* BRACHYCEPHALIC, DOLICHOCEPHALIC.

mesoderm One of the three developmental layers of the embryo, responsible for future connective tissue formation: blood vessels, lymphatics, pleura and peritoneum as well as liver, kidneys and spleen.

mesometrium Suspensory ligament of the uterus covered on both sides with peritoneum; important blood vessels running down it may need ligation during surgical operation; *see also* BROAD LIGAMENT.

mesosalpinx Mesentery carrying the ovarian tubes adjacent to the ovarian bursa.

mesosomes Folds of the cell membrane projecting into the cytoplasm; *see also* CELL MEMBRANE.

mesosternum The body or central part of the sternum; *see also* STERNEBRAE.

mesothelioma Malignant tumour within the thorax derived from cells of the mesothelium.

mesothelium The single layer of cells that lines serous membranes; *see also* ENDOTHELIUM, EPITHELIUM.

mesovarium Suspensory structure that attaches the ovaries to the posterior pole of the kidney capsules; part of the broad ligament but contains the ovarian artery and vein, which may be a source of haemorrhage during 'spaying'.

metabolic Relates to the mainly internal functions of the body.

metabolic acidosis Physiological state caused by alkali loss, as in diarrhoea, or accumulation of carbonic acid; *see also* ACID.

metabolic alkalosis An abnormality of the acid–base mechanism that occurs infrequently but results from loss of acid or accumulation of alkali, e.g. vomiting or after the excessive transfusion of fluids.

metabolic rate Measure of the body energy processes; the **basal metabolic rate** (BMR) is the minimal output of the resting animal, which can be measured.

metabolic toxins Substances that damage normal functions, e.g. phenols, histamine and the ketone bodies produced in acidosis.

metabolic water The involuntary production of water by the body as part of the utilization of ingested food.

metabolism The total amount of chemical and physical processes taking place in the body at one time. **Basal metabolism**

M

is the minimal amount of energy needed for the body to function in a total resting state.

metabolite An end product of some metabolic action in the body.

metabolomics The scientific study of metabolites, the analytic concept that measures mass and relative concentration of all molecules present in a sample.

metacarpus Skeletal structure beyond the carpus or 'wrist' of the foreleg; consists of five parallel small bones that help to form the foot. The innermost digit has several miniaturized bones that can be removed after birth; *see also* DEWCLAWS.

metacestode Developmental stage in the life cycle of the cestode tapeworm parasites of some animal hosts.

metaldehyde poisoning Poisoning from slug bait; now less frequent since the composition of the pellets has been revised; death occurs from respiratory failure following a period of incoordination, hyperaesthesia and convulsions.

metamyelocyte Cell found during the development and maturation of granulocyte (white) cells, the stage before a band neutrophil.

metaphase Second stage of cell division when the nuclear membrane breaks down, then followed by anaphase; *see also* MITOSIS.

metaphyseal osteopathy Severe lameness in growing puppies associated with painful joints and raised body temperature; *see also* BARLOW'S DISEASE.

metaphysis The part of the bone shaft between the diaphysis and the epiphysis region of growth plates in immature animals, situated between the two diaphyses.

metaplasia The reversible process of cell replacement that occurs when one differentiated cell is replaced by another mature differentiated cell, for example replacement of the usual squamous epithelium with columnar epithelium if the distal oesophagus is exposed to chronic gastric acid.

metastasis Spread of tumour cells, often into other organs or structures distant from the primary site; *see also* NEOPLASM.

metatarsus Bones of the hindlimb, distal to the distal row of tarsal bones; four in number connect to the phalanges.

metazoonosis Type of disease transmitted from invertebrates to vertebrate hosts, includes blood parasites such as *Babesia*; *see also* TICK FEVER.

methaemoglobin The iron ion in haemoglobin when oxidized, which prevents the transport of oxygen to tissues by erythrocytes; this toxic damage, due for instance to nitrite poisoning, causes signs such as dyspnoea and muddy-coloured mucous membranes.

methanol Also known as wood alcohol; can cause permanent blindness by brain injury if ingested; *see also* METHYLATED SPIRIT.

methionine Amino acid important in metabolism, may be used therapeutically in the treatment of paracetamol poisoning.

methohexital Anaesthetic agent twice as potent as thiopental and similarly is made up as a solution from the dry powder. Short-acting and considered suitable for greyhounds, etc. Occasional violent recovery stages have led to its replacement by other agents such as propofol.

methoxyflurane Anaesthetic agent based on a halogenated ether; it is environmentally friendly and safe for very small patients.

methylated spirit A mixture containing ethyl alcohol (ethanol) and methyl alcohol (methanol) with petroleum hydrocarbons. As little as 10 ml of pure methyl alcohol will cause blindness in humans if ingested.

methylcellulose Substance used as a bulking agent in the treatment of constipation and sometimes in liquid form as a lubricant jelly.

metoclopramide Medication used for its central effect in suppressing vomiting.

metoestrus Stage of the oestrous cycle when the corpus luteum is still active in the ovary; includes the time up to the development of false pregnancy in the bitch; *see also* PSEUDOPREGNANCY.

metric units of measurement Adopted for all scientific work but not fully used in the USA, etc. The system of measurement with the metre as the basic unit (of length); *see also* SI UNITS.

metritis Inflammation of the uterus; *see also* PYOMETRA.

metronidazole Synthetic compound mainly used against Gram-negative organisms and protozoa.

Metzenbaum scissors Long, slender surgical scissors that can be straight or curved; used for dissection of tissues.

micelle Important in the digestion of fats, a minute globule formed when bile salts join with lipids to produce a fat droplet stable in fluid.

microbiology The study of bacteria, viruses, fungi and protozoa.

microchip Animal identification system using a subcutaneous 'transponder' carrying a unique number for permanent identification.

micrococci Very small bacteria, mainly Gram-positive, found in soil and water.

microcoria Smaller than normal pupils; often a congenital defect found soon after the eyes open at 10 days.

microcyte Red blood cell that is smaller than normal; often associated with certain anaemias, including those caused by iron deficiency (**microcytic anaemia**).

microdontia Underdevelopment of the teeth.

microfilaria Development stage of worms of the Filarioidea family that are residing in the blood. Produced by adult heartworms in dogs, their presence can be detected by fresh blood smears; *see also* HEARTWORMS.

microflora Small organisms that may be found residing in the mouth or the intestine; includes bacteria, viruses, protozoa and fungi.

microglia The parts of the CNS cellular structure that are not nerve cells; may have a phagocytic action.

microgram One-millionth of a gram or one-thousandth of a milligram, written as μg.

microhaematocrit Instrument to centrifuge small quantities of blood in capillary tubes to measure packed cell volume.

micrometer Instrument to measure length or size of small structures; *see also* MICROSCOPE.

micron Smallest unit of measurement in light microscopy, one-thousandth of a millimetre, written as μm.

microorchidia Underdeveloped or very small testes; not necessarily infertile but associated with lower libido in the animal.

microorganism Small organisms, includes bacteria, viruses, protozoa, fungi and algae.

microphallus Smaller than normal penis; may be a hindrance when attempting to catheterize neutered male cats.

microphthalmos Very small eyes, often a congenital defect; may be associated with entropion and epiphora.

micropipette Laboratory instrument for measuring minute quantities of fluid.

microscope Instrument for magnification and measurement, divided into electron and light types; only the light microscope is available in most practice laboratories, known as a compound microscope, it may have binocular eye pieces. The purpose is to magnify very small objects and measurement may be possible using a measuring scale in the eyepiece. A moving stage with a micrometer adjustment can be used to locate objects. A **binocular microscope** is an instrument with two adjustable eyepieces; the ocular lenses are mounted in each eyepiece. A **compound microscope** is a regular microscope with lenses in both the eyepiece and the objective to increase the magnification; an advance on the older simple microscope. An **electron microscope** is a superior method of magnification using electrons to produce the magnified image. A **scanning electron microscope** (SEM) is used to view the surface of the object, which first has to be coated with a fine metallic substance so the electrons can then produce an image. A **transmission electron microscope** (TEM) uses a more complex method whereby the beam of

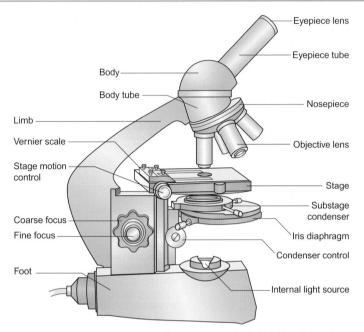

Eyepiece lens
Eyepiece tube
Body
Body tube
Nosepiece
Limb
Vernier scale
Objective lens
Stage motion control
Stage
Substage condenser
Coarse focus
Fine focus
Iris diaphragm
Condenser control
Foot
Internal light source

Figure 33. Microscope. Redrawn with permission from Aspinall V. Clinical procedures in veterinary nursing. Edinburgh: Butterworth-Heinemann, 2003.

the electrons crosses an ultrathin slice of the tissue.

Microsporidia Spore-forming, unicellular obligate intracellular parasites that may be found in most animals, including fish; an example is *Heterosporis saurida* as a pathogen of fish.

Microsporum Genus of fungus causing one form of ringworm of dogs and cats; *M. canis* will infect either cats or dogs. Distinguished by hyphae with conidia and some 50% of samples fluoresce apple–green under ultraviolet light, unlike *M. gypseum*; *see also* WOOD'S LAMP.

microsurgery Delicate surgical work that includes the repair of blood vessels and nerves; involves dissection under the microscope.

microteeth The type of forceps ends used in ophthalmic surgery on forceps

employed to grip the most delicate eye structures.

microtome Laboratory equipment for making the very thin slices of tissue required for biopsy and histological studies.

microtubules Small filaments within the cell cytoplasm that help to maintain its shape.

microurinary calculi Urinary calculi sludge that provides a nidus for bacteria associated with cystitis.

microvascular Involving small blood vessels, as in the techniques to restore blood supply to organs in microsurgery.

microvillus Small folds or finger-like projections to increase surface area and aid absorption in the epithelium of the small intestine.

micturate To empty the bladder.

midbrain The part of the brainstem that carries nerve tracts from the cerebrum to the hindbrain but does not include the pons or the medulla. Contains the visual and auditory centres.

middle ear The nonvisible part of the ear in the tympanic bulla of the skull's temporal bone; it contains the three small bones that connect the ear drum to the inner ear; the eustachian tube connects to the throat; *see also* AUDITORY, EAR.

midges Small biting insects responsible for acute dermatoses and 'hot spots' in dogs.

midline Refers to the central approach, as in an abdominal incision through the linea alba.

migration Movement from an original site, of ova, metal inserts, microchips, etc. Also refers to the protein electrophoresis separation process; *see also* ELECTROPHORESIS.

miliary Refers to small particles the size of a millet seed when describing a nodule or skin lesions; *see also* DERMATOSIS.

milk The fluid of the mammary glands, used to nourish the newborn.

Miller's disease Also known as 'big osteodystrophy' in the horse, causing the face to become enlarged.

milli- One-thousandth of a part; symbol is 'm'.

milligram One-thousandth of a gram, used in medication calculations for dose-rate per kilogram body weight; abbreviated mg.

millilitre One-thousandth of a litre; abbreviated ml. Equivalent to the older 'cc' measurement, which was a cubic centimetre of water.

millimetre One-thousandth of a metre, abbreviated mm.

millimole One-thousandth of a mole, the measure of osmolarity; abbreviated mmol; *see also* FLUID THERAPY.

mineral Group term for essential elements such as iron and calcium; can also include the trace elements such as cobalt.

mineralocorticoid Corticosteroid produced by the adrenal cortex that controls water and salt balance; *see also* ALDOSTERONE.

mineral oil Term used in the USA for the liquid paraffin product derived from petroleum refining; light and heavy grades are available.

minimal inhibitory concentration (MIC) A figure used in measuring the effectiveness of antibiotics, etc.

minimal lethal dose (MLD) A standard once used when testing the safe use of drugs and correct dose rates for therapeutics.

minimum wage The legal minimum wage payable in a country to an individual employee; this varies between countries, but most countries within the United Nations have a legally binding minimum wage.

miotic Substance that constricts the pupils.

misalliance Popular term when a bitch or queen becomes mated by a casual or undesirable male. May be called mésalliance.

miscarriage Popular term for unexpected termination of a pregnancy; *see also* ABORTION.

mismating *See* MISALLIANCE.

Misuse of Drugs Act 1971 States the rules for the possession of 'controlled drugs'. This Act and the Misuse of Drugs Regulations 1985 control the production, supply, possession and dispensing of drugs where there might be abuse by humans.

mite Any small, crawling insect but not including ticks. May cause direct parasitic disease or allergic responses; *see also* DERMATOPHAGOIDES, MANGE.

mitochondria Particles in the cell known as organelles; the mitochondria release energy from food and store it in the cell; *see also* ADENOSINE TRIPHOSPHATASE.

mitosis Stage of cell division when cells duplicate themselves and the nucleus doubles the number of chromosomes before two new cells split.

mitotane Substance used to cause atrophy and necrosis of the adrenal cortex, used therapeutically in Cushing's syndrome; it must be handled with care as it is a carcinogen; *see also* CHEMOTHERAPY.

M

mitotic figure Condition of the nucleus chromosomes when the cell is about to divide. High numbers of mitotic figures in a tissue indicate neoplasia.

mitral Shaped like a bishop's hat – tapered like a mitre. Describes the valve at the entrance to the left ventricle; *see also* HEART VALVE.

Mittendorf's dot Opacity of the posterior lens capsule where the hyaloid artery was attached during the embryonic development of the eye.

mixed mammary tumour One of the commonest neoplasms of the older bitch, resulting from tumour growths of the epithelium, the gland tissue and other connective tissue; frequently found not to be malignant if removed early enough.

MMP Matrix metalloproteinases; zinc-activated endopeptidases that will digest proteins of the extracellular matrix.

modality Term applied to the sense organs; state or condition in respect of a mode or manner.

modes Used in dynamic ultrasound to describe the image produced: **M mode** is for movement mode and **B mode** is brightness.

moist Damp, wet, humid.

moist dermatitis Superficial localized skin response; often the result of insect bite or other allergic response.

moist heat sterilization Describes sterilization by boiling water, now replaced by steam-under-pressure sterilization; *see also* AUTOCLAVE.

moist lung sounds Fluid effusion into the bronchi, often with a productive cough when mucus is expectorated.

molar 1) The type of teeth that fill the posterior part of the upper and lower jaws; *see also* TEETH. 2) Describes the molecular content of a solution; the **molarity** of a volume of a solution is important in fluid therapy.

mole 1) Common term for a black-pigmented skin tumour; melanotic warts are usually nonmalignant; *see also* MELANOMA. 2) The SI unit for the amount of a substance: one mole has a mass equal to the molecular weight in grams, abbreviated mol and containing 6×10^{23} atoms or molecules.

molecular Relating to the composition of molecules; **molecular biology** is used in many investigative procedures in the laboratory.

molecular genetics The study of genes at the cellular or molecular level using microscopy or molecular biological methods.

molecule The smallest portion into which a chemical compound can be divided.

Moller–Barlow disease *See* BARLOW'S DISEASE, METAPHYSEAL OSTEOPATHY.

moniliasis Infection with the small, yeast-like parasite *Candida*.

monitor An instrument that may record multiple parameters such as ECG, O_2 saturation, pulse, respiration or bag movement as an indication of respiratory function. The word can also be applied to the actions of the person overseeing the patient.

monitor lizard Larger reptile occasionally kept as a pet; exercise is important as they would normally have to hunt for their food so may become overweight, with a fatty liver, in captivity; belong to the Varanidae family.

monoblast Precursor cell for the monocyte; its appearance in the blood suggests some leukaemic disorder.

monochromatic Single-colour, used when describing dyes in microbiology. The same word may be used to describe animal vision – a human with complete colour blindness is a monochromat.

monoclonal Describes an antibody produced artificially from a cell clone and thus with a very pure single type of immunoglobulin. Used frequently in many laboratory investigations.

monocular Using one eye; having a single eyepiece, as in the basic microscope.

monocyte One of the granulocytes of the white cell series; phagocytic cells larger than the others in the series. A persisting monocytosis indicates some chronic disorder.

monoestrus The condition of having a single reproductive time in a mating season; the adjective is **monoestrous**; *see also* POLYOESTRUS.

monofilament suture Synthetic material consisting of a single thread, favoured for its strength and lack of capillary action in tissues; *see also* BRAIDED SUTURE.

monogastric Normal state of most pet animals with a simple stomach; *see also* RUMINANT.

monoplegia Paralysis of one limb.

monorchid The presence of only one testis in the scrotum, the 'hidden' testis may be small and soft and found in the inguinal canal or entirely within the abdomen.

monosaccharide Single-sugar substance such as glucose or fructose.

monozygotic twins Two fetuses that developed from a single egg.

monster A fetal abnormality, seen as a congenital defect of the abdomen, limbs or face.

mood-altering drugs Tricyclic antidepressants, benzodiazepines and monamine oxidase inhibitors can all be used to provide relief from chronic pain as they have an analgesic effect as well as their better-known antidepressant use.

morbid Death-like, diseased or in a pathological state.

morbillivirus One of the virus groups, which includes canine distemper and the similar condition of wild seals.

moribund Dying, usually without hope of recovery.

morphine Opioid drug with strong analgesic properties; narcotic and addictive in humans.

morula Early stage of the development of the zygote as a solid ball.

mosquito forceps Name used to describe very fine forceps; *see also* HAEMOSTAT.

motility Used where there is the ability to move, as in the propulsion of intestinal contents; in small organisms' activity, is often the result of flagella (the tail of the sperm).

motions Popular term for the products of bowel evacuation; *see also* FAECES.

motor An adjective used to imply that movement may be expected, e.g. motor nerve.

motor nerve Part of the nerve trunk that runs from the spinal cord to the muscle or other effector organ; dysfunction may lead to rigidity or muscle weakness.

motor neurone Nerve fibril that will cause muscle movement.

mould Fungi seen as fluffy growths on substances, often decaying matter; cause of some inhaled allergies.

mouth Orifice in the head used for ingesting food, vocalization and respiration in times of distress; *see also* BUCCAL.

mouth-to-nose respiration First aid procedure for inflating the lungs with human exhaled air containing additional carbon dioxide as a respiratory stimulant. Equivalent to the 'kiss of life' in human first aid.

mouth rot Necrotic stomatitis in snakes, which can progress to affect the jaw bone and digestive and respiratory systems; requires aggressive management.

MRI Magnetic resonance imaging.

MRSA Methicillin-resistant *Staphylococcus aureus*; an organism of increasing concern in human and veterinary medicine as it is resistant to most antibiotics.

mucilage Gum-like substance in aqueous solution; has a valuable function in natural lubrication.

mucin Glycoprotein or polysaccharide used by the body where lubrication is needed.

mucocele, salivary Distension under the tongue or in the angle of the jaw containing saliva from abnormality or duct leakage; *see also* RANULA.

mucocutaneous junction Relating to the areas where the skin joins the intestinal tract or other mucous membrane.

mucocutaneous system Name used in dermatology when disease affects the skin or the mucosa; *see also* ALOPECIA, PRURITUS, PYODERMA, SEBORRHOEA.

mucoid enteropathy A diarrhoeal disease of rabbits where mucus accumulates in the intestines.

mucolytic Substance that reduces the viscosity of secreted mucus and may allow coughing to remove mucus quicker.

mucometra The state of the uterus that may occur in metoestrus when fluid or 'uterine milk' accumulates in the lumen of the uterus. An ascending or a blood-borne infection may cause the rapid development of disease; *see also* PYOMETRA.

mucopurulent Description of any discharge from the body when infection causes pus to be mixed in with mucus.

mucosa Alternative word for mucous membrane.

mucous The adjective that describes anything that is like mucus or a tissue that secretes mucus. A mucoid internal surface that has some or many goblet cells can cover the surface with a mucus film with valuable lubrication and protective factors.

mucous membrane Protective lining to the body cavities; some are ciliated to move the mucus along with waves of propulsion.

mucus The protein substance produced by the goblet cells of the epithelium.

mud fever Dermatitis caused by the bacterium *Dermatophilus congolensis*, affecting the soft tissue of the equine heel, fetlock and pastern.

müllerian duct Embryonic paramesonephric first stage that forms the uterus, vagina and ovarian tubes or remains as a remnant in the male prostate.

multi- Prefix denoting 'very many'.

multicentric Involving more than one place of development, as in **multicentric lymphoma**, where numerous lymph nodes enlarge simultaneously.

multidisciplinary A group approach by clinical professionals – veterinary surgeons, veterinary nurses, physiotherapists, etc; from more than one clinical discipline such as orthopaedics and dermatology, who work together to provide diagnoses and treatments for patients.

multifactorial Implies that a condition has more than one cause.

multifocal Involving several sites, e.g. in brain trauma, a multifocal injury may lead to coma and death.

multigravida An individual who has been pregnant at least twice.

multilocular ranula Outpouchings filled with saliva that may develop after injury to the salivary duct. The fluid pouches grow between the more rigid structures in the neck and lower jaw area.

multi lumen catheter A catheter with more than one hole and connecting port (can be several) that enables a single catheter to have more than one use.

multiorgan failure (MOF) Generalization in a diseased state, indicating the rapid deterioration of a patient and anticipated death.

multiparous Having had at least two separate pregnancies and births with viable kittens or puppies, etc.

murine Relating to the mouse or rat family. **Murine typhus** causes human disease and deaths.

murmur A noise in the cardiac area caused by turbulence in blood flow, e.g. leaking weak heart valve. Regurgitation of blood occurs to some extent. Anaemic murmurs can be heard when the blood lacks viscosity. Murmurs are graded by their intensity from I–VI, with I being very soft and weak and VI being very loud. Variants may be used to describe the murmur sound, e.g. machinery or musical, while the location is the usual description, e.g. aortic or mitral.

MUS Midstream urine sample.

muscarinic receptors Those nerve receptors that are sensitive to acetylcholine; found at all parasympathetic effector junctions and some sympathetic ones.

muscle Contractile tissue that controls locomotion and movement; divided into three types: smooth, cardiac and voluntary.

muscular dystrophy A degeneration of muscular tissue caused by faulty nutrition. In humans, a genetic cause affects certain young males; the most common form is Duchenne muscular dystrophy. A similar hereditary disorder may occur in golden retrievers.

musculoskeletal Organ system of the body comprising the bones and their attached muscles, responsible for the support and propulsion of the animal.

mustard An emetic that may be advised as a first aid measure when an animal has consumed a noncorrosive poison; two teaspoons in a cup of water.

mustelid Referring to the ferret family, domesticated *Mustelo putorius furo*.

mutagen Any agent, either chemical or physical, that causes DNA mutations.

mutant Change in the genetic composition may occur spontaneously or after damage to the genes from chemicals, radiation or from some viruses.

mutation Process of an alteration in the DNA; usually harmful but sometimes by introducing novel characteristics the individual better competes for survival; characteristics may be transmitted to the next and subsequent generations.

mutilation A harmful change to the body: docking, dewclaw removal and ear cropping are examples often quoted, as the original reason for these procedures has largely been forgotten.

muzzle 1) The part of the face surrounding the nostrils. 2) A device to cover the head and stop the mouth opening so that the muzzled animal cannot bite.

myasthenia gravis Disorder of muscle tissue where there is a lack of acetylcholine production or a loss of acetylcholine receptors at the motor end plate, leading to muscle weakness, exercise intolerance and megaoesophagus.

mycelium Strands of fungal tissue that make up the main visible part of the organism.

mycobacteria Genus of rod-like bacteria, characterized by the 'acid-fast' staining character of the capsule, where the dye is not removed by an acidic solution.

mycoplasma Small organisms lacking a rigid cell wall; found in respiratory tract infections and have been associated with canine distemper. *M. felis* is found in many equine cough infections but can also cause conjunctivitis in cats. *M. haemofelis* is the new name for *Haemobartonella felis*.

mycoplasmosis A common condition of extensively kept chickens, caused by several species of *Mycoplasma*; common

clinical signs include swollen sinuses, nasal discharge, and lethargy.

mycosis A disease produced by a fungus.

mydriasis Dilated pupils, often suggesting blindness; may be induced by drugs used to 'rest' the pupil or allow for a thorough ophthalmoscope examination of the lens and fundus. It may indicate a neurological disease or glaucoma; *see also* GLAUCOMA.

myectomy Removal or excision of a muscle.

myelin Fat-like substance that covers nerve fibrils and allows faster transmission of the nerve impulse; myelin sheaths are produced by the Schwann cells, which lie wrapped around the axon of the nerve.

myeloblast Bone marrow precursor cell responsible for granulocytes; may occasionally appear in the peripheral blood.

myelocyte An immature form of a granulocyte; may differentiate into an eosinophil or a polymorphonuclear cell.

myelofibrosis Disease where normal haemopoietic tissue becomes replaced by fibrous tissue, causing a nonregenerative anaemia, but normal leukocyte and platelet function remains.

myelogram Radiograph after myelography.

myelography A technique involving putting positive contrast media into the subarachnoid space to outline the spinal cord during radiography.

myeloid 1) Referring to the bone marrow. 2) Used as an adjective relating to the spinal cord. 3) May mean 'like a myelocyte cell'.

myeloma Neoplasm of the bone marrow usually diagnosed from haematology and bone marrow biopsy.

myelopathy 1) Pathological disease of the bone marrow. 2) Any functional change or degenerative condition of the myelin in the spinal cord.

myelopathy of the spinal cord Specific and progressive degenerative disease of the German shepherd and some other large breeds; *see also* CHRONIC DEGENERATIVE ADICULOMYELOPATHY.

myeloproliferative tumour Neoplasm of bone marrow with increase of granulocytes, monocytes, erythrocytes, megakaryocytes and mast cells.

myiasis Infestation with fly maggots; rabbits with the cutaneous form can die quickly from toxins absorbed by the subcutaneous blood vessels.

myocardial degeneration Myocardial disease; the early stage of potential heart failure; *see also* MYOCARDIOPATHY.

myocardiopathy Progressive degenerative condition of heart muscle; usually leads to death; *see also* CARDIOMYOPATHY.

myocarditis An inflammatory disease of the heart muscle, the result of an infection – viral or bacterial.

myocardium The muscle of the heart, the middle and strongest layer of the three that make up the heart wall; *see also* ENDOCARDIUM, PERICARDIUM.

myoclonus Repeated small contractions of voluntary muscle groups that persist even when the animal is asleep, often the result of a viral infection; *see also* CHOREA.

myoepithelial cells Contractile epithelial cells found in glandular tissues that help the expulsion of secreted fluids.

myofibril Component of muscle tissue; forms myofilament.

myofilament Actin and myosin combined to form a contractile strand; *see also* SARCOMERE.

myoglobin Substance in the muscle for oxygen transport; similar in structure to the haemoglobin in the blood.

myometrium Smooth muscle tissue of the uterus between the endometrium and the peritoneal outer cover.

myomorpha Suborder of rodents – hamsters, mice, gerbils, rats.

myopathy Any disease of a muscle; some myopathies are inherited, as in the golden retriever breed; some may result from bacterial infections. Myopathies are usually bilaterally symmetrical, but often only one muscle group may be affected, as in **cardiomyopathy**.

myorrhaphy Repair of a muscle by suturing.

myosin The most common protein of muscle tissue, has the ability to contract; *see also* ACTIN.

myositis Inflammation of body muscle, usually with pain and lameness if a leg is affected. **Atrophic myositis** is a chronic progressive disease usually affecting the dog's jaw muscles, eventually making it impossible to open the mouth by more than a few centimetres. **Eosinophilic myositis** is a specific disease of the German shepherd dog usually associated with an eosinophilia in the blood profile. Treatment with steroids is possible, but the cause is unknown.

myotactic reflex Tendon stretch reflex, used commonly when assessing patellar reflex.

myotomy An incision into a muscle.

myotonia Refers to a state where active contraction of the muscle persists after voluntary effort or stimulation has stopped. Muscle stiffness and spasm may be acquired or have a hereditary basis, as in chow chows, great Danes and Staffordshire bull terriers.

myringitis Inflammation of the eardrum; *see also* OTITIS MEDIA.

myringotomy An operation to incise the eardrum to create an artificial opening for drainage; not in common use in animal surgery.

myxo- Prefix denoting 'mucus' or 'mucoid'.

myxoedema A clinical sign of hypothyroidism in humans. It may occur in dogs, with a thickening of the skin, and contribute to a 'tragic' expression.

myxomatosis A viral infection of rabbits characterized by swollen head and closed eyes with profuse oculonasal discharges. Rabbits appear grotesque with swelling from subcutaneous lumps, mainly around the head and genitalia. Mortality rate is near 100%.

n.a.d. No abnormality detected.
Abbreviation used during a clinical examination to denote that no abnormality was detected; it does not rule out the possibility of any 'hidden' disease.

NAD Nicotinamide adenine dinucleotide, a coenzyme; *see also* NIACIN.

NADP Nicotinamide adenine dinucleotide phosphate, a coenzyme; *see also* NIACIN.

naevus A small red area of the skin, popularly known as a birthmark.

nail 1) Keratin structure covering for the claws of an animal. **2)** Intramedullary device used in internal fixation of bone structures.

nailbed infection Infection at the base of the nail; *see also* PARONYCHIA.

nalidixic acid Medication once used for urinary infections; inhibits DNA synthesis.

naloxone Antagonist substance used to reverse the effect of opiates in the narcotic drugs group; an antidote for morphine.

nandrolone Anabolic steroid used therapeutically; has androgenic properties as well.

nanogram A very small measurement of weight, one-thousand-millionth of a gram (10^{-9} g); abbreviation ng.

nanometre The size of a millimicrometre, one-thousand-millionth of a metre (10^{-9} m); abbreviation nm.

naproxen Non-steroidal anti-inflammatory drug (NSAID) used in humans; can be fatal if accidentally swallowed by a dog as it causes gastric haemorrhage, vomiting and melaena.

narco- Prefix that implies a sleep situation or drug-induced stupor.

narcosis State of diminished consciousness or complete unconsciousness.

nares (*sing.* naris) The external nostrils; the opening to the nasal cavity.

Narrowness of the two openings is a problem in brachycephalic breeds.

nasal Relating to the nose.

nasociliary Describes anything in the area of the base of the nose, the eyes and the eyebrows.

nasodigital Describes any condition affecting the tip of the nose and the pads of the feet; hyperkeratosis.

nasogastric tube A fine tube inserted into the stomach through the nose, used for oral fluid administration.

nasolacrimal The tear duct drainage apparatus that runs to the nose, includes the two ducts draining the eye, the lacrimal sac and the nasolacrimal duct.

nasooesophageal tube A tube placed through the nose into the oesophagus for enteral feeding of patients.

nasopharynx (rhinopharynx) The part of the pharynx craniodorsal to the soft palate communicating to the nasal cavity.

nates Anatomically, the buttocks.

National Council for Vocational Qualifications (NCVQ) A central government organization set up in the 1980s for moderating and supervising training in many areas of work, including veterinary nursing and animal care courses. The RCVS is the sole awarding body for Veterinary Nursing Scottish/National Vocational Qualifications (VNS/NVQs).

National Office of Animal Health *See* NOAH.

natural A term widely used when describing treatment or medication, implying that it occurs in nature unaffected by humankind.

natural killer cell Cell involved in fighting infections that recognizes and destroys any cells or antigens without first being required to be sensitized by the target; *see also* IMMUNITY.

nausea A feeling of sickness, often associated with brain stimulation; *see also* VESTIBULAR DISEASE.

navel The umbilical cord attachment point of the abdomen; *see also* UMBILICUS.

navel ill Term used for infection of the umbilicus after birth, usually in horses and farm animals.

navicular bone The sesamoid bone that lies caudal to the P2/3 joint in the foot of the horse.

navicular disease Degenerative condition of the navicular bone; may be the result of impaired blood supply.

NAVTA National Association of Veterinary Technicians in America.

NE Net energy.

near-far-far-near suture Method of suturing that gives a flattened figure-of-eight, used to relieve tension on the wound edges; *see also* MATTRESS SUTURE.

nebula A mild corneal opacity not affecting vision; the same word is used for a very small healed ulcerative opacity in the cornea.

nebulizer An instrument for making a spray; used in oxygen administration to moisten the gases; also used to give medications directly to the respiratory tract.

neck The anatomical area between the skull and the thorax around the cervical vertebrae. The same term is used for any constricted area such as in bones, teeth or the cervical area of the uterus.

necrobacillosis Serious progressive skin infection of rabbits caused by *Fusobacterium necrophorum* that can be fatal.

necropsy Alternative word for a postmortem examination; *see also* AUTOPSY, POSTMORTEM.

necrosis Death of cells or tissue.

needle A pointed object, either with a hollow centre to use for injections or as a solid rod used in suturing or possibly for acupuncture. An **acupuncture needle** is a very fine, long object for inserting into the skin at the points deemed to relate to the condition under treatment. An **aspiration biopsy needle** is a hollow needle to which suction can be applied to obtain a core of biopsy material. **Needle guard** A device attached to a hypodermic needle to resheath it after use to prevent needlestick injuries. **Needle holders** in a variety of patterns are used by surgeons to place needles accurately when suturing skin or other tissues. A **hypodermic needle** is an injection needle originally used for drugs placed beneath the skin; the term is now in general use for any injection or aspiration needle. **Spinal needle** – a needle used with a stylet for accessing the spinal canal to extract spinal fluid or to insert contrast media.

needle stick injury Accidental puncture of the skin of a human with a hypodermic needle or other type of needle; must be reported to a more senior staff member and recorded in the accident book.

negative punishment The removal of an item the animal wishes to have; the result of the action is a decrease in the frequency of the unwanted behaviour.

negative reinforcement Term used in training where a bad experience reinforces unwanted behaviour; an example is trying to clean a dog's teeth for the first time tooth using a brush or finger stall: if the teeth are painful, it often results in the dog resenting the cleaning process for a long time afterwards.

negligence A legal term that implies that there has been a lack of care and attention resulting in harm to the patient; however, in law, if a person has observed normal procedures and there has been adequate supervision, there should be little or no risk to the veterinary nurse working on veterinary premises.

Negri bodies Inclusion bodies recognized under the microscope in nervous tissue – the brain – that are diagnostic of rabies.

nemaline myopathy A rare disease of cats, probably hereditary, that causes twitching. Seen at ages 6–15 months, it may progress to a generalized muscular atrophy; named after the presence of nemaline rods in the skeletal muscles.

nematode Any one of the group of roundworms; the body is not segmented and tapers to a point at both ends; *see also* ASCARID, ROUNDWORM.

neo- Prefix for something new.

neonatal Relating to the period immediately after birth has occurred, usually the first week.

neonatal jaundice A yellow coloration in a newborn animal; may be caused by haemolysis of its own blood or by liver failure.

neonate A newborn puppy, kitten or similar animal at the stage when it cannot survive without its mother or similar intensive care.

neon tetra disease *Pleistophoriasis*; protozoal disease of fish, affects species more widely than just neon tetras; the parasites encyst in the muscle, leading to loss of colour and gradual wasting; there is no cure.

neoplasm New growth; used as a term for cancer or any type of condition with abnormal cell production.

neosporosis Infection with *Neospora caninum*, affecting the CNS, heart, muscles or skin.

neostigmine Medication used for its action in producing a parasympathomimetic effect.

neoteny Some breeds of dog and cat retain infantile or **neotenic** characteristics into adulthood. This characteristic is attractive to some owners as the animal retains many of the characteristics of a child.

nephrectomy Surgical operation to remove a kidney.

nephritis Inflammation of the kidney; *see also* NEPHROSIS.

nephro- Prefix indicating something in the kidney system or the body area in the abdomen under the lumbar muscles.

nephron The active filtering unit of the kidney; composed of glomerulus, Bowman's capsule, proximal and distal convoluted tubules and a loop of Henle.

nephrosis May be any kidney disease but usually implies a degenerative condition rather than an infectious disease.

nephrosplenic ligament The ligament between the spleen and the kidneys in the horse, where bowel can sometimes become trapped (nephrosplenic entrapment), causing colic.

nephrotic syndrome Condition with loss of protein in the urine, often with a fall in albumin in the blood, subcutaneous oedema and ascites; an end-stage disease often the result of a glomerulonephritis.

nerve Collection of nerve fibres, a conducting structure of the body where impulses are carried between effectors, receptors and the whole of the CNS. May be divided into motor, sensory and mixed nerves.

nerve block Method of local analgesia using specific substances to stop nerve transmission, resulting in a loss of sensation or movement of a part of the body. An epidural injection or local infiltration may be used.

nestbox Small enclosed area of a chicken house, often lined with paper, shavings or straw to encourage chickens to lay their eggs inside.

nettle rash A papular eruption of the skin vesicles; *see also* URTICARIA.

neural Relating to a nerve or nerves.

neuralgia Pain, often severe, following the course of a nerve; *see also* TRIGEMINAL NEURALGIA.

neuraxial anaesthesia Anaesthetic injections within the spinal canal; *see also* EPIDURAL.

neurilemma Sheath of connective tissue that surrounds the whole axon formed by a glial cell; *see also* NEURONE.

neurilemmoma (schwannoma) Type of tumour of the peripheral nerve: may be found first as a benign nodule under the skin. Arises from the Schwann cells, which normally produce the myelin to coat the axon.

neuroglia Connective tissue of the nervous system; the packing material around neurones.

neurohypophysis Alternative name for posterior pituitary gland; *see also* HYPOPHYSIS.

N

neuroleptanalgesia A form of chemical restraint close to general anaesthesia. Various combinations of analgesics and neuroleptics may be used.

neurological Relating to the nervous system.

neurological hammer Instrument used for assessing tendon reflexes.

neuromuscular junction The junction of the nerve ending and the muscle it innervates at the specialized motor end plate.

neurone A specialized cell to transmit nervous impulses; may be unipolar, bipolar or multipolar depending on the position of the dendrites through which nerve impulses enter the cell. Afferent and efferent neurones carry impulses to or away from the CNS, respectively.

neuropathic bladder A nonfunctioning urinary bladder where catheterization may be necessary; can be the result of spinal trauma or sometimes associated with bladder neoplasia.

neuropathy Disease state affecting cranial or peripheral nerves, may affect sensory, or motor nerve endings or both; characterized by inflammation and degeneration of the peripheral nerves. **Diabetic neuropathy** is a diseased state of sensory nerves, more common in human diabetics than dogs or cats. **Giant axonal neuropathy** is a hereditary disease of German shepherd dogs; develops when the dog is young; is first seen in the hind legs, progressing to ataxia and megaoesophagus.

neurapraxia Temporary loss of nerve function; may be caused by pressure on the nerve from an intervertebral disc; numbness and weakness result.

neurotmesis Partial or complete severance of a nerve, as may occur in aural ablation surgery affecting the facial nerve – a neurotomy.

neurotoxin An exotoxin produced by bacteria that damages the nervous system – the toxin involved in tetanus is the most common example.

neurotransmitter Chemical substance that is necessary for one neurone to communicate with another neurone or an excitatory tissue (muscle, gland) by altering the transmembrane potential; *see also* TRANSMEMBRANE POTENTIAL.

neuter Common expression for performing a procedure that renders a pet incapable of breeding; *see also* CASTRATION, SPAY.

neutron Particle in the atom with neutral charge; *see also* ATOM.

neutropenia A low white cell count; *see also* AGRANULOCYTOSIS.

neutrophil A granulocyte, one of the white cell series, frequently referred to as a 'polymorph' or leukocyte because of the shape of the nucleus.

Newcastle disease A notifiable disease of poultry and other birds. Acute infections are sudden with a high mortality rate; mild cases show respiratory, intestinal or nervous symptoms with a drop in egg production and an increase in soft shell eggs. Birds can be vaccinated from a day old with live Newcastle disease (ND) vaccine. Revaccination after 14–21 days is necessary.

New Forest Syndrome *See* ALABAMA ROT.

NFA-VPS 'Non-food animal – veterinarian, pharmacist, suitably qualified person', an authorised medicine that can be supplied to non-food animals by veterinarians, pharmacists and SQPs.

niacin One of the vitamin B group; it is an essential component of two enzymes, NAD and NADP, involved in the oxidation/reduction system of carbohydrate, protein and fat.

nicotinic receptors Receptors sensitive to acetylcholine found in autonomic ganglion cells and motor end-plates.

nictitans gland Anatomical structure in the 'corner' or medial canthus of the eye that secretes lubricating mucus to protect the cornea.

nictitating membrane The so-called 'third eyelid', which has a protective function and on its inner surface has lymphoid tissue as well as mucus-producing glands; *see also* MEMBRANA NICTITANS.

nidation Known as 'egg-nesting' or the implantation of the fertilized egg in the endometrium at the very earliest stages of pregnancy before the fetal membranes develop.

night blindness Popular name for progressive retinal atrophy (PRA), where dogs see less well in the half-light of dusk; observed particularly in gun dog breeds with PRA, where the dog misses moving animals; came to public attention when the Irish setter breed had PRA identified in the 1950s as a dominant inherited disorder, which was then bred out of British stock; *see also* PRA, RETINAL DYSPLASIA.

Nipah virus Causes a fatal disease of dogs, cats, people and farm animals. The viral cause is closely related to Hendra virus and is of considerable zoonotic importance in Australia.

nipple Any small protuberance; usually used as an alternative name to teat; the orifice from which milk is obtained in lactating mammals.

Nissl body Found in the cell body of the neuron, stains more darkly because of the density of endoplasmic reticulum and ribosomes; *see also* NEURONE.

nit Popular name for the egg of the louse, which can be found adhering to the hairshaft, only just visible to the naked eye.

nitrofuran One of the synthetic antibacterial substances used for treating urinary and respiratory tract infections, now superseded by more advanced medication.

nitrogen balance Measurement of the body's ability to absorb and process protein from the diet and excrete nitrogenous waste products, mainly in the urine.

nitroimidazoles A group of synthetic substances used against protozoa including *Giardia*; *see also* METRONIDAZOLE.

nitroscannate An anthelminthic used against tapeworms.

nitrous oxide Anaesthetic gas used in circuits mainly for its analgesic properties; it has a diluting effect on oxygen as a carrier gas; cannot be used in a closed anaesthetic circuit.

NMDA receptor antagonist A type of drug used for the control of pain acting on the *N*-methyl dopamine receptors.

NOAH A trade organization, the National Office of Animal Health; the UK national body that represents manufacturers of veterinary products, etc.

no-blame meeting A meeting held with a group of people to investigate how a problem has arisen and how it can be avoided next time, rather than looking to apportion blame; this encourages employees to report incidents.

Nocardia A genus of Gram-positive, acid-fast staining, soil bacteria associated with nonhealing nodules and ulcers on dogs' legs.

nociception The way an animal experiences pain through the brain's cerebral cortex 'feeling' any unpleasant peripheral stimuli.

nociceptive Noci- as a prefix means 'harmful', the word describes nerve fibres, endings or pathways concerned with the conduction of pain.

noct- Indicates a night-time occurrence or activity. **Noctambulation** describes an animal that moves about at night.

node Any small grouping or protuberance of tissue may be called a node. The **A–V (atrioventricular) node** is the point in the heart muscle where cardiac fibres lying between the septa of the atria delay the impulse originating in the S–A node. Waves of electrical activity then spread from the A–V node to the ventricles. **Lymph nodes** are part of the defence mechanism of the body: lymphoid tissue is grouped at strategic points to filter or otherwise deal with infections, etc. The **S–A (sinoatrial) node** is an area of specialized cardiac tissue situated on the wall of the right atrium where the electrical impulse originates to set the heart rhythm; *see also* BUNDLE OF HIS. **Nodes of Ranvier** are points along the nerve fibres where there are gaps in the myelin sheaths. Ionic exchanges take place to reinforce the nerve impulses.

N

nodule A collection of tissue smaller than a node; a term often used to describe small lumps in the skin, etc.

nonaccidental injury (NAI) A term used in nursing where it is believed that injuries to the body may be the result of the activity of the patient's 'carers'. A similar situation in animals may be caused by abusers and other deviants.

nonambulatory The inability to be mobile.

noninvasive tumour Benign tumour or a tumour that does not spread locally or by metastasis; *see also* BENIGN.

nonprotein nitrogen (NPN) Sources of nitrogen that are not proteins. Urea and ammonia are two examples.

nonspecific Indicates there is no one recognizable cause, or it may be used to show that the effect of the condition is general, throughout the body, rather than specific to 'target' areas.

non-steroidal anti-inflammatory drugs (NSAIDs) Chemical compounds that have a similar effect to cortisone in suppressing inflammation; they work by suppressing prostaglandins and have activity against pain (analgesic) and fever (antipyretic) as well as their anti-inflammatory effect.

nonunion fracture Term used where fractured bone ends fail to unite; may result from excess movement, insufficient blood supply or infection at the ends of the bone.

noradrenaline (norepinephrine) One of the two hormones secreted by the adrenal medulla, with a sympathomimetic effect; *see also* ADRENALINE.

norethisterone A progesterone-like hormone produced synthetically; *see also* PROGESTOGEN.

normoblast A developmental stage of erythrocytes; they still have nuclei, having developed from the erythroblast; found in certain anaemias, as are reticulocytes, which are one further stage in the red blood cell's development; *see also* ERYTHROGENESIS.

normocyte An erythrocyte that is normal in size, structure and function.

normothermia Having a normal body temperature.

nose Anatomical structure of the head carrying the external nares.

nose pad Also known as rhinarium; was thought to be of use in identifying dogs, similarly to the use of fingerprints in humans. It is a thick keratinized structure free of body hair surrounding the external nares, usually kept moist by the tongue.

North American Veterinary Licensing Examination (NAVLE) National examination that must be taken by any veterinarian wanting to practice in North America.

nosocomial pneumonia Lung infection acquired during hospitalization; it may be fungal or bacterial; associated with the lowered resistance of inpatients of a veterinary hospital. Gram-negative infections, e.g. *Pseudomonas*, may be a problem.

nostril External opening of the upper respiratory tract; muscular activity can dilate or close the size of the openings, especially in the rabbit.

notarium A single bone in a bird's thoracic region formed by a fusion of vertebrae, it helps to protect the lungs.

notch A depression, usually on a bone surface. The **acetabular notch** is the indentation on the medial surface of the rim of the acetabulum or 'cup' of the hip joint. The **cardiac notch** is the area of the thorax where the lungs do not obscure the heart sounds, used when auscultating the heart during a clinical examination. The **vertebral notch** is the area at the base of the vertebral arch, above the centrum, that gives room for nerves to run through an intervertebral foramen.

notifiable disease One of a number of listed diseases that have to be reported to statutory authorities such as DEFRA in the UK. Usually, they are zoonotic diseases, although some large animal diseases are reportable because of the potential economic losses involved.

notochord A stage in the embryonic development of the skeletal system; its main significance in veterinary nursing is that remnants become the nucleus pulposus of the intervertebral discs; *see also* INTERVERTEBRAL DISC.

notoedric mange A fairly uncommon type of mange found on the head of cats, especially in and around the ears, and caused by *Notoedres cati*.

noxious stimulus A stimulus that causes pain; may be used when testing for nerve paralysis in the feet, etc.

NPO 'Nil by mouth', from the Latin *nil per os*.

NR Neurosensory retina, which is separate from underlying retinal pigment epithelium; *see also* RETINAL DETACHMENT.

nuchal Relating to the area of the neck or the crest; the head is supported by the **nuchal ligament**, which runs from the occipital bone of the skull and the neural spine of the axis bone to the first thoracic vertebra's neural spine.

nuclear medicine Therapeutic and diagnostic use of radioactive sources. *See also* HYPERTHYROIDISM.

nuclease An enzyme produced by the pancreas that breaks down RNA and DNA, also known as nucleotidase.

nucleic acids High-molecular-weight nucleotide polymers; *see also* DNA, RNA.

nucleolus, *pl.* nucleoli Found inside the nucleus of the cell; a spherical structure responsible for the manufacture of ribosomes.

nucleotidase Enzyme from the acinar glands of the pancreas that breaks down nucleotides; *see also* NUCLEASE.

nucleus, *pl.* nuclei The control centre of the cell; contains the chromosomes and one or more nucleoli.

nulliparous Not having given birth to any young.

nurse A person who has undergone professional training and is qualified and authorized in his/her country to practise nursing.

nursing process This requires modules for the formulation, organization and carrying out of a diagnostic or therapeutic plan for an animal. The process is divided into four stages: Assessment, Planning, Implementation, Evaluation.

nutrient That which nourishes, usually a food; includes water, minerals and vitamins.

nutrition A state when substances are taken into the body from the alimentary canal that leads to the correct function of cells and promotes life. Scientific study of this process and the interaction of components for optimal health is of importance to all those caring for animals. **Intravenous nutrition** is feeding by the intravenous route; it includes crystalloids, colloids and various protein, carbohydrate and fat emulsions, often with additional vitamins. **Parenteral nutrition** is feeding by routes other than by mouth, mainly by the intravenous route, but the subcutaneous and the intraperitoneal routes may also be used.

NVQ National Vocational Qualification.

NVQ Assessor Someone who has gained a Level 3 Assessor qualification and can assess student nurses to ensure they meet the required occupational standards.

nylon Synthetic plastic substance used for suture and other forms, such as mesh, for surgical repair. Monofilament nylon is used more frequently than braided nylon.

nymph Juvenile form of some insects, ticks, lice and mange mites, of special interest in nursing animals.

nystagmus Unusual flicking movement of the eyeballs, most easily recognized by using the ophthalmoscope to examine the fundus. May be caused by disorders of the parts of the brain controlling the eyesight and the balance. **Congenital nystagmus** is present from birth; 'wandering' may be a sign of blindness as the retina can never 'fix' on one distant spot, or it may be from a benign injury to the nerve pathway to the brain. **Horizontal nystagmus** is a side-to-side movement most often seen in a cat or dog with vestibular disease. The fast component always 'kicks away' from the side of the brain where there is a lesion; then this is followed by a slower return phase. **Jerk nystagmus** is one of the signs of vestibular disease. **Labyrinthine**

N

nystagmus is a jerking movement caused by disturbance to the labyrinth or the adjacent vestibular nucleus. **Pendular nystagmus** appears as a to-and-fro eye movement where there is no fast phase. **Rotatory nystagmus** involves more violent movement of the eyeball and usually indicates more severe brain damage. **Vertical nystagmus** is rapid eyeball movement on a vertical axis; more severe brain damage is suggested than with horizontal nystagmus.

nystatin An antibiotic substance usually applied in the form of an ointment in the treatment of yeast and fungal infections.

obedience training System for training dogs, usually involving the owner in the training and giving rewards in the form of praise and food. Methods used make the dog a better companion as well as being able to compete in tests at shows, etc.

obesity A condition of excessive fat accumulation that is detrimental to health.

object–film distance In radiography, the distance between the object being imaged and the film; usually the closer the better.

objective Refers to the lens situated at the lower end of the microscope closest to the object being examined.

obligate 'Bound to' or 'has to be'.

obligate parasite One that spends all its time on or inside the host and has no free-living adult existence.

oblique Slanting; a radiographic view where the beam is aimed at the object passing through at an angle may be described this way; or a fracture where the broken ends are at about a 45°-angle to the perpendicular.

oblique muscle Refers to the muscles running diagonally across the abdomen, known as the internal obliques and the external obliques.

observational learning Learning that occurs passively through watching others, used in dog training where it is also known as social learning.

obsessive–compulsive disorder (OCD) A behaviour pattern that develops most frequently in confined animals; repetitive actions are often performed for no obvious reason; *see also* AGGRESSION, STEREOTYPIC.

obstetrics The branch of science concerned with care in pregnancy, the birth process and the immediate postparturient weeks. In veterinary terms, it is often limited to dealing with problems during birth; *see also* DYSTOCIA.

obstetric ultrasound Scanning in pregnancy (usually at 28 days in bitches) for the confirmation of viable fetuses; scanning is also performed after dystocia; *see also* ULTRASOUND.

obstipation A severe form of constipation.

obstruction The condition of being blocked; may occur in the intestines, the uterus, the bladder or the respiratory tract. **Intestinal obstruction** causes severe disease characterized by vomiting and complete loss of appetite, with gas seen on X-ray film; commonly caused by a foreign body, neoplasia or severe constipation. In **urethral obstruction**, calculi are the most frequent cause; *see also* UROLITHIASIS.

obtund Dull or deadened; a description used for brain-damaged puppies or kittens after anoxia at birth. The sense of smell may be obtunded in an adult animal after brain injury.

obturator From obturate, to stop up; used to describe the muscles and a foramen in the floor of the pelvis. The **obturator nerve** that passes through the opening may be damaged in parturition if the fetus is oversized.

occipital bone A flat bone at the caudal aspect of the skull; carries the occipital condyles for articulation with the first cervical vertebra. Between the condyles is the foramen magnum.

occiput The area at the back of the skull.

occlusion 1) Closing off of a vessel or similar. **2)** In dentistry, the tooth surfaces between the upper and lower sets.

occlusive dressing Impervious wound dressing designed to concentrate a topical application so it will be absorbed through the skin or to protect a wound from outside contaminants.

occult blood 'Hidden' blood; evidence of haemorrhage from a gastrointestinal ulcer or damage to an internal organ from parasites or neoplasia.

occupational exposure standard (OES) The limit to which employees can be exposed to hazardous substances during their work, e.g. inhalation of anaesthetics such as nitrous oxide or halothane.

OCD *See* OSTEOCHONDRITIS DISSECANS, ELBOW DYSPLASIA.

octyl-2-cyanoacylate Tissue adhesive; active bioadhesive that forms a polymer on contact with water.

ocular Relates to the eyes or to vision.

ocular reflexes Nervous system tests to ascertain the function of the eye and the eyelids; *see also* CONSENSUAL LIGHT REFLEX.

oculocardiac reflex A potentially dangerous response to manipulating the eye with a slowing of the heart; the bradycardia may lead to death unless corrective measures are taken.

oculomotor The muscle movement of the eyeball is by six muscles; cranial nerve III is also involved in eye position and the size of the iris.

Oddi, sphincter of Anatomical structure found in the liver for bile outflow.

ODE *See* OLD DOG ENCEPHALITIS.

odonto- Relating to the teeth. Odontology is another term for dentistry.

odontoclast Cell that resorbs tooth material.

odontoclastic resorptive lesion (ORL) Dental condition of root resorption found in cats and occasionally in dogs that usually results in loss of teeth.

odontogenesis The formation of the teeth, whether temporary or permanent dentition.

odontoid Any bony process thought to resemble a tooth, especially the odontoid peg of the axis bone.

oedema Excessive accumulation of fluid in the body, usually in the tissues and the body cavities; *see also* ASCITES, ANASARCA, HYDROTHORAX.

Oedipus complex Repressed sexual feelings of a child for the parent of the opposite sex and sometimes rivalry with the same sex parent; made famous by Freud; has no veterinary equivalent because of the earlier independence from the dam.

oesophageal Relating to the oesophagus, part of the digestive tract connecting the pharynx to the stomach.

oesophageal stethoscope Flexible, atraumatic instrument that can be inserted into the oesophagus during anaesthesia and connected to the stethoscope for monitoring heart and respiratory sounds. Can also contain a temperature measuring device.

oesophageal tube A tube placed through the neck into the oesophagus to provide enteral nutrition.

oesophagoscope Instrument to inspect the interior lining of the oesophagus, especially an obstruction, may be a rigid or a fibre-optic instrument.

oesophagostomy Surgical procedure to open the oesophagus with an incision through the neck or via a thoracotomy, usually to retrieve a foreign body.

oesophagus Part of the alimentary canal lined with mucous membrane and with striated muscle to propel food from the mouth to the stomach, this muscle layer is especially important for floor-feeding animals.

oestradiol Natural female hormone responsible for receptivity to the male during the oestrous cycle; formed in the follicle of the ovary, but some is also produced by the adrenal cortex.

oestriol One of the weaker female sex hormones; like oestrone produced by the ovary.

oestrogens The group of steroidal sex hormones responsible for female behaviour and preparing the lining of the vagina, etc. for coitus and the uterus for reception of fertilized eggs. In the male, oestrogens may be produced by the testes retained in the abdomen; *see also* SERTOLI CELL TUMOUR.

oestrous cycle The repetitive changes in behaviour and the reproductive tract separated by short or long times without sexual activity. The secretion of hormones from the pituitary and negative feedback are responsible for female breeding patterns, which vary with the species. Note that primates have the equivalent of a menstrual cycle, which is a different way of preparing the lining of the uterus for the reception of fertilized eggs.

oestrus The noun that describes the most receptive part of the breeding cycle in animals. Adjective, **oestrous**.

Official Veterinarian (OV) A private practitioner who is authorized by the APHA to carry out statutory work on behalf of an EU member state; their work is usually required by law, e.g. meat inspection.

-oid Suffix indicating 'like something else'; *see also* SARCOID.

oil contamination A major problem for animals in coastal and any inland waterway where fuel oil may be spilt. Domestic pets may be contaminated through oil spilt in garages and motor repair yards.

ointment A pharmaceutical description of a cream or stiff paste, semisolid and greasy; usually insoluble in water but easily removed by licking; *see also* OCCLUSIVE DRESSING.

old dog encephalitis (ODE) Degenerative brain disorder of dogs, sometimes associated with canine distemper virus; *see also* ENCEPHALITIS.

olecranon The bony projection at the head of the ulna; helps to stabilize the elbow joint.

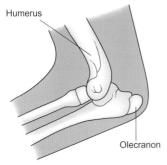

Humerus

Olecranon

Figure 34. Olecranon process of the elbow.

olfaction The process of smelling; olfaction is important in hunting animals to locate food sources.

olfactory bulb End of the olfactory tract that joins the CNS below the cerebral hemispheres; *see also* OLFACTORY NERVE.

olfactory nerve The first cranial nerve, originates from the olfactory bulb and the cerebrum caudally.

oligaemia Shortage of circulating blood; *see also* DEHYDRATION, PCV.

oligo- Prefix meaning 'few' or 'scant in number'.

oligogalactia Sparse or insufficient milk secretion; a problem in nursing bitches and queens.

oligosaccharides Simple sugars formed into chains of 3–10 monosaccharide molecules.

oliguria The production of an unusually small quantity of urine. If fluid is available to drink, it is a sign of renal damage. Also known as hypouresis.

Ollulanus tricuspis Worm that occurs in the stomach of foxes, some cats and pigs.

-oma Term for a growth or tumour.

omega Last letter of the Greek alphabet (ω); encountered in describing fatty acid chains: **omega-3** (fish oils) and **omega-6** (seeds).

omental leaf A method of attaching part of the omentum to the intestine or the prostate to provide an increased blood supply and more antibodies to an area of weakness or bacterial contamination.

omentopexy Method of fixation of the omentum to a site, such as an enterotomy, to improve the repair potential and bring a rich supply of blood containing white cells and antibodies.

omentum Anatomical structure in the cranial abdomen arising as a fold in the peritoneum, but its lace-like structure allows it to pass anywhere in the abdomen: it can be used to assist surgically in repair. The **greater omentum** is the fold that arises from the greater curvature of the stomach that can be stretched as far as the pelvic cavity. The **lesser omentum** is a small structure

O

attaching the duodenum to the shorter and inner concave stomach surface known as the lesser curvature.

omnivore Animal that eats whatever is available whether it be animal or plant.

omnivorous Eating a wide range of animal and plant origin foodstuffs.

omphal- Prefix relating to the umbilicus; *see also* NAVEL.

omphalocele A hernia, when an abdominal organ protrudes through the unclosed umbilicus in the newborn animal. Emergency repair is called for; *see also* UMBILICAL HERNIA.

Onchocerca A parasite spread by microfilaria when flies bite the host; affects deer, cattle and horses; not known in small animals.

onco- Prefix referring to a cancer or a tumour.

oncogene A gene in viruses and mammalian cells that can cause cancer.

oncology The study of tumours and cancers.

oncovirus Virus that may cause cancer; *see also* LEUKAEMIA.

one-eyed cold Disease of birds, with periocular swelling and discharge affecting usually just one eye; may be due to chlamydial infection, see ORNITHOSIS.

One Health Initiative A worldwide strategy for expanding interdisciplinary collaborations and communications in all aspects of healthcare for humans, animals and the environment, so that synergism will advance healthcare by accelerating biomedical research discoveries, enhancing public health efficacy, expanding the scientific knowledge base and improving medical education and clinical care.

on heat Terminology for prooestrus combined with oestrus in the bitch's breeding cycle; breeders incorrectly perceived a raised body temperature as an indication that the bitch was receptive to the male.

ontogeny The developmental time of an individual from the fertilized egg to maturity.

onych- Prefix referring to the nail.

onychectomy The excision of a claw or a nail in its nail bed. Carried out in domestic cats for social reasons.

onychomycosis A fungal infection, such as ringworm, affecting the claws.

oo- Prefix referring to the egg or ovum.

oocyst A resistant stage in the life cycle of organisms such as Coccidia; *see also* COCCIDIOSIS.

oocyte An immature egg in the ovary undergoes meiosis to become the ovum. The maturation of the oocyte after its release from the ovary is necessary for successful fertilization.

oogenesis The production of mature eggs in the ovary from oocytes that develop in the fetus; eventually the cells lining the graafian follicle mature at the time of ovulation.

oophorectomy Alternative word for the surgical removal of the ovaries, as in spaying.

opacity A lack of transparency to light, as found in a corneal opacity.

opaque The inability to see the other side of a structure or situation; part of the body may be opaque to X-rays, which is called radiopacity; *see also* CATARACT.

open-angle glaucoma Raised pressure in the anterior chamber of the eye when there is no blockage of the drainage channel by the iris but there is some defect in the drainage mechanism.

open fracture A fracture when the broken bone penetrates the skin. High risk of complications, including infection. Requires immediate attention; also called compound fracture.

open pyometra Disease of the female reproductive tract where blood, mucopus or green-to-yellow thick purulent matter originating in the endometrium is discharged from the vulva; *see also* OVARIOHYSTERECTOMY.

open-rooted teeth Those that continue to grow throughout life, as are found in rabbits and herbivorous rodents.

open wound An injury that is exposed to the air and thus subject to contamination and infection; *see also* ABRASION, INCISION, LACERATION, PUNCTURE.

operable Term used by surgeons for a condition where there is a justifiable chance of a full recovery or a clinical judgement that the situation will be improved by undertaking a surgical procedure.

operant conditioning A type of learning where behaviours are altered or changed primarily by manipulating the consequences that follow them see also REINFORCEMENT.

operation Action performed on the body with the hands and the use of surgical instruments.

operculum The covering to an opening; the plug of mucus that covers the cervical canal during pregnancy.

ophidian Member of the snake family.

ophthalm(o)- Relating to the eyes.

ophthalmencephalon Nerve tissue that includes the retina, the optic nerves and the visual cortex of the brain.

ophthalmia Inflammation of the eye, especially the conjunctiva; the term is antiquated. Horses suffered with periodic ophthalmia or 'moon blindness'.

ophthalmia neonatorum Conjunctivitis occurring in the newborn animal; previously thought to be caused by infection within the vagina during the birth process.

ophthalmologist A person who has made a specialized study of eye disorders and their correction.

ophthalmoscope An instrument projecting light onto the eye and into the fundus so that the structure can be examined; lenses are used to focus at various depths of the orbital structures.

-opia Indicates a defect of the eye or vision.

opiate A morphine-type substance to induce sleep, provide analgesia or sedate an animal.

opistho- Prefix indicating backwards, dorsal or posterior direction.

opisthotonus Relates to posture where the head, neck and spine are arched back, as

seen in toxaemias and other neurological problems.

opportunistic An organism that happens to take advantage of a 'niche' to multiply; used for infections with organisms that are not usually pathogenic; may be a sequel to immunosuppression.

OpSite Incise Trade name of a sterile disposable drape used for preparation of a sterile field for the surgeon to operate in.

Opsite Film Waterproof adhesive dressing to aid wound healing.

optic Concerned with the eye or vision and sight.

optic chiasma Part of the eye structure at the base of the brain where the optic nerves cross like an X, allowing fibres to distribute to both sides of the brain and to both eyes.

optic disc (papilla) Colourless spot in the fundus where all the nerve fibres collect before leaving the orbit to form the optic nerve, accompanied by blood vessels; examination is important in the diagnosis of progressive retinal atrophy.

optic nerve The second cranial nerve, originating in the sensory receptors of the rods and cones; the nerve is entirely sensory with the motor component absent; the autonomic nervous system controls the pupils.

oral Relating to the mouth, as when suggesting the route of communication; unwritten rules are oral traditions. Some medicines should be administered by the oral route.

oral administration The most common method of administering therapeutic substances; *see also* PER OS.

oral cavity The area inside the mouth behind the lips.

orbicularis oculi The muscle that closes the eye.

orbicularis oris The muscle that closes the mouth.

orbit The cavity in which the eyeball lies; the bony orbit of the skull is made of several bones.

orchi- Prefix denoting the male's testis or testicle.

orchidectomy Castration, or the removal of male gonads; in some European countries 'castration' would also include female neutering as in the UK 'spay' operation, so this term is more specific.

orchiectomy Alternative term for excision of the testes.

orchitis Inflammation of the substance of the testis.

Orem The universal self-care requisites based on experiences of the USA nurse in developing the theory of human nursing practice; the Orem's model is composed of the eight self-care requisites, which are activities that must be performed in order to achieve self-care for the patient. Central to Orem's concept of self-care is that care is being initiated voluntarily and deliberately by an individual. Principles have been adapted to apply to veterinary nursing.

orf Viral infection of sheep; it is a zoonosis as persons may become infected and develop nodules on their hands, which should resolve spontaneously.

organ Independent structure composed of various tissues to fulfil a specific function.

organelles Small microscopic structures inside the cell but not part of the nucleus; includes mitochondria, lysosomes, reticular structures and the Golgi complex.

organic compound A compound that is carbon-containing. Often used to refer to products derived from or containing products from living organisms.

organizational structure An organization's framework or model in which employees and functions are organized. It informs people of how an organization works and where responsibilities lie.

organism An individual plant or animal, often microscopic.

organochloride Chemical substances previously widely used for skin parasite control; their use is much restricted because of toxicity problems in the food chain.

organ of Corti The spiral sense organ within the cochlea of the ear.

organ of Jacobson A taste or sense organ (vomeronasal) that communicates between the roof of the mouth and the nose in rabbits.

organophosphate Chemical compounds used for internal and external parasite control; recently fallen out of favour or much restricted in their use because of nerve toxic changes; *see also* ACETYLCHOLINE.

orgasm The climax of sexual excitement; some pet owners describe seeing this in animals but it is not known to occur during animal breeding.

orientation Obtaining a sense of place or direction; important in surgical technique.

orifice An opening in any anatomical area of the body; *see also* OSTIUM.

origin Usually the beginning of anything, anatomically, the muscle origin is the fixed attachment of the proximal part; *see also* INSERTION.

ornithosis Disease of birds that is zoonotic; *see also* CHLAMYDIOSIS, PSITTACOSIS.

oro- Prefix referring to the mouth.

orogastric route Used in stomach tubing through the mouth; *see also* GASTRIC LAVAGE.

oropharynx The cavity of the mouth beyond the soft palate, into the pharynx chamber and up to the hyoid bone.

orphan virus A term for a recently discovered or emerging virus that has no specific disease known to be caused by it.

ortho- Prefix meaning 'straight' or 'normal'.

orthodontics The branch of dental science concerned with malocclusions and providing straighter teeth.

orthopaedics The science of correcting deformities of the skeleton, often by operating on joints or bones; *see also* BONE.

orthopnoea Breathlessness, with the ability to have a normal breathing pattern only while standing or if the thorax is lifted up. The animal sits or stands with neck extended and elbows abducted.

Ortolani's sign Test used in human infants for hip joint laxity by lifting the head of the femur out of the acetabulum; a click can be felt or heard on return into the joint cavity; *see also* HIP DYSPLASIA.

Oryctolagus cuniculis See RABBIT.

os 1) The oral area or any body opening; *see also* MOUTH. 2) A bone; *see also* HIP.

OSCE Objective, structured, clinical examination; part of the training and examination process for the occupational standards for veterinary nurses; a modern examination and assessment technique designed to test practical clinical skills.

oscheitis Inflammation of the scrotum, may be caused by chemical scalds or trauma.

oscillating saw A rotating saw that rapidly alternates its direction of cut so it appears to vibrate; will not harm underlying soft tissue structures when cutting.

oscilloscope Traditional name for a cathode ray tube or 'screen' in computers.

oscillotonometry Method of measuring blood pressure in animals by attaching a special cuff with a sensor to the tail or a limb.

-osis Word for a generalized disorder or disease state; *see also* ORNITHOSIS.

Oslerus osleri Species of tracheal worm of dogs previously known as *Filaroides osleri*, named after the Canadian surgeon Sir William Osler.

osmolarity The osmotic power of a solution expressed in osmoles per litre of solution (osmolality is per kg solution); *see also* HYPERTONIC.

osmosis The passage of fluid or 'solvent' from a low-concentration liquid to a high-concentration one; *see also* SEMIPERMEABLE MEMBRANE.

osmotic diarrhoea An important cause of fluid loss from the body when osmotic substances are present in the intestinal lumen; the result of a digestive failure or villus atrophy; *see also* MALABSORPTION.

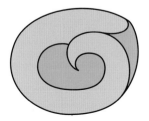

Figure 35. Oslerus osleri egg.

osmotic pressure The pressure by which water is drawn into a solution through a semipermeable membrane; the greater the concentration or strength, the larger the pressure.

os penis Remnant of the splanchnic skeleton found as a fine bone in the penis of the dog, the ferret and the cat.

osselet Extra bone growth in the equine fetlock causing joint inflammation, pain and lameness.

osseous Relating to a bony structure; most often applied to a type of bony substance.

ossicle A bony nodule, especially the three that form a chain across the middle ear.

ossification The process of producing, by osteoblasts, normal bone in the growing animal; if pathological, the results may be seen on a radiograph as bony slivers appearing in tendons near their insertions.

ostectomy Cutting away part or all of a bone, an osteotome may be used.

osteitis Inflammation of a bone; *see also* PERIOSTITIS.

osteoarthritis A degenerative disease of joint cartilage where damage to the underlying bone may cause pain and immobility.

osteoarthropathy Disease of the joints and the bone; *see also* DEGENERATIVE JOINT DISEASE.

osteoblast A cell that forms bone.

osteochondritis dissecans (OCD) A disease is which the thickness of the cartilage in joints becomes so great that slivers of cartilage form flaps or become detached and ulcerated areas of the cartilage remain; may be seen as defects on radiographs of young dogs. Part hereditary, part environmental.

osteochondroma A benign but slow-growing tumour of long bones.

osteochondrosis A developmental disease of articular cartilage with poor differentiation during growth of the long bones, principally the elbows, shoulders and hocks; *see also* ELBOW DYSPLASIA.

osteoclasts Cells that remove bone.

osteocytes Cells in the bone matrix within the lacunae responsible for bone integrity; form part of the haversian system; *see also* LAMELLA.

O

osteodystrophy Disease of bone during its development and growth. **Nutritional secondary osteodystrophy** is seen in growing puppies and kittens when there is a lack of available calcium, often because of feeding an all-meat diet or excess cereal in the diet, when phytates 'lock up' the calcium. **Canine hypertrophic osteodystrophy** is a condition occasionally seen in rapidly growing larger breeds of dog where there is lameness from swollen joints; *see also* BARLOW'S DISEASE. **Renal secondary osteodystrophy** is a disorder seen in advanced kidney disease when phosphates are retained and calcium is withdrawn from the bones, especially from the lower jaw; *see also* RUBBER JAW.

osteogenesis The formation and development of bone.

osteoma A benign bone tumour.

osteomalacia A disease of the skeleton caused by inadequate intake of bone-forming elements in the diet or a deficiency of vitamin D; *see also* RICKETS.

osteomyelitis Inflammation of the bone, usually a deep-seated and persisting infection; involves both the cortex and the medulla. Caused by infection or by trauma, foreign bodies or surgical implants.

osteon The basic unit of bone consisting of the haversian canal and the Volkmann canal in the concentric lamellae of compact bone as found in the cortex; *see also* CORTEX, HAVERSIAN SYSTEM.

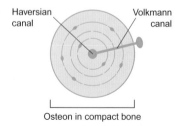

Haversian canal　　　　　　Volkmann canal

Osteon in compact bone

Figure 36. Osteon in compact bone showing the Volkmann canal.

osteopathy Any disease of bone in the skeleton. **Craniomandibular osteopathy** is a specific disorder of the West Highland white terrier and similar terrier breeds with enlargement of the skull bones and lower jaw, often limiting the width of the mouth opening. **Secondary hypertrophic osteopathy** (Marie's disease) is associated with neoplasia and lung changes; the peripheral limb bones swell as a result of periosteal bone deposited, especially above the carpal region.

osteophyte Spicule of bone seen on radiograph near a joint capsule; a sign of osteoarthritis; *see also* EXOSTOSIS.

osteoporosis A loss of bone density, resulting in bones that are brittle and liable to fracture.

osteoprogenitor cell Forerunner of cell that develops as the osteoblast in the formation of bone.

osteosarcoma Malignant bone tumour; secondaries (metastases) are common, and the lungs should always be radiographed before treatment is given.

osteotome Surgical instrument for cutting bone.

osteotomy Surgical procedure that involves the removal of bone. **Bulla osteotomy** is removal of the tympanic bulla to drain the middle ear, used in the treatment of otitis media. **Pelvic osteotomy** is one of the possible treatments for hip dysplasia, where the pelvis is realigned to stabilize the hip joint.

ostium A specialized opening, such as the **ostium abdominale,** where the oviduct from the uterus opens into the abdominal cavity but within the ovarian bursa.

-ostomy Description of any operation where a permanent surgical opening is made, often to allow drainage; *see also* URETHROSTOMY.

ostrich Bird with long legs and long neck, farmed commercially for meat, leather and feathers. Herbivores; males can run very fast before attacking intruders to their paddocks. Females are more docile but easily frightened.

otitis General term for ear inflammation.

otitis externa Inflammation of the outer ear tube and pinna; may be detected by violent shaking, scratching with the back leg and the head held down on one side.

otitis interna Inner ear infection. Inflammation extends to the balance centre; *see also* COCHLEAR.

otitis media Middle ear infection; may follow otitis externa or infection from the throat via the eustachian tube.

oto- Prefix relating to the ear.

otoacariasis Infestation of the ear canal with mites; *see also* OTODECTES CYNOTIS.

Otobius lagophilus Species of tick that may be found on rabbits.

Otodectes cynotis Species of mite found not infrequently in cats' ears; when present in dogs' ears, usually causes severe irritation.

otolith (otoconium) Part of the balance mechanism of the inner ear; calcium carbonate particles float in fluid in the macula of the utricle and saccule of the inner ear.

-otomy Description of any operation where a temporary surgical opening is made, often to allow drainage.

otorrhoea Any discharge from the ear, usually a sign of otitis externa.

otoscope Instrument for examining the outer ear canal and the tympanic membrane; *see also* AURISCOPE.

ototoxic Compounds that are potentially toxic to the hearing and balance organs, aminoglycosides need careful use in animals and can cause neuromuscular blockade.

outbreeding Planning a mating to have as few common ancestors in recent generations as possible; a way of breeding out an undesirable trait or reducing recessive gene problems that have resulted from inbreeding.

outcome The end result, as after head trauma in an RTA; the eventual degree of recovery cannot always be predicted.

outpatient Attending on a daily basis, an alternative to hospitalization as an 'inpatient'.

output, cardiac The aortic blood flow may be measured with Doppler equipment; regurgitation occurs if valves do not close completely in systole.

oval window The communication from the middle ear to the inner ear where the stapes bone transmits sound waves.

ovari(o)- Prefix relating to the ovary, often used as a surgical operation prefix.

ovarian Adjective: part of the ovary.

ovarian bursa Membranous layer of peritoneum that almost envelops the ovary of the bitch, helping the eggs released from the follicles to be wafted into the oviducts.

ovarian cycle The reproductive cycle, controlled by the hormones of the pituitary gland and the ovary.

ovarian cyst Structure like a very large follicle in the ovary, often associated with excess oestrogen production and one form of pyometra.

ovariohysterectomy The surgical operation to remove all of the uterus and both ovaries, commonly known as spaying.

ovary, *pl.* ovaries The endocrine glands of the female, also responsible for release of ova to perpetuate the genes after male fertilization. There are two ovaries in the abdomen, normally found in the area of the kidneys.

overdose (OD) Usually an accidental act of drug administration, caused by misreading the instructions on the label, or in some cases, miscalculating an animal's weight; *see also* POISONING.

overexposure In radiography, a lack of definition or all-over greyness of the plate that may be a result of incorrect technique; the areas covered by metal markers still remain white in overexposure faults.

overhydration Undesirable complication of fluid therapy; fluid may accumulate in the lungs and pulmonary oedema reduces respiratory function; a moist cough may be the first sign during the administration of intravenous fluids.

overriding fracture Complex fracture in which the ends of the bone overlap each other; reduction is essential before fixation of the fracture.

overshot jaw State of the mouth when the lower jaw is short so that the maxilla protrudes and the teeth of the upper jaw are in advance of the teeth of the lower jaw.

O

over-the-counter (OTC) medicines
Nonprescription medicines; some may not have undergone safety evaluation, especially if of herbal nature.

over-the-needle catheter A type of cannula used in fluid therapy; a cut-down on the vein may be needed to prevent the catheter being dragged back by the animal's skin during insertion.

oviduct Delicate structure connecting the fimbriae in the ovarian bursa to the lumen of the uterus; of importance as it is the site for fertilization of ova; *see also* FALLOPIAN TUBE.

oviparous Egg-producing; refers to egg-producing reptiles or birds.

ovoviviparous Giving birth to living offspring from an egg retained in the body, as occurs in certain reptiles, lizards and amphibians.

ovulation The release of ova (or a single ovum) from the follicle in the ovary. Spontaneous in the bitch but induced in the female cat by the mating procedure; *see also* OESTROUS CYCLE.

ovum, *pl.* **ova** Egg; carries the genetic material of the mother and if fertilized goes on to form an embryo.

owner compliance Requirement that the pet owner faithfully carries out instructions issued. 'Need' is an essential requirement, 'like' is a preference expressed; *see also* DIET.

oxalate calculi Concretions composed of calcium oxalate that may form in the urinary tract, characterized by a sharp knife edge to the 'stones', often causing haematuria. Diet changes make these more common than struvite calculi in cats.

OXF Potassium oxalate with sodium fluoride; an anticoagulant used in specimen containers for glucose estimation. It kills the cells, preventing further oxidation of the glucose in the sample.

oxidase Enzyme occurring widely in nature; specific interest is in monoamine oxidase inhibitor drugs, used in behaviour modification.

oximeter Pulse oximeter is an instrument of value in anaesthetic monitoring; it measures the percentage of haemoglobin oxygen saturation.

oxygen Colourless gas in common use for anaesthetic circuits as a carrier and a life-support agent. High-pressure cylinders are black with a white top in the UK. Can also be stored as liquid in tanks and the gas piped to areas of the hospital where it is needed.

oxygen cage A controlled environment cage allowing oxygen to be piped through to aid breathing.

oxygen debt Negative state of anaerobic respiration that can build up but then needs to have oxygen replaced by 'panting' air into the body.

oxygen saturation A measure of tissue oxygen availability; the haemoglobin content can be measured in the laboratory.

oxygen therapy Any form of administration by oxygen cage, mask or tent to relieve hypoxaemia in shock or after blood loss.

oxyhaemoglobin The carriage of oxygen from the lungs to the body tissues is dependent on the ability of the haemoglobin in the red blood cells to make up this molecule.

oxyntic cell Cells of the stomach wall that secrete hydrochloric acid and intrinsic factor.

oxytetracycline Broad-spectrum antibiotic widely used in veterinary medicine.

oxytocic Describes any medication that aids contractions of the uterus.

oxytocin Hormone produced by the posterior pituitary and responsible for contraction of the smooth muscle of the uterus and also for milk letdown in the lactating female.

Oxyuris Parasitic worm, mainly of equines. Nurses may be asked about 'pinworms' that are causing itching and tail rubbing in ponies, but the worms do not infect dogs and cats. The smaller animal pets have oxyurid parasites: *Passalurus ambiguus* in the rabbit, or *Syphacia obvelata* in the hamster; *see also* THREADWORMS.

PABA Para-aminobenzoic acid.

pacemaker Small electrical device implanted under the skin, with electrodes that run to the heart to control the heartbeat.

Pacheco's disease Cause of sudden death in psittacine birds, caused by a marked fatty hepatitis.

pachy- Prefix denoting 'thickening'.

pachydermia Thickening of the skin.

pachymeningitis Inflammation and thickening of the dura, which is otherwise known as the **pachymeninx**.

pacing Form of stereotypic behaviour, as seen in a dog walking in a kennel run repeatedly performed in the same pattern. **Cardiac pacing** electrical stimulation of the heart by a pacemaker to regulate cardiac rhythm.

pacinian corpuscle Encapsulated sensory mechanoreceptor found in the skin; sensitive to deformation; consists of a number of capsular layers wrapped around a sensory nerve ending.

packed cell volume See PCV.

pad Skin covered in cornified epithelium on each toe, may be black pigmented or pale colour; see also PODODERMATITIS, HYPERKERATOSIS.

paediatrics The branch of medicine dealing with disease in children (pediatrics in the USA); in the veterinary sphere, it may be used to describe disease in young animals.

PAF Platelet aggregating factor.

pain An unpleasant physical and emotional experience, associated with potential or actual tissue damage and a cause of stress. Also referred to as nociception.

palatability 1) A measure of how much an animal likes a food. **2)** Nutrition term used to describe the attractiveness of a food: texture, smell and protein percentage are all important.

palate The structure that forms the roof of the mouth, separating the oral and nasal cavities. It is in two parts, the more rostral **hard palate** is formed by the horizontal parts of the palatine, maxillary and incisive bones; this is continued caudally as the **soft palate**, a flap of muscle covered by mucous membrane; see also PALATORRHAPHY.

palatine Relating to the palate, e.g. the **palatine arteries**.

palatoglossal Relating to the palate and tongue.

palatorrhaphy Surgical repair of a congenital cleft palate or acquired break in the palate; involves carefully mobilizing the soft tissues around the defect and suturing them in place.

palliative Symptomatic treatment that will improve quality of life but will not cure the underlying disease, e.g. adequate pain relief for animals that are terminally ill.

pallor Paleness, lack of skin colour.

palmar The undersurface of the front paws, as in the human palm; see also PLANTAR.

palmigrade Abnormal stance where the caudal aspect of the carpus contacts the ground; causes include carpal hyperextension injuries in animals that have fallen from a height, carpal luxation, etc.

palpable Able to be detected by touch, e.g. palpation of superficial lymph nodes, such as the prescapular and popliteal.

palpate Investigate by touch; a cornerstone of clinical examination.

palpation Careful investigation using the hands; commonly used for pregnancy diagnosis in the bitch at 28 days postmating, the time when any conceptuses are most likely to be palpable.

palpebra An eyelid.

palpebral fissure The opening of the eye; the gap between the upper and lower eyelids.

palpebral reflex The closing of the eyelid when the corner of the eye or the eyelid is lightly touched.

palpitation Sudden, irregular, rapid pounding of the heart.

pampiniform plexus The tortuous plexus formed by the testicular vein, lying within the mesorchium just proximal to the testis.

pan- Prefix meaning 'across', 'throughout'.

pancarpal arthrodesis Surgical fusion of all levels of the carpal joint, i.e. the antebrachiocarpal, intercarpal and carpometacarpal joints; the treatment of choice for most carpal hyperextension injuries. Technique involves removal of all articular cartilage, packing the joints with cancellous bone graft and rigidly fixing with a bone plate.

pancreas Both an endocrine and exocrine gland, lying close to the stomach and duodenum; the exocrine acinar cells secrete amylase, lipase and trypsinogen into the duodenum via the pancreatic ducts. The endocrine function is carried out by the beta cells of the islets of Langerhans, which secrete insulin into the bloodstream; *see also* DIABETES MELLITUS, EXOCRINE PANCREATIC INSUFFICIENCY, PANCREATITIS.

pancreatic amylase Enzyme from the acinar cells for the breakdown of carbohydrate started by salivary amylase.

pancreatic lipase Enzyme from the pancreas for the breakdown of fats to fatty acids and glycerol.

pancreatic peptidases Enzymes from the F cells for the breakdown of polypeptide chains to produce free amino acids.

pancreatitis Inflammation of the pancreas; causes anterior abdominal pain and affected animals may adopt a 'praying' stance; may recur in bouts, and can lead to EPI and/or diabetes mellitus; *see also* DIABETES MELLITUS, EXOCRINE PANCREATIC INSUFFICIENCY.

pancuronium bromide (Pavulon) A potent nondepolarizing neuromuscular blocking agent; standard doses provide about 20 minutes' blockade, and the effects can be reversed with neostigmine.

pancytopenia Reduction in the number of all cells (red, white and platelets) circulating in the blood, e.g. caused by bone marrow suppression.

pandemic An infection that spreads across a whole country, or even the world, e.g. influenza can be pandemic.

panleukopenia Abnormally low numbers of all the circulating white blood cells (neutrophils, eosinophils, basophils and lymphocytes); *see also* FIE.

panniculitis Inflammation of the subcutaneous fat to form hard nodules that may drain out on to the skin surface. The condition is usually idiopathic but may be secondary to bacterial and fungal infections; single lesions may be surgically excised; multiple lesions usually respond to steroids.

panniculus reflex The skin twitch response; when the skin along the trunk is pinched or the hair coat is lightly touched the animal responds by twitching the skin of that region. The reflex is brought about by the cutaneous trunci muscle and is particularly well developed in the horse and cow, where the muscle continues into the neck and across the loins. Used during the diagnosis of intervertebral disc protrusion.

Pannus 1) A chronic progressive keratitis and vascularization of the cornea; most common in the German shepherd dog; aetiology is unclear but an autoimmune component is likely; most cases respond to topical steroids or cytotoxic agents. The disease is likely to reoccur; severe cases require superficial keratectomy; *see also* UBERREITER'S SYNDROME. **2)** Growth of hyperplastic synovial membrane across the articular cartilage of a joint; the result of chronic joint inflammation; the cartilage is destroyed by degradative enzymes released from synoviocytes and inflammatory cells; synovectomy may be required.

panophthalmitis Inflammation of the eyeball and all its contents.

panosteitis Inflammation of intramedullary tissues as a sequel to focal areas of fat necrosis; a common cause of pain and lameness in young dogs of the large breeds. It most commonly affects the humerus but is also found in the radius, ulna, femur and tibia; has a characteristic radiographic appearance, with mottled thumbprint lesions; may reoccur in bouts and cause a shifting lameness but responds well to analgesics and has a good prognosis.

pansteatitis Discoloration and inflammation of fat deposits within the body; caused by high intake of unsaturated fats in the diet and inadequate levels of the antioxidant vitamin E; rarely seen, but occurs in cats who are fed solely on fish; signs include pyrexia, lethargy, hyperaesthesia, and pain on handling, and a stiff gait; treatment involves correcting the diet and supplying vitamin E.

pant Rapid, shallow breathing; a normal body response in the dog to hyperthermia, as evaporation from the upper respiratory tract helps cooling; may also occur in shock. In contrast, mouth breathing in the cat is always abnormal and is a sign of severe respiratory distress.

pantothenic acid Part of the B vitamin complex; *see also* VITAMIN B.

panzootic Affecting all the animals within a given area.

papilla, *pl.* papillae A nipple-like bud; describes anatomical structures with this form, e.g. the **optic papilla** where the optic nerve enters the eye.

papillary muscle The muscular columns that attach the chordae tendineae to the walls of the ventricles of the heart, preventing the A–V valves from everting.

papilloedema Swelling of the optic disc.

papilloma Benign neoplasm of stratified squamous epithelium; a small, pedunculated growth, often referred to as a wart.

papillomatosis The growth of many benign papillomas, predominantly on the limbs, head and in the mouth; usually caused by viral infection; spontaneous recovery occurs in most cases; surgical removal may be required, depending on the exact location of the growth.

papilloma virus Virus causing warts; *see also* PAPILLOMATOSIS.

papular Having papules.

papule Small, solid, raised skin nodule; may be a precursor to a pustule if infection becomes established.

para- Prefix meaning 'near to', 'through' or 'beside'.

paracentesis The aspiration of fluid, usually from the abdomen. An area in the midline at the lowest point of the abdomen should be prepared aseptically; the tap can usually be performed with a hypodermic needle and requires minimal restraint or sedation; *see also* FELINE INFECTIOUS PERITONITIS.

paracetamol A widely available human analgesic; other licensed veterinary products are preferred for animals. Care is required if paracetamol is given to animals by their owners as it can be hepatotoxic.

paracloacal spur Sexual organ of the snake, representing a remnant of the pelvic limb.

paracostal incision Surgical approach commencing at the xiphisternum through the abdominal wall following the line of the rib arch but just caudal to it.

paracrine Describes hormone effects that are limited to a localized area.

parafollicular cells Cells in the thyroid gland that produce calcitonin, the hormone that lowers levels of blood calcium; *see also* CALCITONIN, PARATHORMONE.

parainfluenza virus A myxovirus causing acute upper respiratory disease; *see also* KENNEL COUGH.

paralysis Complete loss of function of an area of the body; when applied to a limb, the term means that the animal is unable to make any stepping movements, even if aided; the most common cause of paralysis is intervertebral disc disease; *see also* INTERVERTEBRAL DISC DISEASE, LARYNGEAL PARALYSIS, PARAPLEGIA, PARESIS, QUADRIPLEGIA, TETRAPLEGIA.

paralytic ileus Tympany and stasis of the intestines, owing to a lack of the normal peristaltic waves; may occur after intestinal surgery or if there has been severe distension of the gut; *see also* ILEUS.

parameter A vital sign that should be monitored regularly in hospitalized patients to chart their progress, e.g. temperature, pulse rate and respiratory rate.

paramyxovirus An RNA virus causing Newcastle disease, a notifiable disease mainly of pigeons; common signs include diarrhoea, upper respiratory sounds, poor plumage and nervous signs; a vaccine is available but not compulsory.

paranasal sinuses These large sinuses, which are extensions of the nasal chambers, are located within the bones of the skull; there are maxillary and frontal sinuses, which are subdivided into communicating compartments.

paraneoplastic syndrome Associated with neoplasia but not directly caused by the space-occupying effects of the primary tumour or metastases; includes hormonal, neurological and metabolic imbalances leading to hypercalcaemia, Marie's disease, glomerulonephropathy, DIC, etc. Paraneoplastic neuropathies can occur.

paraphimosis Constriction of the prepuce around an engorged penis so that the penis cannot be retracted back into the prepuce; common in the dog; surgical correction or manipulation under anaesthesia may be required if the penis cannot be replaced; if neglected, gangrene of the tip may result.

paraplegia Paralysis of the hindlimbs.

paraprostatic cyst Large, fluid-filled sacs that develop in the tissues adjacent to the prostate; may be a precursor of prostatic hypertrophy; usually requires surgical drainage/removal or marsupialization.

paraquat A weedkiller whose toxic effects include vomiting, lethargy and progressive respiratory distress, caused by marked interstitial oedema, leading to death within 3–10 days. There is no specific antidote, but support therapy may be tried.

parasite An organism that lives on the surface of (ectoparasite) or within (endoparasite) another organism.

parasitology The scientific study of parasites, their life cycles and the diseases they may cause.

parasympathetic nervous system Part of the autonomic nervous system that has a craniosacral outflow and produces involuntary effects such as slowing the heart, pupil constriction and peristalsis; *see also* AUTONOMIC NERVOUS SYSTEM, SYMPATHETIC NERVOUS SYSTEM.

parasympatholytic A drug, such as atropine, that reduces the effects of the parasympathetic nervous system.

parasympathomimetic Drugs, such as acetylcholine and pilocarpine, that act to increase the effects of the parasympathetic system.

paratenic host A species that is not the normal host for a parasite but that may be used opportunistically by the parasite.

paratenon The connective tissue immediately surrounding a tendon.

parathormone One of the hormones secreted into the bloodstream by the parathyroid glands; it acts to elevate blood calcium levels by increasing resorption from bone and uptake from the gut while promoting renal phosphate excretion; *see also* CALCITONIN.

parathyroid glands Four small glands, as two pairs, situated close to the lobes of the thyroid gland; they secrete parathormone and calcitonin to provide regulation of blood calcium levels.

paravertebral anaesthesia The injection of local anaesthetic solution adjacent to the spinal nerves where they emerge between the transverse processes of the lumbar vertebrae. The technique is used in cattle to provide analgesia over the abdomen to allow procedures such as rumenotomy and caesarean section.

parenchyma The tissue substance of a gland.

parenteral Any route of drug administration that does not involve the gastrointestinal tract, e.g. subcutaneous, intramuscular, intraperitoneal or intravenous.

paresis Muscle weakness with neurological deficits, but the animal can still make coordinated walking movements if the body weight is supported; *see also* PARALYSIS.

Pareto principle The 80–20 rule, applicable in many situations, for example 20% of your clients account for 80% of your business.

parietal Close to the body wall, e.g. the **parietal pleura** is applied to the inner wall of the chest while the visceral pleura covers the lung tissue.

paronychia Inflammation of the nail beds, often with ulceration; may be caused by bacteria, fungi, or diseases such as demodicosis and pemphigus.

parotid duct transplant A surgical procedure involving relocating the distal end of the parotid duct to the conjunctiva to provide moisture to treat dry eye (keratoconjunctivitis sicca).

parotid salivary gland Salivary gland located at the base of the vertical ear canal.

parous Having produced live offspring; *see also* MULTIPAROUS, PRIMIGRAVIDA, UNIPAROUS.

paroxysmal Term used in pathology for an increase in severity of a disease; *see also* TACHYCARDIA.

partial carpal arthrodesis Surgical fusion of the intercarpal and carpometacarpal joints, sparing the antebrachiocarpal joint, where most of the movement occurs; *see also* PANCARPAL ARTHRODESIS.

particoloured Describes the coat colour where the coat has two or more distinct colours, as in the Irish red and white setter breeds.

partnership Common set-up in veterinary businesses, where a group of business partners share responsibility for the business.

parturition The process of giving birth.

parvovirus A small DNA virus that causes acute gastroenteritis in many species; the canine parvovirus is thought to have mutated from the feline form; it causes severe vomiting and diarrhoea, which can be fatal in young pups. The virus is resistant to many disinfectants and can spread rapidly through susceptible populations; faecal and serological tests can be used to confirm the diagnosis; the virus can also replicate in heart muscle, causing an acute myocarditis and sudden death. Multivalent canine vaccines have a component that offers effective protection against the disease.

passerine Term used to describe birds that perch.

passive movement Gentle flexing and extending of the limb joints, with the animal in recumbency; part of physiotherapy and important in the nursing of paraplegic patients.

pastern Part of the equine leg between the fetlock and the coronary band.

Pasteurella Genus of Gram-negative bacteria causing respiratory disease and septicaemia in many species. *P. multocida* is associated with cellulitis and infection from dog and cat bites or scratches.

patella The knee cap; a sesamoid bone within the tendon of the quadriceps muscle mass.

patellar ligament The ligament running from the distal pole of the patella, inserting on the tibial crest.

patellar luxation Displacement of the patella, a congenital abnormality with a genetic component in many dog breeds; the displacement is medial and is often associated with displacement of the tibial crest too in toy dogs and terriers, particularly those with bow legs such as the Staffordshire bull terrier and Jack Russell. It is most often lateral in the Labrador retriever and other large breeds; affected animals show signs of intermittent or persistent hindleg lameness; surgical treatment involves sulcoplasty (deepening of the trochlear groove), releasing the joint capsule on one side and tightening it on the opposite side and transplanting the tibial crest back to its correct midline position.

patellar reflex A sudden contraction of the anterior muscles of the thigh, caused by a sharp tap on the patellar tendon with a neurological hammer.

patent Open, having a lumen.

patent ductus arteriosus (PDA) Failure of the ductus arteriosus to close within the first few days after birth, thus allowing left-to-right shunting of blood from the aorta to the pulmonary artery; clinical signs include poor growth, exercise intolerance, rapid heart rate and a machinery murmur. Surgical ligation of the duct via a thoracotomy is the treatment of choice.

pathogen Any living microorganism that can cause disease, e.g. bacteria, viruses and protozoa.

pathogenicity The ability to cause disease.

pathognomonic A finding that is specific to a certain disease; presence of this finding allows the disease to be diagnosed, e.g. hyperkeratosis of the pads and nose in distemper.

pathology The scientific study of the causes and effects of disease.

pathophysiology Disease process as it affects various body organs.

patient The subject of medical or surgical nursing care.

patient safety The prevention of avoidable errors that have the potential to cause harm to patients.

paw Lower part of the foot that includes toes, toenails, pads and associated structures.

PCV Packed cell volume. The percentage of the circulating blood volume that is taken up by cells, as opposed to fluid; PCV can readily be determined in the laboratory by spinning a blood sample at 5000–10000 rpm for 5 minutes. The red and white blood cells will settle to form a solid column, the platelets will form a cream-coloured band above this (the buffy coat) and the straw-coloured plasma will be on the top. A raised PCV may indicate dehydration; a low PCV indicates shock, anaemia, excessive rehydration, etc.; see also BUFFY COAT, HAEMATOCRIT.

PDA Patent ductus arteriosus.

PDGF Platelet-derived growth factor; a protein factor that controls cell division, especially during angiogenesis.

PDH 1) Pituitary-dependent hyperadrenocorticism; see also CUSHING'S SYNDROME. 2) Police dog handler.

pectinectomy Surgical removal of a portion or all of the pectineus muscle; used as a treatment for hip dysplasia in young dogs; it is thought to relieve tension on the joint capsule of the hip, and thus, reduce pain.

pectus excavatum A rare congenital abnormality of the chest wall where the caudal sternebrae and xiphisternum curve inwards towards the spine.

pedal reflex The withdrawal or flexor reflex; when the animal is placed in lateral recumbency and the toe or web is pinched, the foot should be withdrawn from the noxious stimulus.

pedicle A stalk.

pedicle graft A portion of skin and underlying subcutaneous tissue that retains an attachment to the body (and a vascular supply) via a pedicle of tissue; the skin flap can be transposed and used to close tissue defects.

pediculosis Irritation and hair loss caused by lice infestation; see also LOUSE.

pedicure Nail trimming.

pedigree The family line or ancestry of an individual.

peduncle A stalk or pedicle.

peer review An evaluation process used by experts in the subject field to decide if an academic paper or research report reaches the required standards before publication.

peg teeth Small conical teeth that are supernumerary to the normal dental array.

PEG Percutaneous endoscopic gastrostomy. See PEG TUBE.

PEG tube Percutaneous endoscope-guided feeding tube. An enteral feeding tube placed directly into the stomach via the abdominal body wall; can be made by modifying a Foley catheter. For placement, the animal has to be anaesthetized and an endoscope is required; the tube is well tolerated and can be left in situ for several weeks.

pellagra Name for vitamin B complex deficiency in humans.

pelvis The girdle of bone connecting the lumbosacral spine to the hindlegs; two symmetrical halves, each comprising the ilium, ischium and pubis; organs contained within the pelvis include the bladder (when empty or partially filled), nongravid uterus and rectum.

pemphigus An autoimmune complex disorder characterized by the formation of skin vesicles; diagnosis is confirmed by immunohistochemical staining of biopsy material from the blisters; treatment is based on immunosuppression with glucocorticoids; adjunctive therapies such as gold salts or cytotoxic drugs may also be used.

pemphigus erythematosus A condition in which bullous lesions appear over the nose and ears, made worse by sunny weather; may be confused with the solar dermatitis seen in breeds of dog such as the collie and German shepherd dog.

pemphigus foliaceous The most common autoimmune skin disease, affecting mainly the head and feet, although lesions may occur elsewhere.

pemphigus vegetans Rarest form of pemphigus, with the formation of crusts and scabs.

pemphigus vulgaris The second most common form of pemphigus, with vesicles appearing around the nailbeds and at mucocutaneous junctions.

penicillin A bacteriocidal antibiotic originally derived from *Penicillium* spp. mould but now made synthetically.

penile Relating to the penis.

penis Part of the external genitalia of the male and the organ of copulation; it is composed of erectile tissue that becomes engorged with blood prior to mating; the urethra runs through the penis. In the nonerect state, the penis is retained within the prepuce; in the cat the penis is caudally directed when not engorged and carries papillae on the surface; *see also* MICROPHALLUS.

Penrose drain Pattern of drainage tube for passive removal of fluid, mainly relying on capillary action and wound fluid seepage.

pension A regular payment a person may be entitled to when they reach retirement age; in the UK a person is entitled to a state pension when they reach retirement age. A company pension is one to which a person has contributed to throughout their working life.

pentobarbitone sodium A barbiturate commonly used for euthanasia, although it has also been used at lower concentrations as an induction agent or in the treatment of status epilepticus.

pen torch Slim torch that is useful for testing pupillary light reflexes during eye examinations, placing endotracheal tubes, etc.

pentosan polysulphate Disease-modifying osteoarthritis drug (DMOAD); given as a series of subcutaneous injections in dogs and intramuscularly in horses ; *see also* DEGENERATIVE JOINT DISEASE.

penumbra The area of half-shadow or blurring around the edges of an object that is placed within a beam of X-rays. Penumbral blurring on the finished radiograph can be minimized by using a small focal spot; *see also* FOCAL SPOT.

pepsin One of the key digestive enzymes; secreted as the precursor pepsinogen by the chief cells of the gastric mucosa, pepsin hydrolyses the peptide bonds in ingested proteins.

pepsinogen The precursor of pepsin; *see also* PEPSIN.

peptic ulcer An ulcer of the inner wall of the stomach caused by the action of gastric juices on the susceptible mucosal lining; may be related to stress or infection with *Helicobacter pylori*; seen sometimes in racehorses.

peptide A compound containing two or more linked amino acids.

peptide bond Joining of two amino acids, the carboxyl group of one linked to the amino acid of the next.

peptone Soluble peptides often added to bacterial culture media.

per Through, via or most.

peracute Having an extremely rapid onset.

percuss To tap with the hand or a percussive instrument to determine the density of a part.

percutaneous endoscope-guided gastrotomy (PEG) tube See PEG.

perforation An abnormal opening.

perfusion 1) Fluid with soluble contents passed over or through a vessel or organ. 2) Glomerular blood flow (perfusion) is a measure of renal function.

peri- Prefix meaning 'around', 'in the region of'.

perianal Around the anus.

perianal fistula Blind-ending, necrotic tracts opening to the skin around the anus; occur almost exclusively in German shepherd dogs; see also FURUNCULOSIS.

periapical abscess An abscess that develops around the root of a tooth, usually necessitating removal of the tooth to allow drainage; see also MALAR.

periarticular Around a joint.

pericardial effusion Collection of fluid within the pericardial sac; causes include spontaneous haemorrhage, bleeding from haemangiosarcomata, infection and oedema fluid from congestive heart disease. The effusion leads predominantly to right-sided heart failure; pericardiocentesis is required to type the fluid and drain the pericardium; if there is recurrence of idiopathic effusion, a window may be surgically cut in the pericardium to allow drainage.

pericarditis Inflammation of the pericardium.

pericardium The double-layered (visceral and parietal layers) membranous sac that encloses the heart and the start of the great vessels.

perichondrium Limiting membrane-covering cartilage (but absent across the articular surface of cartilage in joints).

perilymph The fluid contained within the scala tympani and scala vestibuli of the inner ear; see also EAR, ENDOLYMPH.

perimysium The fibrous membrane around skeletal muscle fibres.

perinatal Relating to the period around birth, covering the first 2–3 days.

perineal Relating to the region around the perineum.

perineal hernia Rupture of the perineal musculature (the pelvic diaphragm), allowing protrusion of fat and abdominal contents. The urinary bladder may also retroflex into large perineal hernia defects; often associated with chronic straining, e.g. prostatic hypertrophy or constipation. Males are far more commonly affected than females; requires careful surgical replacement of the contents and closure of the defect;

castration is also recommended in the male animal.

perineal reflex Used in the assessment of anaesthetic depth by watching for a contraction of the anal sphincter.

perineum The region extending from the ischium, between the hindlegs to the pubis; includes the anus, vulva and scrotal sac.

perineurium The connective tissue sheath around nerve fibre bundles.

Period of Supervised Practice (PSP) Time spent by a nurse returning to clinical veterinary practice in order to refresh his or her skills before rejoining the Register; aim is to work with a named mentor to update knowledge and skills; requires a minimum of 595 hours within one year in an RCVS-approved training practice or an accredited practice.

periodontal membrane The tough fibrous membrane anchoring a tooth to the gum.

periodontitis Inflammation of the periodontal membrane; usually caused by the build-up of plaque and calculus within the pockets around the tooth and the start of gingivitis; if left untreated the gums will recede and the tooth will eventually be lost.

periople The outer layer of the hoof.

periorbital Region around the eye.

periosteal proliferative polyarthritis (PPP) An erosive polyarthritis seen in the cat; in addition, there is marked proliferation of bone spreading away from the joints; it affects mainly the tarsal and carpal regions; diagnosis is confirmed by radiography.

periosteum The tough, fibrous membrane that surrounds the outer surfaces of bones; important as the blood supply to the outer third of the cortex runs in the periosteum, which is also rich in nerve endings.

periostitis A bone disorder where there is inflammation of the periosteum, the outer cover of the bone. Dental periostitis may be caused by tooth infection.

peripheral Away from the centre.

peripheral nervous system (PNS) The cranial and spinal nerves that run from the brain and spinal cord to the other parts of the body; most nerves are mixed, carrying sensory information towards the CNS, motor information away from the CNS and also carrying fibres from the autonomic nervous system.

peristalsis The coordinated muscular contractions that sweep along the gastrointestinal tract to mix the food and move it along the tract.

peritoneal dialysis Injection of relatively large volumes of fluid into the abdomen and withdrawal of the fluid after allowing time for waste products in the blood to diffuse across the peritoneum into the fluid.

peritoneum The membrane lining the inner wall of the abdomen and covering the viscera; *see also* EPIPLOIC FORAMEN.

peritonitis Inflammation of the peritoneum; a painful abdominal condition.

perivascular Around a blood vessel; it is important that irritant intravenous substances, such as thiopental or vincristine, are not injected into perivascular tissues by accident as they can cause tissue necrosis.

permanent teeth Teeth present in an adult mouth.

permeable Able to allow molecules through.

pernicious Indicates a harmful disease, such as **pernicious anaemia**.

peroneal Relating to the fibula.

per os Via the mouth.

perosis A nutritional disease of young birds where there is shortening of the limb bones and displacement of tendons; possibly caused by manganese deficiency but may be exacerbated by poor flooring and overcrowding.

peroxide H_2O_2; a bleaching agent; may be used diluted to flush abscesses but can be toxic to tissues.

persistent hyperplastic primary vitreous (PHPV) Congenital condition affecting the vitreous body, where the fetal blood supply to the lens fails to regress; fibrovascular tissue forms on the posterior surface of the lens that may cause blindness if extensive. An inherited defect in the Dobermann and Staffordshire bull terrier.

persistent right aortic arch (PRAA) Congenital abnormality in the formation of the aortic arch, so that the aorta lies on the right of the trachea and oesophagus rather than to the left; this creates a ring around the oesophagus as the ligamentum arteriosum passes round to the pulmonary artery. The signs of oesophageal constriction become apparent at weaning when solid food is regurgitated; surgical sectioning of the ligamentum may resolve the problem, although some degree of oesophageal dysfunction may remain.

Perthes' disease One of the names for avascular necrosis of the femoral head; *see also* LEGG–CALVÉ–PERTHES DISEASE.

pervious Open.

pervious urachus Congenital defect resulting from failure of the urachus to close and regress after birth; urine dribbles constantly from the umbilicus; surgical correction is required.

pessary A medicated vaginal suppository.

PEST (STEP) analysis A business analytical tool used to identify the key factors at work in a particular market, covering the four areas Political, Economic, Social and Technical, see also SWOT ANALYSIS.

pes varus Term used for congenital deformity of the hock, found in some dachshunds as a result of malformation of the distal end of the tibia.

petechia, *pl.* **petechiae** A tiny area of haemorrhage.

pethidine An opiate analgesic, about one-tenth as potent as morphine; may also be used as a premedicant and has some spasmolytic properties; a controlled drug.

petit mal Minor epileptiform seizure, without loss of consciousness; may be a transient lack of awareness of surroundings; *see also* EPILEPSY, MAL.

pet passport Documentation required to enable an animal to travel between member states of the Pet Travel Scheme.

PET scan Positron Emission Tomography. These scans are able to produce three-dimensional images of internal organs and tissues that can be used as a

P

diagnostic tool, especially in cancers, as well as in planning complex surgery.

petri dish A shallow plastic dish with a lid; used in the laboratory as a bacterial culture plate, etc.

pétrissage A kneading movement used in massage to increase circulation and warm the tissues in preparation for more intense massage techniques.

petroleum jelly A commonly used lubricant gel.

PETS Pet Travel Scheme; introduced to the UK in March 2000; designed to allow dogs and cats to enter the country from European and other safe areas but to exclude the introduction of rabies by planned vaccination, identification and certification; *see also* RABIES.

-pexy Surgical fixation.

Peyer's patches Aggregates of lymphoid tissue within the wall of the small intestine.

pH A scale used to measure acidity, ranging from 0 (most acidic) to 14 (most alkaline), with 7 being neutral; may be measured with probes, or more roughly, with colour-change strips based on litmus paper; *see also* LITMUS PAPER.

phacoemulsification The use of high-frequency ultrasound to break down a cataract so that it can be removed with minimal disturbance to the eye. Early referral while the cataract is immature is advised; *see also* IMMATURE CATARACT.

phaeochromocytoma A rare tumour of the chromaffin cells of the adrenal medulla, giving rise to signs such as weakness, vomiting, diarrhoea and tachycardia.

phagocyte A scavenger cell that can ingest bacteria, foreign material and other cells.

phagocytosis The processes of ingestion and digestion of substances by phagocytes.

phalanx, *pl.* **phalanges** A toe.

phallus Penis.

pharmacodynamics The study of the therapeutic effects an individual drug has on the body.

pharmacokinetics The study of the absorption, distribution, metabolism and excretion of an individual drug.

pharmacology The study of drugs, their effects and uses.

pharmacy A place where drugs are dispensed.

pharmocovigilance The process of recording all occurrences of suspected adverse reactions when administering medicines. The purpose of the process is to ensure that the balance between benefits and risks of using authorized medicines remains favourable.

pharyngeal Relating to the pharynx.

pharyngostomy Creation of a surgical opening into the pharynx via the skin of the throat region; most commonly to allow placement of a feeding tube; iatrogenic damage can be caused during this procedure, and the tube is poorly tolerated by patients.

pharyngostomy tube A feeding tube surgically placed into the pharynx; *see also* PHARYNGOSTOMY.

pharynx The cavity at the back of the mouth leading to the oesophagus and trachea; divided into the (lower) oropharynx and (upper) nasopharynx.

phenobarbital A sedative anticonvulsant used in the control of epilepsy; *see also* EPILEPSY.

phenocopy Abnormality that appears to be a genetic defect but is actually the result of some toxin or environmental change.

phenol A group of potent disinfectants toxic to cats.

phenotype The outward appearance of an animal, reflecting the genetic make-up; *see also* GENOTYPE.

phenylbutazone The standard non-steroidal anti-inflammatory drug (NSAID); used widely for chronic locomotor diseases, such as osteoarthritis, and as an analgesic.

phenytoin An anticonvulsant used to treat epilepsy.

pheromone Chemical substances secreted by an animal and used in communication; appeasement pheromones are used in behaviour modification, other pheromones are important in courtship and mating. Used therapeutically to stop 'spraying' by cats, etc.

philopatry The tendency for animals to stay or return to their home area; of significance in primate behaviour.

phimosis Narrowing or constriction of the prepuce; *see also* PARAPHIMOSIS.

phlebitis Inflammation of a vein.

phlegm Excessive amounts of mucus produced from the respiratory tract.

phobia Any irrational or fearful response, often to a seemingly small or innocuous stimulus. When of emotional origin, may lead to antisocial behaviour in pets.

phosphaturia Increased phosphate in the urine, common finding in many renal disorders, leads to osteomalacia; *see also* FANCONI'S SYNDROME.

phospholipid A lipid molecule containing phosphorus; such molecules are important constituents of cell membranes.

photoelectric effect Generation of electricity from the action of light.

photophobia Avoidance of light; associated with painful ophthalmological conditions such as glaucoma and uveitis.

photoreceptor A cell that is sensitive to light, e.g. the rods and cones of the retina.

photosensitization Sensitization of the skin to the effects of sunlight.

photosynthesis The process plants use to build complex molecules from water and carbon dioxide, using chlorophyll and driven by the action of sunlight.

phototaxis Movement of an organism in response to a light stimulus.

phrenic Relating to the diaphragm.

phthisis bulbi A shrunken, blind eye.

phylum A taxonomic division used in the classification of plants and animals.

physiology The study of how the normal body functions.

physiotherapy Physical treatments designed to speed healing and recovery.

physis The epiphyseal plate or growth plate; the cartilage zone at the epiphysis of long bones that allows lengthening of the bone in immature animals; *see also* ENDOCHONDRAL OSSIFICATION.

physitis Enlargement of the physeal areas of growing long bones in horses, causing lameness.

phytin Calcium and magnesium salt of phytic acid.

phytomenadione Medication used in anticoagulant toxicity (alternative name vitamin K); *see* VITAMIN K.

phytotoxin Poisons of plant origin, may cause severe signs 4–12 hours after ingestion.

pia mater Literally 'tender mother'(L.); the innermost of the three meningeal layers, a delicate membrane that is closely applied to nervous tissue of the brain and spinal cord.

pica Depraved appetite.

picornavirus Group of small RNA viruses that includes feline calicivirus.

pigment Coloration.

pill A small, round object; *see also* TABLET.

pilocarpine Parasympathomimetic drug used to treat intestinal stasis and atropine overdosage; *see also* PARASYMPATHOMIMETIC.

piloerection Raising of hairs caused by the action of piloerector muscles; the hair coat may stand on end to trap an insulating layer of air to prevent excessive loss of body heat in cold environments. The same effect is used when animals 'raise their hackles' to make themselves appear bigger and more threatening.

pimobendan Positive inotrope and myocardial stimulant.

pinch graft Skin grafting technique where a punch is used to collect numerous 4- to 5-mm diameter plugs of skin from a clipped donor site; the plugs have the subcutaneous fat trimmed away and are then pressed into small pockets cut into the recipient site; *see also* STAMP GRAFT.

pineal gland Pine cone–shaped structure within the midbrain; its exact function remains poorly defined but it influences growth and seasonal patterns of behaviour.

pinealocytes Cells in the pineal gland that secrete melatonin; *see also* PINEAL GLAND.

pin firing Contentious treatment formerly commonly used for tendon strains in horses.

pin fitment The arrangement of pins and pinholes that allows only the correct gas cylinder to be fitted to the port of an anaesthetic machine.

pinioning Surgical removal of one wing tip in young birds, to prevent flight; it is permanent, unlike clipping of flight feathers.

pinna The external ear flap.

pinocytosis The process by which a cell forms invaginations along its outer membrane; the invagination forms a vesicle that gets pinched off, trapping external molecules that are then taken into the cell.

pins Metal implants used for internal fracture fixation; the pin is inserted into the medullary cavity of the fractured bone; pinning is best used for long, oblique fractures. In humans, the pin is commonly removed after fracture healing; in animals the pin is usually left in situ.

pinworm See *OXYURIS*.

piperazine A common worming preparation formerly used to treat ascarid infestations.

pipette A piece of laboratory equipment for accurately measuring out volumes of fluids; mouth pipettes should no longer be used because of the possible danger of swallowing toxic chemicals.

piroplasmosis Acute or chronic illness caused by *Babesia canis* following tick bites; see also *BABESIA*.

pituitary dwarf Congenital abnormality of the anterior pituitary, which fails to secrete sufficient levels of growth hormone; affected animals are stunted and retain their soft, juvenile hair coat; most commonly affects German shepherd dogs, where it is inherited as an autosomal recessive trait. Seen in Siamese and exotic cat breeds also.

pituitary gland An endocrine gland, also known as the hypophysis, lying ventral to the optic chiasma on the base of the brain. The pituitary is divided into two lobes, separated by Rathke's cleft; the anterior lobe (adenohypophysis) secretes growth hormone, prolactin, thyroid-stimulating hormone, follicle-stimulating hormone, luteinizing hormone, ACTH and lipotrophin; the posterior lobe (neurohypophysis) secretes oxytocin and antidiuretic hormone (vasopressin); see also HYPOTHALAMUS.

Pityrosporum canis Previous name for *Malassezia canis*.

PKD See POLYCYSTIC KIDNEY DISEASE.

placebo A harmless substance given as a medicine and commonly used in drug trials as a comparator for the active treatment. In humans, there may be a placebo or psychological effect associated with taking medication, even if it contains no active drug – this effect is not seen in animals.

placenta The highly vascular membranous structure that allows attachment of the developing fetus to the uterine wall; allows the transfer of nutrients and oxygen from the mother to the fetus and the transfer of fetal waste products in the opposite direction; see also AFTERBIRTH.

placentation The formation of the placenta into one of three types, depending on the distribution of the chorionic villi: diffuse (mare, sow), cotyledonary (ruminants) or zonary (dog, cat).

placing reflex The normal reflex when an animal is held up and brought towards the edge of a table, so that the limbs are extended, ready for weight bearing; visual placing may be tested in this way, and tactile placing can be tested by covering the animal's eyes with your hands during the test.

plane A surface, real or theoretical, along which any two points can be joined by a straight line, e.g. a **transverse plane** cuts across the long axis of the body at right angles and the **median (vertical) plane** cuts the body into two equal sides.

plantar Relating to the undersurface of the paws on the hindlegs; see also PALMAR.

plantigrade Abnormal stance where the hock and caudal aspect of the metatarsus contact the ground; causes include rupture of the common calcaneal tendon and tarsal luxation; *see also* PALMIGRADE.

plaque The sticky film that builds up on the teeth, eventually hardening to form tartar; the initial film consists of a mixture of saliva, food debris and bacteria; plaque formation leads to periodontitis and may necessitate descaling.

plasma The fluid component of the blood, including the clotting proteins; may be obtained by taking a blood sample into an anticoagulant and spinning it so that the cells settle out. The fluid therapy of choice to treat haemorrhagic shock; *see also* SERUM.

plasma cell Cell that is stimulated to secrete specific antibody in the presence of the trigger antigen; derived from B lymphocytes.

plasma membrane Alternative term for the cell membrane.

plasma proteins Albumin, globulins and other enzymes, clotting factors, hormones and carrier proteins normally found within the blood; commonly measured as 'total protein'. Commonly increases in total protein (hyperproteinaemia) are associated with dehydration, immune-mediated and chronic diseases; hypoproteinaemia may be caused by liver disease, nephrotic syndrome, burns and protein-losing enteropathies.

plasmid A length of DNA that carries a number of nonessential genes and can be transmitted from one bacterium to another; this can have clinical implications, e.g. if the plasmid encodes antibiotic resistance. Plasmids in gene therapy are denoted by the prefix 'p' and often described in the form p-promoter gene expressed.

plasminogen A precursor of plasmin, a potent fibrinolytic enzyme.

plaster of Paris (PoP) Powdered calcium sulphate, derived from gypsum; it is used to coat white open-wove bandage, which then hardens when wetted; used to make casts and splints. The material is cheap, easy to apply and can be removed with plaster shears; setting time is long, allowing time to construct complex casts; disadvantages include the long setting time (during which the animal should

not bear weight on the cast), the heavy weight and the fact that the cast must be kept dry or it will soften.

plastron Ventral shell of a tortoise; see SCUTES, CARAPACE.

platelet Thrombocyte; small cell fragments found in the circulation derived from megakaryocytes; platelets stick to areas of damaged endothelium, and in conjunction with fibrin, form a clot.

plate out Laboratory technique for preparing colonies of bacteria by streaking them across the surface of a shallow culture plate, using a platinum loop, and then incubating the plate (usually at 37°C for 24–48 hours); the loop is sterilized between each of the streaks, gradually reducing the concentration of bacteria so that separate colonies can be grown; different patterns are required if the plate is to be used for antibiotic sensitivity testing; *see also* PETRI DISH, PLATINUM LOOP.

platinum loop A fine wire loop with a handle; used for plating out bacteria for culture; the loop can be repeatedly sterilized by holding it in the hottest part of a Bunsen flame until it glows red.

platyhelminth A flatworm or fluke; *see also* TREMATODE.

-plegia Muscle weakness; *see also* PARALYSIS, HEMIPLEGIA, QUADRIPLEGIA.

plenum Anaesthetic gas vaporizer, calibrator with compensation devices for flow or temperature variations.

pleiotropic Having more than one effect, e.g. a pleiotropic gene will have more than one phenotypic effect, so an alteration in the gene may have multiple phenotypic effects.

pleura The serous membranes lining the thoracic cavity; the **parietal pleura** is closely applied to the inner surface of the chest wall, while the **visceral pleura** covers the lung tissue. There is a small, fluid-filled space between, which means that the lungs follow the movements of the chest wall during respiration.

pleural effusion Collection of fluid in the pleural space between the visceral and parietal layers of the pleura; the fluid may be a transudate, exudate,

P

blood, pus, chyle or associated with neoplasia. Clinical signs include progressive dyspnoea, with tachypnoea and unwillingness to remain in lateral recumbency; radiography usually confirms the diagnosis and thoracocentesis is used to type the fluid; affected animals require careful handling and should not be stressed unnecessarily.

pleural fluid Normal lubrication fluid over lung surface, may become excessive in disease, etc.; *see also* PLEURISY.

plexus A network of blood vessels or nerves; *see also* BRACHIAL PLEXUS, LUMBOSACRAL PLEXUS, PAMPINIFORM PLEXUS.

plication Surgical technique making tucks or folds in a tissue or organ to make it smaller.

Pneumocystis Genus of bacteria that cause pneumonia; may occur as opportunistic pathogens in immunocompromised animals.

pneumocystogram The introduction of air as a radiographic negative contrast agent into the bladder; may be used to demonstrate calculi, tumours, etc.

pneumomediastinum The presence of free air within the mediastinum of the chest; usually a result of damage to the trachea.

pneumonia Inflammation of the lung tissue; causes include bacterial or viral infection, allergy, aspiration of gastric contents and paraquat poisoning.

pneumoradiography The use of air as a negative contrast agent.

pneumothorax The presence of free air within the thoracic cavity; usually the result of trauma to the thoracic wall but may also result from tracheal rupture, overinflation of the lungs during intermittent positive pressure ventilation (IPPV), lung lobe torsion, etc.

PNKA Test kit available for testing blood clotting time, stands for 'protein induced by vitamin K assessment'.

pododermatitis Inflammation of the skin around and between the toes; causes include demodectic mange, hookworm and grass seeds; *see also* INTERDIGITAL CYST.

poikilocyte Irregular, pear- or teardrop-shaped erythrocyte seen in some cases of chronic anaemia. Poikilo- means 'many-coloured' or 'many varied'.

poikilotherm A cold-blooded animal; having a body temperature that varies according to the environmental temperature.

point of lay Term used to describe an adult female bird that is about to start laying eggs.

points Acupuncture points were first located on humans; the points have been adapted for animals undergoing veterinary acupuncture; the horse has 361 acupuncture points.

poison A harmful or toxic substance; possible sources of poisoning include insecticides, rodenticides, weedkillers, paints, antifreeze, plants (such as yew, rhododendron and deadly nightshade), fungi, heavy metals, bites and stings, drug overdosage or misuse of human medicines for animals. Clinical signs vary according to the type of poison; first aid measures include administering an emetic if a noncorrosive poison has been ingested, giving mild purgatives, removing skin contamination and administering specific antidotes if appropriate. Poisons advice for veterinary practices in UK can be sought from the Veterinary Poisons Information Service (VPIS).

polar Type of cataract where the opacity is first seen in the centre of the lens.

polarized 1) Describes cells that have a transmembrane potential. **2)** To give magnetic properties to either end of a metal bar; *see also* DEPOLARIZATION.

polioencephalomyelitis Inflammation of the grey and white matter of the brain; a rare condition in animals of undefined aetiology.

pollakiuria Producing small amounts of urine frequently.

poly- Prefix meaning 'many'.

polyamide Nylon; synthetic, nonabsorbable suture material; high tensile strength and fair knot security, although the larger diameters can be stiff to handle and difficult to tie, have low tissue reactivity and the ends of the suture may irritate; widely used as a skin suture.

polyarteritis nodosa Inflammation of a number of small arteries, with distension and bulging of the vessel walls; an autoimmune condition that may also be associated with a polyarthritis; rare.

polyarthritis Inflammation of several joints.

polyarthritis/polymyositis syndrome Inflammation of joints and muscles; a rare syndrome reported in dogs; affected animals have a stiff gait and muscle atrophy may be marked; thought to be immune-mediated; treatment with prednisolone and cytotoxic drugs may be tried.

polychromasia Varied pattern of staining; term used to describe the staining of immature red blood cells.

polycystic Containing many fluid-filled cysts; used to describe multiple cysts in the kidney, for example.

polycystic kidney disease (PKD) An inherited condition of cats, affecting the Persian breed most commonly, although it may be found in many other kittens.

polycythaemia Increased number of circulating red blood cells; *see also* PCV.

polydactyl Having more than the normal number of toes; a common congenital deformity in the cat and usually of no clinical significance.

polydioxanone Synthetic monofilament suture material (PDS) of high tensile strength, handles well and ties good knots; removed by hydrolysis, retains up to half its strength for 30 days and takes 180 days for complete absorption; widely used for internal sutures where strength is needed.

polydipsia Increased thirst; a common clinical sign and often associated with polyuria. The causes include dehydration, hyperthermia, restricted access to water, diabetes insipidus, diabetes mellitus, renal disease, liver disease, pyometra, Cushing's disease, Addison's disease, hyperthyroidism, etc.

polyester Braided, synthetic, nonabsorbable suture material, may be coated; has very high tensile strength and moderate ease of handling and knot security.

polyglactin Coated, braided, synthetic, absorbable suture material (Vicryl); strong, with good knot security and handling; absorbed by hydrolysis; shorter-lasting than polydioxanone.

polyglycolic acid Braided, synthetic, absorbable suture material that may also be coated (Dexon-Plus); strong, with good handling and knot security; absorbed by hydrolysis; shorter-lasting than polydioxanone.

polymeric diets Balanced liquid diets that can be used for meal replacement; because of their small particle size they can be fed through small-diameter nasogastric tubes.

polymorph Nucleated white blood cell (leukocyte) with a multilobed nucleus and granular cytoplasm; adult neutrophil; *see also* LEUKOCYTE, NEUTROPHIL.

polymyopathy Any disease affecting multiple muscle groups; may be inflammatory, degenerative or metabolic; associated with conditions such as Cushing's disease and hypothyroidism; specific inherited myopathies have been reported in the Labrador and golden retriever and some spaniel breeds, an idiopathic form occurs in cats; *see also* MYASTHENIA GRAVIS, POLYMYOSITIS.

polymyositis Inflammation of several muscles; associated with diseases such as toxocariasis (visceral larva migrans), clostridial infection and toxoplasmosis.

polyneuritis Inflammation of nerves.

polyneuropathy Widespread nerve disorder affecting sensory and then motor nerves, may be immune-mediated. May be associated with neoplasia; *see also* PARANEOPLASTIC SYNDROME.

polyoestrus The condition of having more than one reproductive time in a mating season; the adjective is **polyoestrous**.

polyp Benign, pedunculated growth arising from a mucous membrane, e.g. nasal polyps may enlarge behind the soft palate in the cat, causing increasing dyspnoea and nasal discharge; treatment is usually surgical removal.

polypeptide A chain of three or more linked amino acids.

polyphagia Increased appetite.

polypharmacy Use of several drugs to treat a condition; the drugs may be given separately or may be available within the same product; this approach should be based on careful clinical judgement as it may be effective but associated with an increased risk of developing resistance.

polyploid Having more than twice the usual haploid number of chromosomes in a cell, e.g. triploid cells have three times the haploid number; *see also* DIPLOID.

polyradiculoneuropathies Inflammatory diseases that affect nerve roots; *see also* NEOSPOROSIS.

polysaccharide Large carbohydrate molecule consisting of several linked simple sugars; starch, glycogen and cellulose are all examples.

polysome Group of ribosomes linked by a molecule of RNA; the ribosomes move along the RNA strand to synthesize a specific protein; *see also* RNA.

polytocous Normally producing more than one offspring, e.g. a litter.

polyunsaturated fatty acid (PUFA) A fatty acid containing more than one double bond.

polyuria Increased production of urine; often associated with polydipsia; causes include diabetes insipidus, diabetes mellitus, use of diuretics, etc.; *see also* POLYDIPSIA.

polyvalent Term used to describe a vaccine that contains more than one antigenic agent, e.g. combined flu and enteritis vaccine for cats.

POMR Problem-orientated medical records.

POM-V Prescription only medicine – veterinarian; an authorized medicine that can only be dispensed by a veterinary surgeon.

POM-VPS Prescription only medicines – veterinary surgeon, pharmacist or suitably qualified person; veterinary medicinal product drugs that can only be supplied by a responsible qualified person (RQP), defined as a registered veterinary surgeon

or a registered pharmacist or a registered suitably qualified person (SQP).

pons Part of the brainstem; the bridge of tissue between the medulla oblongata and the midbrain; a major relay centre.

popliteal Relating to the calf region of the hindleg, behind the stifle, e.g. popliteus muscle, popliteal sesamoids, popliteal lymph node.

porous Containing pores or minute openings that will allow molecules to pass through.

porphyria Elevated levels of circulating porphyrins, usually caused by a metabolic defect; excess porphyrins are excreted via the urine and faeces. Urine colours are unusual.

portal Relating to the venous blood system, which takes blood rich in dietary nutrients from the intestine to the liver.

portocaval The portal vein that drains blood from the spleen, stomach and the anterior mesentry. It connects to the posterior vena cava after the blood has passed through the liver by a short vein; also spelled **portacaval**.

portocaval shunt Abnormal anastomosis between the hepatic portal vein and the caudal vena cava; usually congenital but may be acquired following liver cirrhosis. Blood is diverted away from the liver, affecting the metabolism of many products. The clinical signs include weight loss, lethargy, stunted growth and nervous signs (hepatic encephalopathy) that are often most pronounced soon after feeding; laboratory tests show low plasma urea but elevated ammonia and bile acids. Portal angiography is required to localize the shunt accurately; surgical partial ligation of discrete, extrahepatic shunts may be possible, although intrahepatic shunts may be more difficult to locate and correct; *see also* PORTOSYSTEMIC SHUNT.

portosystemic shunt Any vascular anastomosis between the portal vein and the systemic circulation; most commonly as a result of a patent ductus venosus. The ductus venosus carries fetal blood from the gut and placenta to the vena cava; although the duct runs through the liver, blood bypasses the hepatic sinusoids; this duct usually closes within a few hours of birth.

position Spatial relationship between the spine of the fetus and the birth canal; positions may be dorsal, ventral, right or left lateral; see also POSTURE, PRESENTATION.

positive pressure ventilation Controlled techniques for pushing air into the lungs of patients who cannot breathe for themselves; *see also* INTERMITTENT POSITIVE PRESSURE VENTILATION.

positive punishment A decrease in the frequency of a behaviour that follows an aversive event.

positive reinforcement Process of increasing the frequency of a behaviour by following it with an event or a stimulus the animal wants (food, verbal praise, etc.).

posterior Towards the rear; the caudal surface.

posterior chamber The caudal chamber of the eye, behind the lens; contains the vitreous body and the light-sensitive retinal layers.

posterior pituitary gland Endocrine gland; the hormones oxytocin and antidiuretic hormone are in fact manufactured by secretory cells higher up the brain; *see also* NEUROHYPOPHYSIS.

posterior pole Subcapsular cataract site in lens, appears Y-shaped or triangular as it affects the suture lines within the lens caudal; *see also* MATURE CATARACT.

postganglionic neurone Neurones to the tissues distal to the ganglion.

posthibernation anorexia (PHA) Condition of tortoises where they are reluctant to eat after hibernation; treated by maintaining the correct temperature, fluids, fat-soluble vitamins and appropriate diet.

postmortem 'After death'; usually an autopsy or examination to find out the cause of death.

postoperative Occurring after surgery.

postpartum Occurring after birth.

postprandial After a meal.

posture Position of the fetal limbs, e.g. forelimbs extended; *see also* POSITION, PRESENTATION.

potassium Dietary mineral and intracellular electrolyte. Deficiency causes muscle weakness and may arise following severe diarrhoea, vomiting, end-stage renal disease, prolonged fluid therapy or the use of potassium-losing diuretics. Excess (hyperkalaemia) occurs in Addison's disease, acute renal failure and use of potassium-sparing diuretics; elevated levels of potassium can be cardiotoxic and lead rapidly to cardiac arrest, so prompt treatment with intravenous fluids to dilute the potassium is required; *see also* ADDISON'S DISEASE.

Potomac horse fever An acute enterocolitis of horses that graze along riverbanks in the US; caused by a rickettsial parasite *Ehrlichia rusticii*; common signs are diarrhoea and fever; treated with supportive therapy and antibiotics. A notifiable disease in Australia.

potentiated sulphonamide One of a group of broad-spectrum antibiotics.

Potter–Bucky A type of moving grid housed within the radiography table and used when tissue more than 10 cm thick is being radiographed; as the grid moves rapidly during the exposure, gridlines are blurred and do not appear on the fixed radiograph; *see also* GRID.

poultice A paste (often kaolin-based) that is applied to an area to draw out infection; used more widely in large animal medicine than for small animals.

povidone iodine An iodophor skin disinfectant and surgical scrub solution.

powder feathers Short, blunt feathers that function to provide powder down, necessary for waterproofing.

poxvirus An infection; in pigeons causes scabs and proliferation of beak wattle, oral cavity, etc.; control is by use of vaccine and removing insect vectors.

PPM Persistent pupillary membrane.

PRA Progressive retinal atrophy; a disorder causing loss of sight. Group of different hereditary diseases that all show the same phenotype – progressive degeneration of the photoreceptors of the retina; *see also* RETINAL ATROPHY.

Practice Standards Scheme RCVS scheme to accredit veterinary practices by setting of standards and carrying out of regular inspections.

precipitate Solid particles that settle out to the bottom of a solution.

preclipping Clipping a conscious patient several hours prior to surgery; this allows more efficient use of theatre time and allows loose hairs to be shed outside the theatre; it may need more staff, however, and can be impossible with uncooperative patients or painful surgical sites.

precocial Relatively advanced from an early age.

precursor Something that comes first; may be a substance from which another is formed.

prednisolone Synthetic steroid with a similar action to cortisone; it has analgesic and anti-inflammatory properties; at high doses it is immunosuppressive. Treatment should not be withdrawn suddenly as adrenal insufficiency can occur; dogs should be given the medication in the morning, and cats in the evening, so that the dose pattern follows the normal cortisol peak. The common side effects include polyphagia, polyuria and polydipsia; prednisolone should not be given to pregnant animals.

preen gland Sebaceous gland located at the base of a bird's tail, also called the uropygial or oil gland; the glandular secretion is spread by the bird across its body during preening.

preganglionic neurone Forms part of the autonomic nervous system; arises proximal to a ganglion.

pregnancy diagnosis Confirmation that an animal is carrying one or more offspring; a variety of tests are available, depending on the species and the stage of gestation; tests include abdominal palpation, ultrasound, hormone assays, vaginal mucus smears and radiography. Other signs corroborate: failure to return to oestrus, prominent teats, enlargement of the mammary glands, behaviour changes and significant weight gain.

pregnancy toxaemia Metabolic disorder occurring in late pregnancy, caused by the high demands of the fetus or inadequate nutrition of the mother; rare in small animals but common in sheep.

pregnant mare serum gonadotrophin (PMSG) Hormone produced by mares to help sustain pregnancy; purified PMSG can be used in other species to stimulate the formation of ovarian follicles and spermatogenesis.

prehensile Used for wrapping around and grasping; mainly used when referring to a tail.

premedication Drug given prior to another drug, usually to counter side effects; examples include use of an antiemetic prior to chemotherapy and the widespread use of sedatives, analgesics and antisialagogues prior to anaesthesia.

premolars The teeth in the upper and lower jaws between the canine teeth and the molars; *see also* CARNASSIAL TOOTH.

preparation room The room where animals are prepared for theatre; anaesthesia may be induced here, the patient clipped, the surgical site given an initial scrub, intravenous catheters inserted, etc.

prepatent period The time between infection of a host with a parasite and the excretion of infective forms, e.g. eggs or larvae, by that host.

prepubic hernia Following the tearing of muscles of the abdominal wall after trauma of road accidents, especially seen in cats.

prepuce The sheath that covers the penis.

presbycusis Deafness associated with old age.

prescapular lymph node The palpable lymph node located just cranial to the scapula.

prescribing Writing or giving directions for the medication of animals under the veterinary surgeon's care. Clients must be able to obtain prescriptions as appropriate and they must be told the price of medicine to be dispensed. Itemized invoices must be made available for individual products.

prescribing cascade Veterinary medicines licensed in the UK for use in specific animal species should always be used first; failing that, veterinary medicines licensed for use in a different animal species may be used; failing that, medicines licensed for human use may then be used with owners' written consent. Importation of medicines from the EU and medicines prepared for individual use also form parts of the cascade.

prescription A written legal instruction for a pharmacist or other veterinary practice to supply a certain drug to an owner for treatment of an animal under the signing veterinary surgeon's care; the following must appear – the name, address and telephone number of the prescriber, qualification, name and address of owner, species and name of animal, date, signature of prescriber, name and amount of medicine prescribed, dosage and administration and any warnings.

presentation 1) The clinical signs and symptoms shown by an animal. 2) The relationship between the long axis of the fetus and the birth canal; presentations may be longitudinal, transverse or (rarely) vertical; *see also* POSITION, POSTURE.

pressure bag An inflatable cuff and bladder device used to hold fluid bags that, when inflated, enable the rapid delivery of intravenous fluids to patients with hypovolaemia.

pressure bandage Pad of absorptive material applied firmly with a bandage to control haemorrhage; usually used on the distal limb; should not be left on for more than 24 hours.

pressure sore *See* DECUBITAL, ULCERS.

prevalence The number of cases of a disease within a specified population at any point in time; *see also* INCIDENCE.

preventive medicine Branch of veterinary medicine dealing with the prevention of disease in individual animals or groups; preventive medicine includes the use

of vaccines, control of environmental factors, hygiene, etc.

priapism Prolonged erection of the penis.

primary beam The useful, main part of the X-ray beam that produces the latent image on the film; should be coned down to just the area of interest and staff should never get any part of their bodies in the primary beam.

primary haemorrhage Blood loss immediately following rupture of a vessel.

primidone An anticonvulsant used for the control of epilepsy; *see also* EPILEPSY.

primigravida Describes an animal that is pregnant for the first time.

Principles of Practice As directed by the RCVS Code of Professional Conduct – Five professional responsibilities that all veterinary nurses must fulfil: **1)** Professional competence. **2)** Honesty and integrity. **3)** Independence and impartiality. **4)** Client confidentiality and trust. **5)** Professional accountability.

prions Minute particles smaller than viruses of a protein-like nature that are considered to be the infective agent for bovine spongiform encephalopathy, scrapie and new-variant Creutzfeldt–Jakob disease in humans.

probe A blunt-ended instrument used for assessing the depth of a tract or recess.

probiotics Live natural products given by mouth; bacteria that will improve the normal microflora of the intestines.

process mapping A method of recording the reality of every stage of a patient journey. Used to improve patient care, safety and clinical efficiency.

proctitis Inflammation of the rectum.

proctodeum The common part of the cloaca of the bird where urine and faeces mix.

proctoscopy Endoscopic examination of the rectum.

prodromal Preceding, occurring before, e.g. a **prodromal phase** may be recognized before an epileptic seizure.

proenzyme Inactive form of the enzyme that needs another factor for it to become active; *see* TRYPSINOGEN, PEPSINOGEN.

professional accountability The acceptance of responsibility for one's own actions and quality of work.

Professional Development Phase (PDP) Introduced by the RCVS in 2007, a programme of ongoing development for veterinarians in their first year after qualifying.

Professional Development Record (PDR) Log to record hours spent undertaking Continuing Professional Development activities.

progeny All the offspring of a single animal.

progeny testing Assessing the usefulness of a breeding animal by looking at the quality of their offspring.

progesterone Hormone produced by the corpus luteum, which develops after a follicle has released its ovum; the hormone sustains pregnancy and inhibits return to oestrus.

progestogen A drug with progesterone-like activity, e.g. megestrol acetate.

proglottid The mature, gravid segment of a tapeworm that is released into the faeces; these sac-like structures typically appear like rice grains and contain the eggs.

prognathism Having the lower jaw longer than the upper jaw; undershot.

prognosis The likely outcome of a disease.

progressive axonopathy (PA) A rare giant axonal neuropathy reported in German shepherd dogs and inherited as an autosomal recessive trait; affected dogs show paresis and pelvic limb ataxia, typically at 1 year of age; the disease worsens and there is no cure.

progressive retinal atrophy *See* PRA, RETINAL ATROPHY.

project management The focused use of knowledge, methods, skills, processes and measured resources to achieve a specific objective within a given time frame.

projectile vomiting Propulsive vomiting; may be associated with mechanical abnormalities such as pyloric stenosis.

prolactin Hormone secreted by the anterior pituitary, stimulating lactation.

prolactin-inhibiting hormone Originating in the hypothalamus, it inhibits the release of prolactin. The release of prolactin can also be inhibited by stimulating dopamine receptors by drugs such as bromocriptine and cabergoline.

prolactin-releasing hormone The hormone secreted by the hypothalamus that stimulates the pituitary to produce prolactin.

prolapse The displacement of a structure or organ from its usual location, e.g. prolapsed rectum, uterus, etc.

prolapsed third eyelid Swelling of the free border of the nictitating membrane or third eyelid; may require surgical correction.

proliferative enteropathy A diarrhoeal disease of rabbits caused by *Lawsonia intracellularis*.

pronation Rotation of the paw so that the palmar or plantar surface faces ventrally; the opposite of supination.

prone Position where an animal is lying on its ventral surface, with its back uppermost.

pro-oestrus The phase of the reproductive cycle occurring immediately before oestrus; during pro-oestrus, there is follicular growth and maturation, the uterus enlarges and the endometrium hypertrophies; in the bitch there is vulval oedema and bleeding; *see also* ANOESTRUS, DIOESTRUS, METOESTRUS, OESTRUS.

propatagonum Sheet of muscle and tissue connecting the avian humerus to the carpal joint.

prophylactic A treatment used to prevent a disease.

proprioception The sense of spatial awareness and limb positioning.

proptosis Protrusion of the eyeball.

prostaglandin $F_{2\alpha}$ Luteolytic hormone secreted by the uterine endometrium.

prostaglandins Group of diverse molecules formed from fatty acids; they can have hormone-like effects in the body and can be potent inflammatory mediators; synthetic prostaglandin analogues are used to regress the corpus luteum, leading to abortion or induction of parturition.

prostate The male accessory sex gland situated at the neck of the bladder, surrounding the urethra; it secretes fluid into the urethra for sperm transport.

prostatitis Inflammation of the prostate. **Benign hypertrophic prostatitis** is a common consequence of ageing; enlargement may be associated with a degree of prostatitis and is often subclinical; in some cases the hypertrophy may cause dysuria or constipation, often with tenesmus; steroid hormones may be used to cause the gland to regress, or castration can be performed.

prosthesis An artificial replacement, e.g. a hip prosthesis.

protamine zinc insulin An insoluble insulin preparation with a duration of action of approximately 24 hours.

protein Large molecule made from amino acids; proteins function as enzymes and hormones and are used as structural building blocks for body tissues; there is constant turnover of protein in the body; when fat and carbohydrate reserves are used up, protein can also be catabolized to release energy.

protein-energy malnutrition (PEM) In a chronic illness the cumulative drain on tissues may continue, for weeks and if not corrected, can result in protein-energy malnutrition. During this time, nutritional support becomes a crucial part of the treatment. Protein-energy malnutrition can delay recovery and increase the patient's susceptibility to infection and shock.

protein-losing glomerulonephropathy (PLGN) Kidney disease leading to loss of protein across the glomerulus into the urine; occurs in dogs, with the deposition of circulating antibody–antigen complexes in the glomeruli of the kidney.

proteinuria Presence of protein in the urine; causes include renal disease, inflammation elsewhere in the urogenital tract, haematuria and natural secretions such as semen.

proteolytic Substance that breaks down proteins by severing the peptide bonds.

Proteus Genus of Gram-negative bacteria that are commensals of the gastrointestinal tract and common pathogens.

prothrombin Precursor of thrombin, formed by the liver; *see also* THROMBIN.

proton An elemental particle carrying one positive charge; it is the equivalent of the nucleus of a hydrogen atom and is commonly represented as H1; see also ELECTRON.

protoplasm The cytoplasm or ground substance of a cell.

protozoa Unicellular parasitic organisms such as Coccidia.

proud flesh Exuberant granulation tissue that may be produced during second-intention wound healing; the tissue is vascular but aneural; if the tissue rises above the level of the epithelium, the epithelial cells cannot migrate across to cover the defect; proud flesh can be reduced with astringents such as copper sulphate or may require surgical cutting back.

proventriculus The glandular stomach of the bird with gastric glands; located between the crop and the gizzard.

proximal Towards the centre or origin.

proximal convoluted tube Collecting canal from the glomerulus of the kidney nephron to the loop of Henle.

pruritus Itchiness, irritation of the skin; a common sign in many skin diseases.

pseudoarthrosis A fibrous articulation that develops between two bone ends when the usual articular surfaces are no longer in apposition, e.g. the fibrous joint that allows functional movement of the hip after femoral head excision.

pseudocyesis False pregnancy; *see also* OESTROUS CYCLE.

Pseudomonas Genus of Gram-negative, motile, rod-shaped bacteria found commonly in stagnant water and decaying matter; some species are pathogenic and are associated with urinary, ear, gastrointestinal and wound infections.

pseudopodia Cytoplasmic projections from unicellular organisms that help them to move.

pseudopregnancy False pregnancy; *see also* OESTROUS CYCLE.

pseudorabies Aujeszky's disease, infectious bulbar paralysis or mad itch; acute disease caused by a herpesvirus; the natural host for the virus is the pig, although many other species may be affected; after a 2–10 day incubation period, affected animals become pyrexic, agitated and increasingly pruritic; signs progress rapidly and death usually occurs in 24–48 hours.

pseudotuberculosis Granulomatous disease or enteritis caused by *Yersinia* spp.; the organism is zoonotic, so suspected cases should be handled with extreme care.

psittacine Term used to describe climbing birds, e.g. parrots and budgerigars.

psittacosis Ornithosis, chlamydiosis; disease of psittacine birds caused by the intracellular organism *Chlamydophila felis* (previously known as *Chlamydia psittaci*); signs include ruffled feathers, green/grey diarrhoea and conjunctivitis; the disease is zoonotic, causing a flu-like syndrome in humans that may occasionally be fatal; treatment of affected birds may be attempted, but because of the zoonotic risk, euthanasia is usually performed.

psoriasis An erythematous, scaling skin disease in humans with secondary bacterial infection. No equivalent disease in dogs.

Psoroptes ovis Surface-living mite of sheep that causes intense irritation with scratching and wool loss (sheep scab); sheep scab is no longer a notifiable disease.

PSS Portosystemic shunt.

psychology The study of an animal's behaviour in its normal environment.

pterygae Tracts of a bird's feathers.

ptosis Drooping of the upper eyelid so that the palpebral fissure is narrowed; occurs with lesions of the oculomotor (III) cranial nerve, e.g. Horner's syndrome.

ptyalin The enzyme in saliva that breaks starch down into sugar; salivary amylase.

ptyalism Increased saliva production, also known as hypersialism.

puberty Sexual maturity.

pubic symphysis The joint between the left and right pubic bones of the pelvis; the cartilaginous joint weakens in late pregnancy to aid expulsion of the fetus.

pubis The most ventral bone in the hemipelvis, contributing to the acetabulum and the obturator foramen.

Public Space Protection Orders Measures that can be applied by local authorities in England where a dog is found out of control in a public space; can be used to control dogs' fouling or a dog that regularly escapes and attacks others.

pudendal Relating to the region around the external genitalia.

puerperium The time from birth to the end of uterine involution.

PUFA Polyunsaturated fatty acid.

pulmonary Relating to the lungs.

pulmonary circulation Blood flow from the right ventricle via the pulmonary artery through the lungs and back to the left atrium via the pulmonary vein, which contains freshly oxygenated blood.

pulmonary embolus A small blood clot that lodges within a vessel in the lungs; some may be subclinical while others may cause sudden-onset dyspnoea.

pulmonary oedema Inflammation of lung tissue, with build-up of oedema fluid within the alveoli; the most common cause is left-sided heart failure, although other causes include paraquat poisoning, hypoproteinaemia and smoke inhalation. There is usually dyspnoea and wet respiratory noises; diuretics and oxygen should be administered and stress minimized; the primary cause should be treated and antibiotics may be given to prevent secondary infection.

pulmonary valve The valve of the heart that opens when the right ventricle pumps blood towards the lungs and then closes off the base of the pulmonary artery, preventing backflow or regurgitation. Three cusps close together as a tight seal.

pulmonic stenosis Congenital malformation of the cusps of the pulmonic heart valve, with narrowing of the artery; affected animals are stunted and have poor exercise tolerance. Signs of right-sided heart failure may develop, and there is a harsh systolic murmur; ECG, radiography and ultrasound confirm the diagnosis; dilation of the narrowing (balloon valvuloplasty) or patch grafting may be attempted.

pulpitis Inflammation of the pulp cavity within a tooth.

pulsate Throb.

pulse The palpable thrill that can be felt in a superficial artery where it passes over bone; in the normal animal there is a palpable thrill for each beat of the heart; pulse is usually referred to in terms of the rate (number of beats per minute), rhythm (regular, irregular, galloping, etc.) and character (weak, full, bounding, etc.).

pulse deficit Term used when the number of pulses felt is less than the number of beats of the heart; if there is an arrhythmia, some heart beats will be premature and will occur before the ventricles have filled correctly – the peripheral pulse associated with this beat may be weak or not able to be felt at all; the greater the pulse deficit, the more serious the cardiac abnormality.

pulseless electrical activity (PEA) Term used in assessing cardiac arrest where there is no detectable pulse but the heart has electrical activity.

pulse oximeter A piece of monitoring equipment that works by producing a source of light originating from a probe, which is normally attached to the tongue. The light is partly absorbed by haemoglobin, and the equipment can compute the proportion of haemoglobin that is oxygenated.

pulse oximetry A noninvasive technique of measuring the saturation of haemoglobin with oxygen. Mostly used during anaesthesia and intensive care nursing.

punch biopsy A special instrument used for taking small skin biopsy samples.

punctate Dotted or pitted.

punctum, *pl.* puncta The openings in the upper and lower eyelids for tears to drain into the lacrimal ducts.

puncture Make a small hole with a sharp, pointed instrument, stab.

PUO Pyrexia of unknown origin.

pupa Part of the life cycle of an insect.

pupil The gap in the centre of the iris through which light passes to the retina; the size of the pupil is regulated by the iris.

pupillary light reflex (PLR) When a bright light is shone into the eye, the pupil should constrict (direct response); there is also a consensual response, with the other pupil constricting too. When the stimulus is removed, the pupils should rapidly dilate; the PLR tests the function of the optic (II) and oculomotor (III) cranial nerves.

purgative Agents that decrease gastrointestinal transit time; strong purgatives should be avoided as they may irritate the mucosa, cause pain and can lead to potassium depletion; *see also* LAXATIVE.

purine One of the component bases of DNA and RNA.

Purkinje cell Inhibitory neurone found in the cerebellum; plays an important role in regulating muscle tone.

Purkinje fibres The network of fibres that conducts the waves of depolarization over the heart.

purpura Haemorrhagic condition, thought to be immune-mediated and usually following another illness; ecchymoses, petechiae or areas of haemorrhage and oedema arise spontaneously.

purulent Pus-like; containing pus.

pus Thick liquid composed of bacteria, leukocytes (predominantly dead neutrophils) and necrotic tissue debris.

pustule A small swelling containing pus, often a skin blister.

putrefaction The process of tissue decomposition brought about by bacteria.

PVC 1) Polyvinyl chloride, used in tubing manufacture. 2) Posterior vena cava.

P-wave The electrical wave on the ECG trace that occurs before the QRS complex and represents depolarization of the atria; in the normal trace every QRS complex should be preceded by a P-wave.

pyaemia Severe septicaemia, with the presence of pus in the blood.

pyelitis Pus in the renal pelvis and urine; usually caused by an ascending urinary tract infection.

pyelogram Radiographic contrast study of the kidney.

pyelonephritis Inflammation of the renal pelvis and cortex; caused by infection from the bloodstream or ascending from the ureters.

P

pygostyle Fused coccygeal vertebrae that support a bird's tail.

pyknosis Shrinking and condensing of the nucleus of a cell; often a sign of impending cell death.

pyloric glands Stomach wall glands that produce mucus for protection and lubrication.

pyloric sphincter Circular smooth muscle ring that controls the passage of ingested food from the stomach into the duodenum; *see also* PYLOROPLASTY.

pyloric stenosis Congenital or acquired narrowing of the pylorus, so gastric emptying is delayed; affected animals vomit frequently and may bring up food that they have eaten several days earlier. Vomiting may be projectile; surgical correction is usually required; *see also* PYLOROMYOTOMY, PYLOROPLASTY.

pyloromyotomy The muscle layer of the pyloric sphincter is cut surgically to increase the size of the opening from the stomach into the duodenum; care is required to ensure that the incision does not penetrate the mucosa; the effectiveness of the technique may be limited in the long term because of the development of fibrous scar tissue.

pyloroplasty Permanent surgical correction of pyloric stenosis where a longitudinal incision is made across the pylorus, through all tissue layers; the incision is then closed transversely.

pylorus The canal between the stomach and duodenum; bound by a muscular collar, the pyloric sphincter.

pyoderma Bacterial infection of the skin; may be surface (e.g. moist dermatitis), superficial or deep; a wide range of bacteria have been implicated but the most common is *Staphylococcus intermedius*.

pyogenic Capable of forming pus.

pyometra Presence of pus in the uterus; a common problem in nulliparous bitches and prevented by spaying. Pyometra may be open or closed, depending on the state of the cervix; affected animals are depressed, polydipsic and may vomit; with open pyometra there is a vulval discharge; the animal has usually been in oestrus within the previous 8–12 weeks; treatment is ovariohysterectomy.

pyonephritis Pus in the renal cortex.

pyothorax Pus within the thoracic cavity.

pyrethrum Insecticide based on plant extracts.

pyretic Having a raised body temperature, fevered.

pyrexia Fever; elevated temperature.

pyrexia of unknown origin (PUO) *See* PYREXIA.

pyrogen An agent that produces pyrexia in an infected animal.

pyuria White blood cells in the urine, indicates bacterial infection.

Q fever Zoonotic disease caused by the rickettsial organism *Coxiella burnetii*; affects mainly sheep and cattle and is characterized by pyrexia, abortion or pneumonia.

Qi In traditional Chinese medicine, the force or energy that controls the harmony of the animal body.

q.i.d. Dispensing instruction for a medicine to be given four times daily (L. *quater in die*).

QRS complex Part of the electrical trace on an ECG representing depolarization of the ventricles of the heart.

quadriceps femoris Muscle mass lying cranial to the femur; consists of four separate muscles that arise from the pelvis and proximal femur and insert on the patella; they act to extend the stifle and flex the hip.

quadriparesis Weakness affecting all four limbs, with neurological deficits, but the animal is still able to make stepping movements.

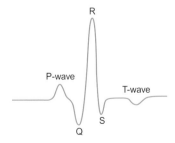

Figure 37. QRS complex.

quadriplegia Paralysis of all four limbs; *see also* TETRAPLEGIA.

quadruped A four-footed animal.

quality assurance Systematic processes of monitoring to ensure specified requirements are being met.

quality control A method of evaluating the accuracy or efficiency of a procedure; should routinely be applied to all practice laboratory tests.

quality standards A set of statements based on clinical evidence designed to drive improvements in patient care.

quarantine Statutory isolation period, usually longer than the incubation period of a disease, for animals being brought into a country or region; *see also* RABIES.

quaternary ammonia compound Group of disinfectant compounds based on ammonium hydroxide; suitable for skin preparation; nontoxic but inactivated by soap or organic matter.

queen Female cat of breeding age.

quidding Condition in the horse where food is taken into the mouth and chewed but dropped out; may indicate dental problems or difficulty swallowing.

quinolone Antibiotic drug occasionally used as nalidixic acid to treat resistant infections. Fluorinated quinolones are derivatives used as antibacterial agents; *see also* CIPROFLOXACIN.

quittor Infection of the lateral cartilage of the hoof, which may discharge above the coronary band.

Q wave The downward phase of the QRS complex on an ECG trace; indicates early contraction of the ventricles.

R

rabbit Small mammal, now the third most popular domestic pet. An efficient digester of cellulose by its almost unique process of caecotrophy. Pet rabbits are prone to dental disease as their nutritional needs are still not fully understood.

rabies Disease of the CNS of mammals caused by a Lyssavirus; transmitted mainly via bites; an important zoonotic disease that is not normally found in the UK; incubation may be as long as 4 months; signs include bouts of hyperexcitability, weakness and difficulty swallowing; the control of stray dogs and routine vaccinations are ways used to control infections overseas.

rachitic Suffering from rickets.

radiation The electromagnetic spectrum of rays such as radiowaves, light, X-rays and gamma rays; the radiation of a short wavelength and high energy can penetrate tissue and ionize molecules.

radiation protection adviser (RPA) Qualified person (e.g. holder of Diploma in Veterinary Radiology) who advises a practice on radiation procedures and safety, in line with the code of practice.

radiation protection supervisor (RPS) Employee of the practice who is responsible for radiation safety on a daily basis.

radiculitis Inflammation of a spinal nerve root, the main presenting sign being pain.

radiculomyelopathy Pathological condition of the spinal nerve roots and white matter of the spinal cord. Probably an autoimmune condition, most common in German shepherd dogs; *see also* CHRONIC DEGENERATIVE RADICULOMYELOPATHY.

radioactive Able to spontaneously emit X-radiation by radioactive decay when the nucleus of the atom loses energy by emitting radiation, e.g. iodine-131.

radiocarpal joint The joint between the distal radius and radiocarpal bone.

radiodense Unable to be penetrated by radiation, e.g. lead; radiopaque; the more radiodense a material, the whiter it will appear on the finished radiograph.

radiograph The developed and fixed X-ray film or digital image, showing the negative image of the object that has been radiographed.

radiographer A technician trained and qualified to take radiographs and often other diagnostic images such as MRI scans and CT scans.

radiography Diagnostic imaging of a part of the body using X-radiation.

radioisotope A molecule that spontaneously emits radiation, losing energy and changing to a more stable form.

radiologist Specialist trained in the interpretation of radiographs and other diagnostic imaging techniques.

radiology The science of the use of radiation for diagnosing and treating disease.

radiolucent Able to be penetrated by X-radiation; the more radiolucent a material is, the darker it will appear on the finished radiograph; gases are the most radiolucent substances.

radiopaque *See* RADIODENSE.

radiotherapy The use of radiation for the treatment of disease, especially neoplasia.

radiotracer A radioactive substance that is delivered to a patient via injection and releases positrons that enable a three-dimensional image to be produced via a PET scan.

radius Main bone of the foreleg, running from elbow to carpus.

rage reaction Instinctive reaction of the queen to attack the tomcat as he dismounts after copulation.

ragwort Common poisonous plant (*Senecio jacobaea*) with small yellow flowers. Fatally poisonous to horses. Horses are most at risk when grazing, especially during hot dry weather when grass is scarce.

RAID Redundant array of independent discs; term used in the storage of digital radiographs.

rain scald Skin disease of horses; see *Dermatophilus congolensis.*

rale A respiratory noise heard on auscultation; may be moist, gurgling, dry, crackling, etc.

ramify Divide into branches.

Ramstedt operation Name given to surgical operation of pyloromyotomy, also known as Fredet–Ramstedt operation.

ramus Anatomical term meaning a branch.

ranula A fluid-filled swelling (mucocele) under the tongue, often caused by obstruction of the duct of the sublingual salivary gland; may be drained surgically or treated conservatively.

raphe A line of union, e.g. the linea alba.

raptor A bird of prey.

rarefaction Becoming less dense.

rate The speed at which something happens.

rationale The scientific reasoning behind the management of a patient.

react To respond to a stimulus.

reactionary haemorrhage Leakage of blood from vessels within 24 hours of an injury or postoperatively; primary haemorrhage occurs immediately after injury, while secondary haemorrhage may develop 7–10 days later.

reactionary Occurring as a fairly rapid response to a situation, such as **reactionary haemorrhage**, which occurs after an animal's blood pressure has risen again following surgery or shock.

reactive Term used in cytology, suggesting neoplasia or an acute inflammatory reaction.

rebreathing circuit Type of anaesthetic circuit that includes a soda lime canister to absorb carbon dioxide from the exhaled gases; thus, the remaining gases can be inhaled again by the patient as long as sufficient oxygen remains. Rebreathing circuits include the to-and-fro type (for animals under 20 kg) and the circle type (for animals over 20 kg). Rebreathing circuits are generally more economic to run but the level of anaesthesia is more difficult to control accurately compared with nonrebreathing circuits.

receptors Sensory nerve endings that respond to specific stimuli.

recessive Genetic term used to describe a trait that is only apparent in the homozygous animal; the trait will not be apparent if other dominant alleles are present.

recipient The patient who receives donated blood, tissues, etc.

reconstitute 1) Return to the original state. 2) Add diluent to a vaccine or sterile water to a powder to make a solution that can be injected.

recovery Return to consciousness after general anaesthesia; recuperation from a disease.

recrudescence Recurrence of a disease after a period of remission.

recruitment The process of recruiting and selecting new employees to fill job vacancies.

rectal prolapse Protrusion of part of the rectal wall through the anal sphincter; results from prolonged tenesmus, e.g. severe diarrhoea, perineal hernia, prostatic hypertrophy. A prolapse may be replaced manually, although a purse-string suture may be required for 24–48 hours to prevent recurrence; if the rectal tissue is not viable, resection and anastomosis is performed.

rectal pull-through Surgical technique for the removal of rectal lesions that could not be removed via the abdomen; a circumanal incision is deepened and the rectum is freed and exteriorized by applying traction to stay sutures.

rectifier Part of the electrical circuit of an X-ray machine that converts the alternating current to a direct current.

rectovaginal fistula Connection between the rectum and vagina, usually caused by tearing of tissues during parturition.

rectrices The tail feathers of a bird, used to control direction during flight.

rectum The terminal portion of the gastrointestinal tract, extending from the colon to the anus.

recumbent Lying down, unable to stand.

recurrent Describes a disorder that returns regularly or frequently at irregular intervals.

red mite *See* DERMANYSSUS GALLINAE.

reduce Put back in its normal anatomical position; term used to describe the realignment of fracture fragments.

reducing valve Valve on an anaesthetic machine between the cylinder and the flowmeter that reduces the pressure of the gas and allows small adjustments in flow rate to be made.

referral The seeking of a second opinion from another veterinary surgeon or specialist. Referral may be suggested by the first veterinary surgeon or may be requested by the owner; it is the ethical duty of the referring veterinary surgeon to provide a case history, and the second vet should not examine the animal without this document or the permission of the referring vet.

reflective practice A process by an individual of consciously making time to think about decisions made, critically analyze practice and use knowledge and evidence to change behaviour and treatments to improve clinical performance and outcomes.

reflex ovulator Term used for induced ovulation following stimulus of coitus; *see also* OVULATION.

reflex An involuntary response to a stimulus, e.g. pupil constriction when a light is shone into the eye, the knee-jerk response when the patellar tendon is tapped.

reflux Backward flow; commonly used to describe the movement of gastric contents back into the oesophagus.

refraction Bending of light rays as they pass through a substance such as a lens.

refractometer An instrument that measures the deflection of light passing through a material; hand-held refractometers are used to measure the specific gravity and total protein levels of liquids such as urine and CSF.

refractory stage A nerve delayed response caused by depolarization of a neurone. Followed by a repolarization – the absolute refractory stage is followed by the relative refractory period.

regional anaesthesia Local anaesthetic technique where conduction in a specific nerve is blocked, providing anaesthesia of the region innervated by that nerve.

Register of Veterinary Practice Premises (RVPP) In the UK, all veterinary practices need to be registered to support the traceability of medicines; this register is held by the RCVS; see VETERINARY MEDICINES DIRECTORATE.

regurgitate 1) Backward flow of blood through incompetent valves. **2)** A passive movement of food from the oesophagus back to the mouth; usually occurs soon after feeding, but may occur up to 24 hours later; associated with megaoesophagus, persistent right aortic arch, oesophageal stricture, etc.; may also be normal in nursing animals, snakes, birds, etc.

rehydration The supply of fluids to a dehydrated patient; *see also* FLUID THERAPY.

relapse The return of a disease.

relaxant A drug that reduces muscle tone; may be used during an anaesthetic protocol to provide good relaxation of skeletal muscle, but as the respiratory muscles will also be affected, the patient will need to be ventilated; *see also* VENTILATOR.

relaxin A hormone secreted by the corpus luteum during pregnancy; causes a softening of the cervix and loosening of pelvic ligaments prior to parturition.

remiges Arrangement of the flight feathers of the bird.

remission Reduction in symptoms; period during which the disease disappears.

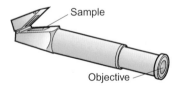

Figure 38. Refractometer.

renin The enzyme that converts angiotensinogen to angiotensin I.

renin–angiotensin system The homeostatic mechanism controlling sodium excretion and water loss from the kidneys; if extracellular fluid and sodium are lost, the kidney produces more renin, which increases levels of angiotensin I; this is converted to active angiotensin II in the lungs and other tissues and stimulates aldosterone production, thirst and vasoconstriction.

rennin Enzyme from stomach of milk-fed animals, rennet is produced commercially from young calves; *see also* CHYMOSIN.

reproduction The process by which animals produce offspring.

reproductive tract The body system in the male (testis, epididymis, vas deferens, urethra, penis, prostate and other accessory glands) and female (ovary, oviduct, uterus, cervix, vagina, vestibule and vulva) that allows reproduction to occur.

RER *See* RESTING ENERGY REQUIREMENT.

rescue breathing Method providing artificial respiration in cases of apparent cessation of breathing; the equivalent of the 'kiss of life' in human first aid.

resection Surgical removal of tissue.

reservoir 1) A source of infection, e.g. **reservoir host**. 2) A bag used in an anaesthesia circuit; the size should match the tidal volume of the patient.

resistance The force opposing the movement of air through the respiratory system.

resorption Removal of tissue by absorption, e.g. bone resorption during disuse; resorption of fetuses during early pregnancy.

respiration The cellular process where molecules are oxidized to release energy and form carbon dioxide and water; on a gross scale, the process also involves breathing and carriage of oxygen to the tissues via the red blood cells.

respiratory acidosis Increased amount of carbon dioxide carried in the bloodstream, resulting in lowering of the pH of the blood; causes include

hypoventilation caused by painful chest trauma, suffocation, etc.

respiratory alkalosis Increase in the pH of the blood, as a result of hyperventilation, e.g. panting.

respiratory centres Hindbrain centres in the medulla oblongata and pons to control all aspects of external respiration; *see also* APNEUSTIC CENTRE.

resting energy requirement (RER) The calculated number of calories (kcal) of energy required for a 24-hour period by the body of a patient during resting conditions. Similar to BMR – basic metabolic rate.

restraint Manual or chemical means of handling an animal.

resuscitation Reviving a patient when respiration has ceased (heart may also have stopped beating); the measures include establishing a patent airway, administering oxygen, external cardiac massage or internal cardiac massage and drug therapy; *see also* INTERMITTENT POSITIVE PRESSURE VENTILATION.

retained afterbirth Failure to expel the fetal membranes soon after whelping/ kittening, etc.; symptoms include pyrexia and an unpleasant vulval discharge.

retained cartilage cores Localized delay or failure of endochondral ossification, resulting in columns of cartilage remaining in some growth plate areas; the distal radius is most commonly affected; the significance of these cartilage cores, which are eventually replaced by bone, remains unclear.

retained meconium Failure of the neonate to pass meconium soon after birth, resulting in abdominal cramps and increased chance of infection; neonates should be observed carefully to ensure that they receive adequate colostrum and pass the meconium.

retch Gagging response, often immediately prior to vomiting.

rete A fibrous network.

reticular activating system (RAS) The thalamic brain centre where fibres in the ascending tract of the spinal cord terminate and cause the animal to

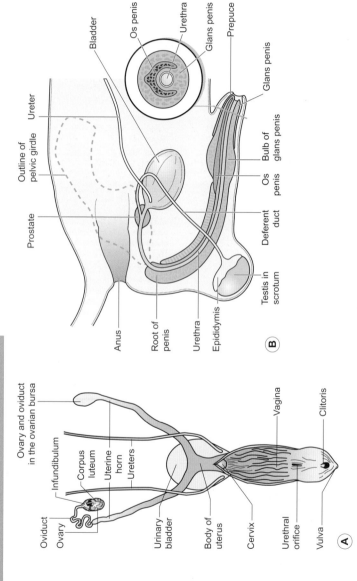

Figure 39. Reproductive tract. (a) Female; (b) male. Redrawn with permission from Aspinall V, O'Reilly M. Introduction to veterinary anatomy and

become stimulated and alert to sensation; *see also* SPINOTHALAMIC.

reticulocyte An immature red blood cell.

reticuloendothelial system Part of the immune system protecting the body with macrophages widely dispersed. The system comprising cells from the bone marrow, spleen, liver and lymphoid tissue; the cells share a common embryonic ancestry and are involved in fighting infection and producing antibodies and blood cells.

retina The light-sensitive membrane lining the back of the eye.

retinaculum A fibrous band of tissue that acts as a retaining strap to hold a tendon or ligament in the correct place.

retinal atrophy Degeneration of the retina, broadly divided into forms affecting the photoreceptors (generalized progressive retinal atrophy (PRA)) and those affecting the pigment epithelium (retinal pigment epithelium dystrophy). The conditions are inherited, with generalized PRA occurring in many breeds, including setters, poodles and retrievers. The first clinical sign is often night blindness and the condition worsens until the animal is totally blind; a control scheme operates in the UK, run by the Kennel Club and British Veterinary Association and annual ophthalmological examinations are required; *see also* RETINAL PIGMENT EPITHELIUM DYSTROPHY.

retinal dysplasia A congenital condition where the retina is thrown into folds or rosettes; breeds affected include the beagle, Rottweiler, Yorkshire terrier, Bedlington terrier, Labrador, cocker spaniel and English springer spaniel.

retinal haemorrhage Bleeding between the retina and the choroid, or sometimes into the vitreous humour. It may be the result of trauma or some hereditary defect, such as the collie eye anomaly, retinal dysplasia, etc. Detachment of the retina also occurs.

retinal pigment epithelium Part of the retina; the single cell layer between the photoreceptors (rods and cones) and the choroid.

retinal pigment epithelium dystrophy (RPED) Disease of the retinal pigment epithelium, where deposits of brown lipopigment build up, leading to destruction of photoreceptors and retinal atrophy; the peripheral retina remains intact and so sight is poor, particularly in bright light, but total blindness is rare; affected breeds include the retrievers, spaniels, briard, sheepdogs and collies.

retractor A surgical instrument used for holding tissues away from the operating site; may be self-retaining or hand-held.

retrobulbar Lying behind the globe of the eye but within the orbit, e.g. **retrobulbar abscess**.

retroflexion Bending back upon itself, e.g. the bladder may be exteriorized and retroflexed during a cystotomy, so that the incision can be made into the dorsal bladder wall.

retrognathia The condition of having the lower jaw shorter than the upper jaw; overshot jaw.

retrograde In the reverse direction.

retrograde urethrography A procedure in which positive contrast agent is injected into the urethra and fills towards the bladder, in the opposite direction to normal urine flow.

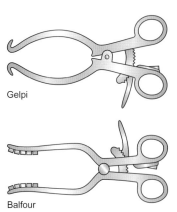

Figure 40. Retractors, two types of self-retaining: Gelpi and Balfour.

retrovirus A family of viruses including human immunodeficiency virus, maedi and visna.

rhabdomyolysis Condition found in racing greyhounds and other dogs involved in vigorous activity. The signs after exercise are painful back muscles and dark yellow-to-brown urine.

rhabdomyoma Benign tumour of striated (skeletal and cardiac) muscle.

rhabdomyosarcoma Malignant tumour of striated (skeletal and cardiac) muscle.

rhabdovirus Formerly a virus in the grouping that included rabies; *see also* RABIES.

rhamphotheca A keratin layer over the beak.

rheumatoid arthritis An immune-mediated, erosive, inflammatory polyarthropathy; cartilage and bone are eroded within affected joints, the condition progressing towards an ankylosed end stage. Treatment options include analgesics, immunosuppressive therapy, cytotoxic drugs and gold injections.

rhexis Rupture of a blood vessel, resulting in frank haemorrhage.

rhinarium The hairless area of the nose around the nares.

rhinitis Inflammation of the nasal mucous membranes within the nasal chambers and sinuses.

rhinotheca A keratin layer over the maxillary beak.

rhinotomy Surgical opening of the nasal passages.

rhodopsin The pigment in the rods of the retina; visual purple; the pigment is bleached by the action of sunlight but is restored in the dark.

rhonchus A musical sound heard during inspiration or expiration when air is passing through constricted bronchi and bronchioles.

rhus tox Homeopathic remedy used for the treatment of muscle and joint pain, itchy and red skin disorders.

rhythm Repetitive pattern such as in the cardiac cycle sounds.

rib Curved bones forming the thoracic wall.

ribonucleic acid *See* RNA.

ribosome An intracellular granule of ribonucleic protein that is the site of protein synthesis.

rickets Skeletal disease occurring in puppies fed a diet lacking vitamin D and phosphorus; rare nowadays; leads to failure of endochondral ossification, with painful enlargement of the growth plates. **Renal rickets** occurs if the conversion of vitamin D to its active metabolites by the kidney is impaired and phosphate excretion is blocked, as in some congenital renal disorders; in these cases, mineral is absorbed from the skeleton, to a degree where the mandibles become soft and malleable (rubber jaw).

Rickettsia Genus of pleomorphic Gram-negative bacteria causing diseases such as Rocky Mountain spotted fever.

RIDDOR The Reporting of Injuries, Diseases and Dangerous Occurrences Regulations 2013; legislation governing the recording of accidents in the workplace, making it the responsibility of the injured person to ensure that the accident book is filled in, although anyone can fill in the book on behalf of the injured person. Under this legislation the employer is responsible for reporting serious accidents/incidents to the Health and Safety Executive (HSE) within a certain time frame.

Rideal–Walker test Measure of the effectiveness of a disinfectant at killing microorganisms.

rigor mortis Stiffening of a cadaver that occurs 1–6 hours after death; rigor mortis then wears off after approximately 24 hours, depending on the ambient temperature.

RIM test A rapid immunological test for feline leukaemia virus, where the p27 antigen is bound by antibody conjugated to colloidal gold.

rima glottidis The space between the two vocal cords at the entrance to the larynx.

ringbone Osteoarthritis of the pastern joints in the horse.

Ringer's solution Isotonic solution, a physiological aqueous solution for fluid therapy; contains sodium chloride, potassium chloride and calcium chloride; used to replace water loss and as a topical physiological salt solution;

see also HARTMANN'S SOLUTION.

ringing The fitting of a uniquely numbered metal band around a bird's leg for identification.

ringworm Fungal skin disease; see also DERMATOPHYTOSIS, MICROSPORUM CANIS, TRICHOPHYTON.

risk management Culture, structure and system that is used to identify potential opportunities and minimize adverse effects.

RNA Ribonucleic acid; a single-stranded, helical molecule consisting of ribose sugars, linked by the purines adenine and guanine, and the pyrimidines cytosine and uracil; **messenger RNA** carries the genetic code from DNA in the nucleus out to the cytoplasm of a cell; ribosomal RNA controls protein synthesis within the cell and **transfer RNA** brings specific amino acids to the ribosomes for protein synthesis.

road traffic accident *See* RTA.

roaring Abnormal sound when air is breathed into the throat of a horse.

Robert Jones bandage A useful first aid and orthopaedic support bandage for the distal limbs; the dressing includes several thick layers of cotton wool or padding, that are then firmly compressed by a bandage; the central toes are left uncovered.

rod Light-receptive cell forming part of the neuroretina; contains rhodopsin and provides night/dusk vision.

rodent ulcer Eosinophilic granuloma; an erosive lesion most commonly affecting the upper lip in cats; possibly has an immune mechanism and generally responds to steroids, although antibiotics may also be indicated if there is secondary infection.

Romanowsky's stain A compound stain containing eosin and methylene blue, used for differential white cell counts and examination of blood smears.

rongeurs Surgical instrument with jaws for cutting and removing bone.

root The part of the tooth below the gum margin where pulp is found; this can be removed in a root filling.

root cause analysis A technique used for identifying the primary cause of a problem/incident so that it can be addressed to prevent recurrence.

rose Bengal A red/pink stain used occasionally in bacteriology.

Rose–Waaler test An immune-based test carried out on a blood sample to help to confirm a diagnosis of rheumatoid arthritis.

rostellum The cranial part of the scolex (mouthpart) of a tapeworm, often carrying a ring of hooks to anchor the parasite to the intestinal wall.

rostral Term used to describe structures on the head that are towards the nose.

rot Term often used to imply a fungal infection, e.g. **fin rot** in ornamental fish.

rotavirus Group of RNA viruses with a wheel-like structure; a common cause of diarrhoea in neonates.

Rothera's test A test for the presence of ketone bodies, where urine is mixed with reagent and develops a purple colour if ketones are present.

roughage The indigestible fibre in the diet.

rouleaux formation Aggregation of erythrocytes in a blood smear to form long columns; a normal finding in the horse and the cat, when it looks like a pile of coins.

round ligament The distinct band of fibrous tissue running in the lateral edge of the broad ligament of the uterus.

roundworm Group of fleshy endoparasitic worms that occur mainly in immature

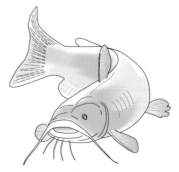

Figure 41. Catfish: fins liable to rot.

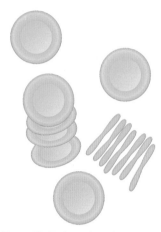

Figure 42. Rouleaux formation.

animals; *see also* ASCARID, *TOXOCARA CANIS*.

Royal Army Veterinary Corps (RAVC) The part of the army in the UK that provides veterinary care for the horses, dogs, etc. used in the armed forces, now part of the Army Medical Service (AMS).

Royal Charter A formal document issued by a monarch to grant powers to a body or corporation; the Royal College of Veterinary Surgeons was created by royal charter in 1844, with the most recent update coming into effect in 2015; this charter also recognizes veterinary nursing as a profession.

Royal College of Veterinary Surgeons (RCVS) The governing body of the veterinary profession. Individuals must be registered with the RCVS to practise in the UK; the RCVS draws up professional codes of conduct, advises the government on legislative issues and oversees veterinary and veterinary nurse training and examination. The RCVS has to maintain a register of veterinary surgeons and veterinary nurses.

Royal Veterinary College (RVC) Founded in London in 1792, the RVC is the oldest and largest UK veterinary school, providing veterinary and paraveterinary courses. In 1999 it became the first UK veterinary school to be accredited by the American Veterinary Medical Association.

RPA *See* RADIATION PROTECTION ADVISOR.

RPS *See* RADIATION PROTECTION SUPERVISOR.

RSI Repetitive strain injury; pain in muscles and tendons resulting from chronic overuse, often work-related, e.g. as a result of long hours at a computer with poor posture. Work-related RSI should be reported to your employer.

RQP 'Responsible qualified person'; person who is permitted to dispense POM-VPS medication. A RQP is defined as a registered veterinary surgeon or a registered pharmacist or a registered suitably qualified person (SQP). Persons qualified to dispense VMP must have been registered with a body that has provided training to them and they must then have passed an examination and be present at each sale of a VMP. The prescribing RQP must be satisfied that the person administering the product (an SQP) has the competence to do so safely.

RTA Road traffic accident; common type of accident suffered by dogs, cats and other animals; any animal that has been in an RTA should be examined as soon as possible to assess the extent of the injuries and should be treated for shock.

rub, pericardial Sound heard on auscultation when the two layers of the pericardium rub over each other.

rub, pleural Sound heard on auscultation when the visceral and parietal layers of the pleura rub against each other.

rubber jaw *See* RICKETS.

rubor Redness; one of the classical signs of inflammation. *See also* CALOR, DOLOR, TUMOR.

rubricyte One stage in the maturation of the red blood cell in which the nucleus is still present; *see also* NORMOBLAST.

ruga, *pl.* **rugae** A fold, particularly in the lining of the stomach.

ruminant Herbivorous animal with a four-chambered stomach, consisting of the rumen, reticulum, omasum and abomasum such as cattle.

rumination Regurgitation of food from the rumen back up to the mouth for further chewing before being swallowed again; an important part of the digestive process in ruminants.

rupture A traumatic tear in the wall of an organ.

ruptured bladder Tearing of the bladder wall caused by trauma or overdistension, e.g. blocked urethra.

ruptured spleen Traumatic tearing of the capsule of the spleen that may result in significant and life-threatening internal haemorrhage; neoplasia is another cause.

Rush pin A metal pin, used as a pair for internal fracture fixation.

R

S

Sabouraud's agar Culture medium used in mycotic disease diagnosis; has a low pH of 5.6 and additional glucose content; *see also* RINGWORM.

sabulous Sand-like, usually referring to calculus material in the cat with urethral obstruction; *see also* CALCIUM OXALATE, FELINE UROLOGICAL SYNDROME, STRUVITE.

sac Term for a purse-like structure; the respiratory system of birds depends on such air-filled cavities.

saccharide Carbohydrate energy source; depending on number of groups present may be mono-, di-, tri-, oligo- or polysaccharide.

saccule Term for a small purse or bag-like structure; the small cavity at the base of the semicircular canals of the ear is the saccule connecting to the utricle.

sacculitis, anal Inflammation of the lining of the anal sacs; causes the production of foul-smelling liquid; irritation to the perineal area may make the dog slide or 'scoot' or bite at the hindquarters; *see also* ANAL SAC DISEASE.

sacral Relating to the area of the back known as the sacrum.

sacral artery The final part of the dorsal aorta continues to the tail as the median sacral artery.

sacral dysgenesis Disease where there is a failure of bone development, sometimes associated with urinary incontinence.

sacrococcygeal Relating to the area posterior to the sacrum running to the coccygeal vertebrae.

sacrococcygeal agenesis A failure of development of the vertebrae of the tail area; seen in old English sheep dogs or 'bobtails'.

sacrococcygeal fusion An extension of the fused vertebrae that make up the sacrum into the first coccygeal vertebra; a condition sometimes seen in radiographs.

sacrococcygeal luxation The result of accidents to the pelvic region; nerve damage is the main complication.

sacroiliac Relating to the articulation of the cranial end of the sacrum with the wing of the ilium on either side; the joint is usually fibrous and may be easily damaged in RTAs; especially liable to such injury is a cat that has been dragged under a vehicle.

sacrolumbar Relating to the articulation of the sacrum with the last lumbar vertebra, often the site of pain on palpation in older dogs; *see also* DEEP PAIN SENSATION.

sacrosciatic ligament The fibrous band that connects the sciatic tuberosity of the ilium to the sacrum.

sacrum The three fused vertebrae at the base of the spine with a narrow triangular shape have this special name, from the Greek word for 'sacred bone'.

safe light Method of illumination in photographic dark room that allows the operator to view negatives without harming the image; the colour of filter used must be suitable for each type of film.

sagittal Like an arrow (L. *sagitta*) cutting an object into two; the **sagittal plane** is, therefore, parallel to the median plane.

SAIDS Simian acquired immunodeficiency syndrome; a virus infection of primates similar to AIDS.

salicylate Salt used medicinally in many products such as aspirin; it has antipyretic and anti-inflammatory properties; the first pharmaceutical discovery made was that willow tree bark was of benefit in rheumatic disorders.

saline (normal saline) Common salt or sodium chloride, widely used in nursing as a solution for flushing wounds and for fluid therapy; normal saline is isotonic at 0.9% solution.

saliva Secretion in the mouth that lubricates the food, maintains a protective coat on the mucous membranes, has some digestive enzyme content, and especially in cats, is a valuable substance for washing and grooming the rest of the body; can be reliably used to measure hormones such as cortisol; *see also* CORTISOL.

salivary Relates to the production of saliva.

salivary amylase Enzyme secreted in very small quantities in the mouth to commence carbohydrate digestion.

salivary ducts The tubular connection of one of four pairs of salivary glands with the mouth.

salivary glands The four paired glands found in the dog and cat are zygomatic, sublingual, mandibular and parotid. They are responsible for the secretion of saliva into the oral cavity via the salivary ducts.

salivary mucocele Leakage of saliva from a damaged duct results in a subcutaneous swelling. The first injury or obstruction of a duct may be unnoticed, but often an enormous nonpainful swelling appears at the angle of the jaws; *see also* MULTILOCULAR RANULA.

Salmonella Group of Gram-negative bacteria associated with enteric diseases. Distinguished on culture as nonlactose-fermenting organisms; *see also* MACCONKEY'S AGAR, ZOONOSIS.

SALP *See* ALKALINE PHOSPHATASE.

salping- Relating to the uterine tubes; **salpingitis** may be a cause of infertility.

salpinx 1) The uterine tube. **2)** The auditory tube.

salt Chemical definition is a combination of a base and an acid. Sodium bicarbonate is an example of a salt. **Bile salts** are substances found in the liver secretion that help in the digestion of fats. **Common salt** is sodium chloride. **Epsom salts** are magnesium sulphate, formerly used for wound lavage, poulticing and for their laxative properties.

Salter–Harris fracture classification Classification system for fractures in skeletally immature animals that involve the growth plate region of long bones.

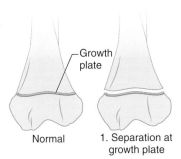

Normal

1. Separation at growth plate

2. Separation above growth plate

3. Separation below growth plate

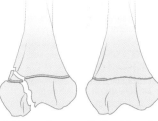

4. Separation through growth plate

5. Crushing of growth plate

Figure 43. Salter–Harris fracture classification.

sample 1) Specimen usually collected for laboratory tests. **2)** Statistically, the number that needs to be analyzed to produce an accurate picture of the whole population.

sand Gritty material with a silica base; may be the cause of irritation to dogs running on sand surfaces – especially racing greyhounds.

sandfly Insect from Mediterranean countries more associated with woodland than sandy shorelines, important as a vector for leishmaniasis.

sanguin(o)- Prefix indicating blood; pus with a pinkish blood tinge is **sanguinopurulent**.

S–A node The sinoatrial node, the microscopic area of the heart muscle that sets the pace of the beat by the discharge of rhythmic electric impulses; situated in the right atrium muscle; *see also* A–V NODE.

saphenous vein Superficial vein on the lateral aspect of the hindleg above the tarsus. Site of venepuncture as an alternative to the forelimb or the neck.

saprolegnia A water mould that can secondarily infect skin lesions in fish.

saprophyte Free-living group of bacteria usually feeding on dead or decaying matter.

Sarcocystis Genus of parasitic protozoon closely related to Coccidia. Dogs are the final hosts for some species and oocysts appear in the faeces; they are not associated with canine disease. The intermediate hosts, such as sheep or humans, may have the disease sarcocystosis.

sarcoid A small tumour on the skin surface, not usually malignant.

sarcolemma The plasma membrane covering the striated muscle fibres.

sarcoma Type of malignant tumour; *see also* LYMPHOSARCOMA, OSTEOSARCOMA.

sarcomere Smallest contractile unit of muscle tissue, made of thin protein fibres of actin and thicker fibres of myosin.

Sarcoptes Genus of external parasites, the cause of pruritus and mange. The mites are usually detected by skin scrapings, which may have to be taken from several sites; sometimes it is necessary to use blood tests to confirm a suspected problem.

sarcoptic mange A type of mange characterized by intense itchiness and caused by *Sarcoptes scabiei*, which may be very difficult to find in skin scrapings. An antibody test is available to examine the blood for exposure to a previous infection with the mite.

SARD Sudden acquired retinal degeneration; sudden blindness occurring over 1–2 days; associated with Cushing's disease.

SARS Suspected Adverse Reaction Surveillance Scheme; the scheme for veterinary medicines is operated by the Veterinary Medicines Directorate. Adverse reactions are reported on the yellow form (MLA 252A Rev 8/01).

sartorius muscle Muscle on the inner surface of the hindlimb, the so-called 'tailor's muscle' from the time when such workers sat cross-legged and the muscle hypertrophied.

SAT Serum agglutination test.

satiety Term used in nutrition to describe the feeling of being filled or fully satisfied; *see also* FEEDING ON DEMAND.

SAVSNET Small Animal Veterinary Surveillance Network; group set up for scanning surveillance to monitor disease trends in companion animals.

saws Used orthopaedically, may be oscillating or wire; *see also* GIGLI SAW.

s.c. Subcutaneous route; **SC** or **SQ** are alternatives.

scab A crust on the skin surface; *see also* SARCOPTIC MANGE.

scabies Human disease caused by *Sarcoptes scabiei*.

scala tympani Part of the cochlea of the ear.

scald Moist heat necrosis of the superficial skin layers, but sometimes deep penetration if the hot fluid unavoidably remains in contact with the skin; *see also* BURN.

scaler Instrument to remove dental calculus; *see also* ULTRASONIC.

scale rot Infectious dermal ulceration; areas of necrotic ulceration on the skin of a snake; treated with antibiotics, supportive therapy and improved environmental management.

scalpel Instrument for cutting tissue; detachable blades of various shapes are available; *see also* BARD–PARKER.

scaly face/leg Red, crusty scales on the unfeathered area of a bird's legs, caused by the mite *Cnemidocoptes mutans*; treated by wiping the area with surgical spirit or covering with petroleum jelly; *see also* CNEMIDOCOPTES.

scan A method of producing an image used diagnostically, as in ultrasound or computed tomography.

scaphoid bone Skeletal bone found in the carpus.

scapula Triangular skeletal bone forming the top of the shoulder and the joint with the humerus; *see also* GLENOID CAVITY.

scar Fibrous contracted tissue, the result of healing after an incision, burn, scald, abscess, etc.

scatter 1) Implies a wide distribution. 2) Incident photons in radiography that may interact with solid tissues. **Back scatter** is a type of diversified ionizing radiation that occurs in X-ray work; cassettes are designed to absorb and reduce this effect; tables must be covered with lead rubber.

scattered or secondary radiation The amount is small in cats, thin patients and whenever a lower kilovoltage is used; it causes blackening of X-ray plates, thus reducing image quality. Always a hazard to personnel and precautions are necessary.

scavenging of anaesthetics Safety measures should be used to remove toxic and hazardous gases from the operating room. Active and passive systems are available.

SCC *See* SQUAMOUS CELL CARCINOMA.

SCFA Short-chain fatty acid.

Schedule 3 Regulation of vital importance in veterinary nursing that gives authority for procedures undertaken by registered veterinary nurses. Amendments to paragraphs 6 and 7 allow for suitably qualified nurses to provide care and treatment for all animal species, not only pets.

Schedule 3 procedures Minor surgical procedures that may be carried out by a Registered Veterinary Nurse under the Veterinary Surgeons Act and do not involve entering a body cavity.

Schiff–Sherrington response Extensor rigidity of the forelegs and a flaccid paralysis of the hindlegs with absence of deep pain sensation; *see also* NEUROLOGICAL SIGNS.

Schirmer tear test Method of measuring tear secretion and flow by the use of prepared strips of absorbent paper suspended from the lower eyelid.

schisto- Prefix denoting 'a split', as in **schistosomus** for a fetus with an open or split abdomen.

Schroeder–Thomas splint A type of external fixation splint used in the treatment of injury to the proximal limb of cats.

Schwann cells Cells that wrap around the nerve axons to form a myelin sheath to increase the speed of conduction; *see also* MYELIN.

SCI (seasonal canine illness) Sickness, diarrhoea and lethargy in dogs that occurs in the summer and autumn within 72 hours of being walked in woodlands; the cause remains unclear.

sciatic nerve The nerve with sensory and motor components that, in conjunction with the femoral nerve, innervates the hindlimb.

scintigraphy Scanning process used to measure gamma radiation released by body tissue after injecting a radionucleotide intravenously; *see also* TECHNETIUM.

scissors Instrument with apposed two-blade action used frequently in surgical procedures. May be curved or straight, blunt or sharp-tipped; *see also* MAYO SCISSORS.

scissor bite Description used for the closure of the incisor teeth favoured by most dog breed standards; a slight overlap of the front teeth of the upper jaw over those of the lower jaw; *see also* OVERSHOT JAW.

sclera The tough outer casing of the sensitive structures of the eye; a continuous globe structure except for

S

the optic nerve exit and the transparent cornea in front.

scleral ossicles Ring of small bones that maintain the eye shape of the bird.

scleritis Inflammation of the sclera; may be a localized raised patch or a general reddening of the 'white' of the eye; *see also* GLAUCOMA.

scolex The head of the tapeworm, which attaches to the host's intestine wall using either suckers or a series of hooks; *see also* ROSTELLUM.

scoliosis Condition of curvature of the spine, usually a lateral displacement of the neck and back. It may be congenital or acquired; *see also* KYPHOSIS.

scooting A popular term used to describe a dog's action of sliding along with hindlegs extended forwards, usually considered as a sign of anal sac impaction.

scope An abbreviated form used to describe the examination of a part of the body with an endoscope.

-scopy Suffix used to describe the examination of a part.

scoring Indicates a method of assessing radiographically the condition of hip or elbow joints; *see also* GRADING.

scours Popular descriptive term for diarrhoea in large animals.

scraping Implies taking superficial or deep samples of skin to detect ectoparasites.

scratching When used radiographically it is a film fault caused by some sharp object or grit damaging the film surface.

screening 1) Term in general use for any series of tests to look for diseases. The Guthrie test was the first such test used on human babies to look for phenylketonuria by testing one drop of urine. 2) Used to include fluoroscopy or dynamic image intensification.

screw Metal fixation device for attaching bone plates or holding fracture fragments in place.

screwtail Inherited condition in the bulldog where the short tail is distorted and presses into the perineum.

Screw worm fly The maggots affect the skin of dogs, cats, sheep and cattle. If left untreated, animals can die in 2 weeks or more; *Chrysomya bexxiana* is a cause of much economic loss and is a notifiable disease in Australia.

scrotal Relating to the sac (scrotum) that contains the male organs for sperm production and the accessory epididymis.

scrub nurse Theatre technician who helps the surgeon by passing instruments, organizing the instrument trolley, swabbing, etc.; the scrub nurse follows the same aseptic technique as the surgeon.

scurf Popular description of skin scales, seen more easily in black- and dark-coated breeds; *see also* CHEYLETIELLA, ZINC.

scurvy Disease of humans associated with vitamin C deficiency. Among animals, only guinea pigs can be affected by a similar deficiency, as other animals synthesize vitamin C.

scutes The keratin shields that form the carapace and plastron of the tortoise.

scybalum A lump or mass of hard faeces.

seasonally polyoestrous Having the reproductive cycle pattern seen in the cat; *see also* OESTRUS.

sebaceous Relating to the production of the greasy skin substance sebum. The **sebaceous glands** are the main sites for finding the parasite *Demodex*.

seborrhoea Skin disorder characterized by excess scaling or sometimes a greasy form is associated with overactive sebaceous glands, masking the keratinization defect.

sebum The oily substance produced by sebaceous glands that helps to seal the skin against water loss and at the same time acts as a bacteria barrier.

second-intention healing Type of healing that occurs where the incision, if sutured, has failed to heal, or as in an open wound, where there has to be granulation tissue formed before the epithelium can cover it over.

secondary Indicates something that develops later.

secondary haemorrhage The type of bleeding that occurs at least some 24 hours after an injury, may be caused by infection of the blood clot or a delayed clotting problem.

secondary radiation *See* SCATTER.

secondary sexual characters Those that develop on maturation; in the bitch and queen, the mammary glands only grow in pseudopregnancy or in pregnancy.

second generation A further development of a drug with improved characteristics, e.g. anticoagulant rodenticides were developed as a safer way of killing rats and mice without harming pets.

secretin Hormone associated with the production of pancreatic and intestinal juice.

section The act of cutting or dividing up. **Caesarean section** is the delivery of one or more fetuses by cutting into the abdominal wall and the uterus; *see also* HYSTERECTOMY, HYSTEROTOMY.

sedation Method of preparing an animal for surgery or helping it to relax during a time of excitement by the use of medication.

sedimentation rate *See* ESR.

sedimentation The settling out of the solid parts of a suspension.

seedy toe A condition in horses where the inner hoof wall becomes separated from the underlying soft tissues, which can cause inflammation and infection because of dirt and debris entering the space; has many possible causes, including chronic laminitis and the yeast *Candida albicans*.

seeing practice Traditional term for veterinary students attending the workplace to learn the art as well as the science of their veterinary duties; *see also* EXTRAMURAL STUDIES.

seizure General term used for an epileptic fit.

selenite broth An enriched culture medium used in the identification of *Salmonella*.

selenium Chemical element used in the treatment of conditions such as muscular dystrophy, often combined with vitamin E.

self-care The practice of activities that will maintain life and health and will promote well being; *see also* OREM.

self-trauma Damage done to an animal by its own actions of biting, scratching or

rubbing at a painful or irritating part; *see also* PRURITUS.

semen White fluid ejaculated from the penis during reproductive activity, rich in spermatozoa.

semen diluent Buffered solution used during the preservation of collected semen. **Frozen semen** is a method of preserving genetic material in liquid nitrogen at $-197°C$, to be used for artificial insemination at a later date.

semicircular canals The balance centre of the inner ear, contained in the bony labyrinth.

semilunar Describes either of the two heart valves shaped like half moons that allow the forward flow of blood from the ventricles; *see also* AORTIC VALVE, PULMONARY VALVE.

semimembranosus muscle A muscle of the group that occupies the caudal aspect of the thigh known as the 'hamstring group'.

seminiferous tubule Structures in the testis where the formation of sperm takes place; *see also* EPIDIDYMIS.

seminoma Testicular neoplasm often associated with cryptorchidism, the hormonal effects are less oestrogenic than others; *see also* SERTOLI CELLS.

semipermeable membrane A separating layer that only allows water and small molecule-sized particles to pass through. Diffusion across the membrane is governed by osmotic pressure, a process with many examples in physiology.

semitendinosus muscle Muscle of the hindleg group that occupies the caudal aspect of the thigh known as the 'hamstring group'.

senile The state of physical and mental deterioration that is part of the ageing process.

sensible losses Losses of fluids that are roughly equivalent to the urine output and any vomit; *see also* INSENSIBLE LOSSES.

sensilla Part of the communication system in insects where sensory hairs are used in olfactory and tactile message giving.

sensitization An alteration in the reaction of the body to the introduction of a foreign substance.

S

sensory Relating to the part of the nervous system that carries the receptors and the transfer of this received information to the spinal cord and the brain.

sensory nerve An afferent nerve conveying information of stimuli received.

sentient Describes an animal that is able to feel, and in some people's minds, is also able to be sensitive, with emotions.

sentinel In the case of dogs, refers to guard dogs; other sentinel animals are also used in the detection of diseases as they spread, e.g. foot-and-mouth disease.

separation anxiety Situation where an animal becomes anxious or distressed when isolated from members of its pack or, more commonly, from its owner.

sepsis The presence of infection in tissues or the blood causing inflammation and tissue destruction; *see also* BACTERAEMIA, TOXAEMIA.

septal Relating to a division or dividing membrane.

septal cells Found within the lung alveoli, secrete surfactants.

septal defect Usually a congenital fault, as in a hole between the two ventricles or atria of the heart.

septicaemia Condition where bacteria are multiplying in the bloodstream; toxins add to the problem; *see also* TOXAEMIA.

septum A dividing wall, as in the nose or heart.

sequelae After-effects; any disorder or pathological condition that follows a disease.

sequestration Formation of a dead or separate part, especially after bone injury.

sequestration, feline corneal Seen as a black, raised spot in the cornea; this is an avascular response to injury.

seroconversion Part of the production of the immune state, measured by the change in the titre of antibodies following the use of a vaccine or possibly after an infection.

serology Study of components of blood serum, e.g. for antibody and antigen presence; may be used diagnostically; *see also* ANTIBODY.

seroma An accumulation of fluid, usually under the skin, following surgery or an injury; may appear on the outside as a tumour-like mass; *see also* HAEMATOMA.

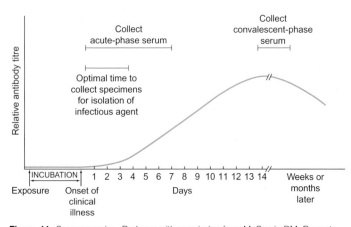

Figure 44. Seroconversion. Redrawn with permission from McCurnin DM, Bassert JM. Clinical textbook for veterinary technicians, 6th ed. St Louis: Elsevier Saunders, 2006.

seropurulent Describes a discharge that is thinner in constituency than normal pus and may indicate a foreign body or a recovery stage after infection.

serosa The name for any serous membrane.

serotonin Hormone and neurotransmitter, also known as 5-hydroxytryptamine; found in many tissues and may be associated with sleep.

serotype The characteristic of a bacterial group recognized by its antigens; *see also* MOLECULAR.

serovar A bacterial variant, as occurs with *Leptospira interrogans*.

Sertoli cell A specialized cell in the testicular tissue that helps the spermatids to mature; may become neoplastic in the older dog, with the production of oestrogens; *see also* CRYPTORCHID.

Sertoli cell tumour Neoplastic growth within the testis that may produce oestrogens, causing feminization. This is a particular risk with the intraabdominal retained testes of the cryptorchid.

serum Biological fluid noted for its antibody content but containing all the liquid elements of plasma (once fibrinogen and the blood cells have been removed in the clot). Usually obtained by taking a blood sample in a plain (preferably glass) container and allowing it to stand long enough to clot. The cool part of a room or a 5°C refrigerator may help the clot to retract and free the serum.

serumal Relating to the production of serum.

serum alkaline phosphatase (SAP) A labile enzyme used in estimation of liver damage and bone activity.

service 1) The physical act of mating; term most used in large animals but occasionally used by dog breeders. **2)** Any provision of supplies or procedures, e.g. a **laboratory service**.

sesamoid Small bone that lies within a tendon, often at a joint flexure point.

sesqui- Infrequently used prefix meaning 'one-and-a-half'.

sessile Flat or adherent, close to the surface.

seta, *pl.* setae Hairs found on insects, used in communication; *see also* ATTENATION.

sevoflurane A volatile liquid anaesthetic gas administered with oxygen or a combination of oxygen and nitrous oxide to induce and maintain anaesthesia. It is a nonflammable, highly fluorinated methyl isopropyl ether with the second fastest onset and offset of anaesthesia after desflurane.

sex 1) The basic difference in the gametes produced by an organism, used in reproduction of the species. **2)** To determine future development into male or female and therefore whether suitable for breeding as pairs, e.g. in birds, kittens and puppies, etc.

sexarche The age at which an individual first becomes involved in breeding.

sex-linked Describes a characteristic or a disease associated with a gene located on a sex chromosome, usually the X chromosome.

sex pili Cell wall structures occurring in Gram-negative bacteria that allow them to stick to the lining of the host's intestinal, respiratory or urinary system; also the manner in which bacteria reproduce by conjugation, passing DNA from donor to recipient cell.

sexual Relating to breeding or to secondary sexual characteristics and behaviour.

sexual behaviour Any usual or unusual activity associated with reproduction.

sexual cycle Oestrous cycle or a pattern of behaviour occurring in some male animals, such as deer in the rutting season.

sexual maturity The time when breeding is possible; may be delayed in some male animals when there are no external signs of maturation.

SG Specific gravity.

SGOT Serum glutamic-oxaloacetic transaminase; used as a liver damage test; *see also* AST.

SGPT Serum glutamic-pyruvic transaminase; used as a test for degree of liver cell damage; *see also* ALT.

shaft 1) The portion of a long bone between the two epiphyses; *see also* DIAPHYSIS. **2)** The hair's main length.

S

shampoo A suspension of detergent and medication used in grooming and for the medical treatment of skin diseases.

shaping Training technique employing successive approximations to a desired end goal; a gradual way of developing the intended behaviour.

sharps Term used for any sharp disposable item such as surgical blades, needles, pins, wires, etc. that must be disposed of safely in specially designed and approved plastic waste bins to prevent injury or contamination.

sheath 1) The outer covering, as used in the microscopic structure of the hair; nerves have myelin sheaths and synovial sheaths cover tendons. 2) Popular word used to describe the male's prepuce.

shell 1) Part of the exoskeleton of the tortoise, consists of a carapace and a plastron. 2) The outermost protection layer of the egg in birds and reptiles.

shell gland Part of the bird's oviduct responsible for producing the tough outer shell of the egg.

Sherman bone plate Traditional form of implant used in fracture repair by internal fixation; the weakness is the narrow part between each screw hole.

shock Profound physiological change in the body with circulatory collapse as the result of trauma, bacterial toxins or allergic response; *see also* FLUID THERAPY.

short-chain fatty acid (SCFA) Important in the production of the watery faeces associated with many diarrhoea conditions.

shoulder The first joint of the proximal limb, between the scapula and the humerus.

shunt A passage connecting two anatomical channels or a diversion. A **left-to-right shunt** is a diversion of the blood from the left side to the right side of the heart, usually caused by a defect in the septum. A **portosystemic shunt** is a congenital disease seen in growing puppies where blood from the intestines passes directly to the right atrium without being processed in the liver.

s.i.d. Dispensing instruction for a medicine to be given once or a single time each day.

sidebones Calcification of the lateral cartilages in the hoof of the horse.

side effect The effect of a drug that happens in addition to the intended effect.

sialagogue A drug that promotes the secretion of saliva.

sicca Term denoting dryness; *see also* KERATOCONJUNCTIVITIS SICCA.

sign Objective, outward evidence of disease e.g. a temperature of 104°F; *see also* SYMPTOM.

signalment Means a visible sign or signs to distinguish; used when taking case histories to record age, sex, breed, etc.

significant event Any undesirable or unexpected event associated with the clinical care of a patient.

silent heat An unobserved breeding period; accounts for presumed anoestrus in bitches, etc.

silicea Used as a homeopathic remedy; it is derived from quartz. Used to expel foreign bodies, such as grass seeds, and in the treatment of sinuses.

silk suture Traditional fine permanent material used for suturing eyelids, etc.

silver Metallic element, also used to describe the coat colour of some breeds.

silver halide Part of the photographic developing process; involves the conversion of exposed particles of silver bromide into black particles of metallic silver, which remain on the final plate.

silver nitrate Prepared in sticks, it may be used as a chemical cautery to control bleeding or treat superficial warts.

simian Describes a member of the ape and the monkey family.

sinoatrial node *See* S–A NODE.

sinus 1) A blind-ended infected tract or drainage channel. 2) Term used anatomically for any air- or fluid-filled cavity.

sinus arrhythmia During the pulse measurement of the normal patient, the pulse rate increases on inspiration and decreases on expiration; a normal variation.

sinusitis Inflammation of one of the sinus cavities of the skull, often the result of an upper respiratory tract infection.

situ At that site.

situs invertus The right-to-left inversion of the body organs, e.g. heart and liver, a rare genetic fault affecting thorax and abdomen disposition.

SI units A standard of 'Système International' units; replaced many of the traditional units of measurement.

skatole A protein breakdown product that causes one of the characteristic odours of fresh faeces.

skeletal muscle The voluntary muscles under control of the nervous system; *see also* STRIATED.

skeleton The bony framework that supports the body and largely determines its shape. .

ski slope Term used in radiological diagnosis to describe the shape of the anconeal process when affected by osteophytes; *see also* OSTEOCHONDROSIS.

skin The outer covering, and therefore, the largest organ of the body. Variously covered with hair, feathers and scales and carrying pigment; *see also* CUTIS, DERMIS, EPIDERMIS.

skin glue *See* DERMAL ADHESIVE.

skin tenting The reduced rate at which the skin returns to its normal position after being pulled up and released. This can be a late indication of dehydration; also known as skin turgor.

skull The skeletal structure of the head, made up of many fused bones; the mandible is the only articulating structure.

skyline view One used radiographically to get an angled or silhouetted view.

SLE Systemic lupus erythematosus; an autoimmune disease characterized by chronic skin changes; *see also* LUPUS.

sleep A natural state of unconsciousness in which brain activity is not apparent. '**Put to sleep**' is a lay term for euthanasia; it is difficult to be certain about the intention – a signed authority is best obtained to avoid the possibility that the owner thinks it is a form of anaesthesia that is being described. **Rapid eye movement (REM) sleep** describes a stage of sleep where the muscles of the eye are in constant motion, equated with dreaming.

sleeper disease State of immobility in hamsters, that may mimic death, arising when the room temperature is too high.

sleeping sickness Eastern equine encephalitis, a viral disease of horses on the coastal eastern plains of North and South America; transmitted by mosquitoes, causing a high fever and paralysis leading to death; vaccines are available.

slide A piece of glass used in examination under the microscope. An **acetate tape slide** is used in obtaining superficial parasites of the skin for transfer to the laboratory.

slime disease Deposition of a layer of mucus over the body of a fish, often reflecting poor water quality and caused by protozoa.

sling A support for an injured part of the body; helps to promote rest; *see also* EHMER SLING, VELPEAU SLING.

slit lamp A piece of ophthalmic equipment that focuses a high-intensity slit light beam at the anterior structures of the eye while the examiner looks through a magnifying scope.

SLOB 'Same lingual opposite buccal' term used in dentistry to describe X-ray positioning for the three roots of the carnassial tooth.

Slocum plate Orthopaedic implant used in triple pelvic osteotomy.

slough A piece of dead tissue, often peels away from the living tissue underneath. **Anaesthetic slough** is a necrotic area of skin and underlying vein caused by perivascular injection of an irritant such as thiopental.

slow Not rapidly developing; some infections are caused by a slow virus; *see also* LEUKAEMIA, PRIONS.

small A diminutive term as used in small bowel or smallpox.

small intestine Includes the duodenum, jejunum and ileum.

S

smear A method of examining a specimen under the microscope by spreading a film across a glass slide.

smegma Greasy substance found outside the vulva in overweight bitches. Occurs also in the prepuce of horses.

smell Odour or fragrance detected by the receptor cells of the mucous membrane covering the ethmoturbinate bones of the nose.

smoke injury Animals involved in fires may cough only slightly at first but then develop pneumonia and pulmonary oedema caused by the inhaled smoke particles becoming attached to the lower bronchial airway, even into the alveoli.

smooth muscle Type of muscle without conscious control, opposite of voluntary muscle. Found in intestine, bladder, iris of eye, etc.; *see also* INVOLUNTARY MUSCLE.

smothering One cause of neonatal death, resulting from overcrowding of puppies and kittens.

smudge cells Seen in blood smears as indistinct cells with pale eosinophilic nuclear material lacking shape; a sign of degeneration or excessive pressure being applied when the slide was made.

snake Reptiles are often kept as pets; the nurse should ask the attendant whether the patient is poisonous before handling it; large pythons will crush their victim and a second person should always be present in case of injury.

snoring Reverberating noise from the soft palate and pharynx on inspiration or exhalation; adjusting the head position may reduce the noise produced.

snuffles Nasal sound produced by cats after sinusitis; small mammals with upper respiratory tract infections also breathe like this.

social Relating to animals living in a community.

social behaviour Behaviour of a domestic animal that is not harmful to its fellows, especially those in the same group or locality.

social distance The spacing out of animals such as birds on a telephone line or cats in suburban gardens.

socialization Process of adapting to living with other animals or humans; one of the necessary duties of a 'puppy walker' is to introduce the recently weaned animal to human carers and other external experiences.

social order The hierarchy that allows animals to coexist without constant fighting; depends on dominant and submissive behaviour patterns.

soda A salt containing sodium, often associated with the release of carbon dioxide. Old (flat) soda water is a first-aid drink for dogs that have vomited frequently. **Baking soda** is sodium bicarbonate, used for teeth cleaning or in dilute solution as a skin wash. **Washing soda** is sodium carbonate; a large crystal makes an effective emetic for a dog.

soda lime Used in anaesthetic circuits to absorb carbon dioxide; consists of a colour indicator for the combination of sodium hydroxide and calcium hydroxide, together with silicates to reduce dust.

sodium Chemical element; symbol Na for natrium, hence hyponatraemia for low serum level.

sodium bicarbonate A salt used in first aid and as an antacid.

sodium carbonate Washing soda; used as an emetic; *see also* VOMIT.

sodium chlorate Cause of severe poisoning in dogs that have accidentally ingested weedkiller.

sodium chloride Common salt, used in emergency oral fluid therapy.

sodium cyanide Poisonous substance used in certain chemical plants, sometimes causing fish to die in contaminated watercourses.

sodium hydroxide Caustic soda used in degreasing; strongly alkaline.

sodium hypochlorite Mild antiseptic used for sterilizing feeding bottles, etc.

sodium lactate Compound included in Hartmann's solution to provide bicarbonate.

sodium pump Cell-regulating mechanism to maintain the isotonic state.

soft palate The caudal part of the pharynx that can be used to seal off the nasopharynx, oesophagus and larynx.

solanine Toxic compound found in green potatoes.

solar Relating to the sun. **Nasal solar dermatitis** is crusty dermatosis known as 'collie nose'.

solar burns Dermal necrosis, especially caused by ultraviolet radiation.

solid phase immunoassay Diagnostic method often using microtitre wells, dipsticks or immunofiltration solid-phase assay kits; based on specific monoclonal antibodies.

solute The dissolved part when a solution is made up from a solid and a solvent.

solution A mixture in which a solid is evenly distributed in the liquid solvent.

solvent The liquid in which another substance is dissolved to form a solution; some propellant and volatile liquids have been used for their stimulatory effects on humans; *see also* POISON.

soma The entire body, excluding the germ cells.

somatic Describes cells that relate to the animal's body; *see also* NERVE.

somatostatin Hormone secreted by the pituitary and the islets of Langerhans in the pancreas; inhibits the production of insulin and glucagon.

somatotrophin Growth hormone.

soporific Sleep-inducing substance.

sore A name for any abrasion or ulcerating area. A **bed sore** is a pressure sore, usually on the elbow or bony prominences; *see also* DECUBITUS. **Pressure sore** is a general term for any skin damage in a recumbent animal, most often on the elbows but can occur on the shoulders or hindlegs of greyhounds.

sore hocks Common condition of rabbits where hair loss, thickening and ulceration occur on the plantar aspect of the hocks; requires improved environmental conditions.

sour crop Candidiasis of the crop, there is often a pungent smell and the crop can feel soft; treated with ketoconazole; see CROP.

space Any unfilled area. **Dead space** is a surgical term for a cavity left after an excision, liable to fill with serum or blood. The **epidural space** is the space outside the spinal cord membranes, usually containing fat; used for filling with an anaesthetic substance; *see also* REGIONAL ANAESTHESIA. The **intercostal space** is the space occupied by muscles between two ribs and provides an access point to the chest. The **subarachnoid space** is the space between the arachnoid mater and the pia mater, the membranes around the brain and spinal cord; contains the CSF.

spasm A sustained involuntary muscle contraction, most serious when it restricts a channel such as the airway; *see also* BRONCHOSPASM, LARYNGOSPASM.

spasmolytic Medication that relieves spasms of smooth muscle.

spastic Characterized by spasms.

spavin Osteoarthritis in the hock joint of the horse.

spay From an early English word meaning to neuter the female; *see also* GELD.

specialist A person who, by special studies, concentrates on one species of animal or one particular branch of his/her profession. Only veterinary surgeons currently listed can call themselves 'RCVS specialists'. Other veterinary surgeons can call themselves 'specialists' provided they can substantiate their claim. If a practice indicates that it only deals with one particular species or is mainly restricted to a particular species, it must ensure that specialist status is not implied where this is not the case.

specific Particular, one that is clearly distinguishable from others.

specific drug A medicine that has particular properties to cure a disease.

specific gravity The relative density of a liquid.

specimen 1) A sample usually obtained from the animal patient. **2)** May mean an unusual or unique sample.

spectinomycin Broad-spectrum antibiotic used mainly against Gram-negative bacterial infections.

spectrum, broad Describes a medication with a wide band of activity against microorganisms.

S

speculum An instrument, usually trumpet-shaped, for examining or dilating a body orifice to see inside.

sperm *See* SPERMATOZOON.

spermatic cord Suspensory ligament structure of the testis that contains an artery, a vein, a nerve and a muscle as well as the vas deferens.

spermatid A juvenile or developing spermatozoon produced by meiotic division, one developmental stage before the functioning spermatozoon.

spermatocyte The germ cells produced by the spermatogonium.

spermatogenesis The process of maturation of spermatozoa that takes place within the testis; the cells lie in the seminiferous tubules, eventually passing into the epididymis. Reduction division or meiosis is an important stage in the development so that only one copy of the genetic information is available for the fertilization of the ova; *see also* MEIOSIS.

spermatogonium Cells that line the seminiferous tubules of the testes and are responsible for producing immature sperm or spermatids by meiosis.

spermatozoon, *pl.* **spermatozoa** The mature male sex cell. The tail allows for movement by swimming in a fluid medium, and the head (acrosome) allows for penetration of the ova, when fertilization may take place. In the dog, the spermatozoa can survive for 5 days in the fallopian tube of the bitch after mating.

spermaturia Reflux into the bladder of spermatozoa remaining in the prostate area of the vas deferens.

spermiogenesis The second stage of maturation where the spermatids are developed to form spermatozoa.

spey Alternative spelling for neutering procedure; *see also* SPAY.

sphenoid bone The bone at the base of the skull behind the eyes, so-called because of its wedge shape.

spherocyte 1) Immature red blood cell, often seen with anaemia. 2) Erythrocyte of small size as found in feline blood samples.

spheroma Any tumour shaped like a sphere or ball.

sphincter A circular muscle whose function is to keep an orifice closed until such time as the contents need to be discharged from within; in the case of the pupil, the iris dilates to allow more light to reach the retina.

sphincter mechanism incompetence (SMI) A common cause of urinary incontinence that may occur in 16% of spayed bitches during their lifetime.

sphincterotomy An incision into a sphincter to allow easier passage of contents.

sphygmo- Prefix relating to the pulse in the animal's circulation.

spica bandage A bandage wound around repeatedly in a figure-of-eight pattern so a series of V-marks appear on the outside surface of the bandage.

spicule A small fragment, often spike-shaped.

spiculosis Skin disorder of the Kerry blue terrier where keratin sticks out from the hair follicles, more so on the hindlegs.

spider Member of the Arachnida, an invertebrate; some are terrestrial, some aquatic, some aerial.

spider monkey Small monkey from the New World group, with long legs and a long tail as they are active tree climbers.

spigot Small peg or pin, usually plastic or metallic, used to regulate the flow of liquid from a catheter.

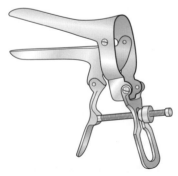

Figure 45. Cusco vaginal speculum.

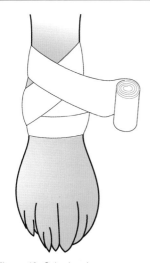

Figure 46. Spica bandage.

spike 1) A sharp point. **2)** The trace on an encephalogram of brain cell activity; *see also* EPILEPSY.

Spilopsylla cuniculi The most common rabbit flea; acts to spread the myxomatosis virus, *see* VECTOR.

spina bifida Developmental fault of the neural tube where part of the spinal cord of the newborn is unprotected by vertebrae.

spinal Relating to part of the CNS and bony vertebral column.

spinal anaesthesia Regional anaesthesia for certain segments of the spine; *see also* EPIDURAL.

spinal column The vertebrae that make up successive parts of the spine.

spinal cord The nerve tissue that occupies the spinal column; *see also* CNS.

spinal muscular atrophy Rare inherited disease affecting movement, with eventual paralysis.

spinal nerve Paired nerves that run from the spinal cord to various structures, exiting between the vertebrae.

spinal reflex A reflex action that involves the nerve impulses passing through localized segments of the spinal cord.

spinal shock Paralysis that develops above and below an injury to the spinal cord accompanied by many of the other circulatory signs of shock.

spindle cell tumour Neoplasm of skin structures; may be malignant in the vertebrae.

spine 1) A sharp prominence; in reptiles a modification of the skin. **2)** Anatomical feature of the skeleton such as the ridge down the scapula or the whole length of the backbone.

spinosad Insecticide used to control flea infestations in dogs and cats; rapid kill within 30 minutes and effect lasts 4 weeks.

spinothalamic tract Main pathway for the transmission of pain sensation, the sensory fibres in the ascending tract of the spinal cord terminate in the thalamus and brainstem; *see also* RAS.

spinous process Bony prominence, well developed in the thoracic vertebrae and less strongly developed in the cervical and lumbar regions.

spirit An alcohol-based liquid; industrial methylated spirit has been used as a disinfectant and for topical application to unbroken skin.

spironolactones A group of potassium-sparing diuretic substances that act on the distal tubule.

splanchnic Relating to the abdominal contents or viscera. The **splanchnic nerves** are part of the sympathetic nervous system; *see also* AUTONOMIC NERVOUS SYSTEM.

splanchnic skeleton Any bone that develops in tissue rather than being part of the axial or appendicular skeletons; *see also* OS PENIS.

spleen One of the abdominal viscera; lies adjacent to the stomach. Its main function is to act as a reservoir for erythrocytes.

splenectomy Surgical removal of the spleen; may be necessary for gross enlargement, e.g. tumour, or uncontrollable haemorrhage, e.g. rupture of the spleen after trauma.

splenomegaly Enlargement of the spleen; causes include neoplasia, gastric torsion

S

or the action of some drugs, e.g. barbiturates.

splint 1) A supporting structure, used in first aid for fixing displaced or fractured bones. **2)** The very slender second and fourth metacarpal/tarsal bones in the horse. **3)** Hard, bony exostoses arising on the cannon bones of horses.

spondylo- Prefix relating to the spine or vertebrae.

spondylosis The production of bony spurs along the ventral borders of the vertebrae, resulting from chronic instability.

spongiform encephalopathy A degenerative condition of the brain characterized on postmortem examination by softened or spongy areas; *see also* BOVINE SPONGIFORM ENCEPHALITIS, CREUTZFELDT–JAKOB DISEASE.

spontaneous abortion Loss of the fetus(es) without apparent external or infectious cause; indicates a hormonal or autoimmune problem.

spontaneous ovulator Normal reproductive pattern where an ovum or ova is/are released at a set point in each reproductive cycle; the cat is an exception, remaining seasonally polyoestrous until mated; *see also* COITUS, REFLEX OVULATOR.

sporadic Indicates an irregular or once-only event; sometimes meaning at distantly placed locations.

spore Resistant form of a bacterium, such as *Clostridium*, or of a fungus.

sprain Injury to a ligament caused by sudden overstretching; *see also* STRAIN.

spray freezing Type of cryosurgery when liquid nitrogen is jetted onto a surface until an ice ball forms.

spraying Undesirable behaviour in cats when urine is used to mark territory, including the living areas of the house; *see also* PHEROMONES.

sprite Spayed female rabbit.

spur veins Veins on the lateral surface of the thorax that lie subcutaneously and can inadvertently be punctured when giving vaccines or other injections by the subcutaneous route. The name comes from similar veins on the horse that can be damaged by a rider's spurs.

sputum Expectorated mucus from the bronchial tubes and lungs, rarely produced in dogs as there is a tendency for such material to be swallowed.

SQP Suitably qualified person; a person suitably qualified for dispensing veterinary medicinal products (VMPs) must have registered with a body that has provided training to him or her and have passed an examination and must be present at each sale of a VMP medicine. Although a clinical assessment of the animal is not a prerequisite, the prescribing Registered Qualified Person must be satisfied that the person administering the product has the competence to do so safely.

SQ ('sub q') An abbreviation for the subcutaneous route for giving drugs or an entry point for a drain or feeding tube.

squab An immature pigeon, often poorly feathered.

squamous Involving a thin, plate-like layer.

squamous cell carcinoma A type of malignant tumour, not uncommon as a cause of cancer in the cat's mouth often treated by radical surgery; *see also* HEMIMANDIBULECTOMY.

squint Angulation of the eyes; seen in some cats; may be divergent or convergent.

SRM Steroid-responsive meningitis.

S–T segment The part of the electrocardiogram trace at the end of each cycle that represents the repolarization of the ventricles.

stabilization Term used in fracture treatment for aiding healing by stopping undue movement between fragments.

stain Substance used to delineate a structure; may be used in microscopy or for a corneal ulcer.

stamp graft Pattern of skin grafting where minute squares are implanted in a postage stamp pattern; *see also* PINCH GRAFT.

standard Regular or normal level.

standard deviation 1) Statistical estimation of the variation found in a number of determinations of the same parameter. **2)** Normal variation allowed in a healthy population of animals for biochemical and other parameters.

standard operating procedures Health and Safety regulations in the UK require these to be written and followed for anything involving a hazard to humans; a written protocol detailing how processes should be performed; *see also* COSHH.

stapes One of the three small bones that form a chain across the middle ear, this one being stirrup-shaped.

staphylo- Prefix relating to the bunch-of-grapes appearance of the causal organism.

Staphylococcus Important genus of Gram-positive bacteria, often the cause of severe skin infection and food toxin illnesses; *see also* MRSA.

staphyloma The exception to 'staphy-' indicating bacterial infection, as it is the swelling of the eye sclera or cornea caused by injury or raised intraocular pressure.

staple A metal fastener used to hold layers of tissue together while they heal; mostly used in skin and gastrointestinal surgery.

stapling The process of using metal staples to hold tissue layers together. Staples are inserted using a surgical stapler. Stapling is most commonly used in skin, intestines and lungs and is a much faster way of closing wounds than traditional suturing.

starch Carbohydrate compound used in storage; enzyme action (ptyalin and amylase) is needed to release sugars.

starvation Either enforced or voluntary deprivation of food; may have irreversible long-term consequences.

stasis Lack of flow, as with an intestinal obstruction; *see also* ILEUS.

State Board examination The examination held by any state in the US that allows a veterinarian to work in that state.

static A form of electrical discharge that can mark undeveloped X-ray film, caused by the films in storage being agitated.

stationary anode The part of the X-ray tube that produces the ionizing radiation.

stationary grid Device used in radiography to reduce scatter when X-rays are directed at thicker parts of the body, more than 10-cm thick.

status epilepticus A severe form of epileptic attack where the body remains in a constant spasm rather than the usual tonic–clonic convulsions of fits; *see also* EPILEPSY.

steatitis An inflammation of fatty tissue, often followed by softening with necrosis; *see also* PANSTEATITIS.

steatorrhoea Excessive fat in the faeces, making them pale-coloured and greasy.

Steinmann pin An intramedullary pin used for fracture fixation.

stem cell Bone marrow haematopoietic cell that is the precursor of both red and white cells.

stem cell therapy A relatively new and developing treatment of collecting and reintroducing stem cells to regenerate damaged tendons, ligaments and joints in horses.

stenosis Narrowing or contraction of an opening; mainly used in describing blood vessel narrowing, e.g. PULMONARY STENOSIS.

Stensen's duct Anatomical name for the duct that drains saliva from the parotid gland to the mouth.

stent A tube or mesh device placed in the body to keep a channel patent, where a blockage or narrowing has occurred, e.g. arterial and urethral stents.

stercus Another word for faeces. Often the adjective is used, as **stercorous**.

stereotypic Describes a behaviour pattern with constant repetition of what may be a quite complicated action. Seen in animals confined in cages for a long time.

sterile 1) Aseptic, incapable of producing microorganism growth. **2)** Infertile or barren, may be applied more commonly in males than females.

sterilization The process of removing all microorganisms and spores using methods such as steam heat, dry heat, chemical(cold), gas plasma or radiation.

sternal Relates to the lower surface area of the thorax over the sternum.

S

sternal recumbency When the animal lies on its chest with limbs equally placed on either side.

sternebrae The chain of sternal cartilages that forms the lower side of the thoracic cavity.

sternocostal Relating to the area where the ribs join the sternum.

sternum Flat structure in mammals made of eight cartilaginous structures (sternebrae) that receive the ribs to support the thorax but allow for flexibility while breathing.

steroid An organic four-ring compound produced naturally by the adrenal cortex; as hormones have potent effects. Steroids are also synthesized and used medically, and one form is used as a cat anaesthetic; *see also* ALPHAXALONE.

stertor Difficult respiration with a characteristic snoring sound.

steth(o)- Prefix relating to the chest area.

stethoscope Instrument for listening to the heart and lung sounds.

stifle The complex joint between the femur and the tibia and fibula and the associated sesamoid bones and cartilages; also known as the knee.

stilbestrol Synthetic oestrogen formerly used as a milk suppressant and for mésalliance. Has benefits in some forms of urinary incontinence but is no longer available.

stillbirth When a fetus is born but there is no evidence of life.

Stille shears A pattern of shears for cutting plaster casts.

stimulant Any medication that stimulates reflex activity, appetite or demeanour.

sting Injury by the proboscis of an insect or a silicone-tipped plant, usually followed by intense irritation.

stippling Speckled body colour pattern; also appears in the haematological examination of red cells as an indicator of anaemia.

stirrup Popular name for the stapes bone found in the middle ear; *see also* ANVIL, STAPES.

stitch Knotted fibre or suture used in repairs.

stitch abscess A reaction to slow-dissolving soluble suture material, sometimes associated with wound infection.

stock control Maintenance of sufficient supplies to cover day-to-day and emergency use.

stoma An orifice; may be natural, like the mouth, or surgically produced; *see also* URETHROSTOMY.

stomach Storage organ of the alimentary tract; can distend in carnivores; acidification and digestion of swallowed food should occur in it; *see also* GASTRIC TYMPANY.

stomatitis Inflammation of the mucous membranes of the buccal cavity.

-stomy Suffix used for procedures that produce a permanent hole, often for drainage of contents.

stone It was the hardness of phosphate calculi that was the origin of this name; *see also* CALCULUS.

stool Word used in human nursing for faeces outside the anus; originally from a 'close stool' or wooden seat used by persons in the production of the product.

storage diseases Includes a group of conditions with defects in enzyme function, leading to metabolic errors; genetic in origin; *see also* METABOLIC.

strabismus Squint, deviation of the pupil direction.

straelensiosis Skin disease caused by a parasitic mite, seen as nodules induced by the invasion of the dog's hair follicles by *Straelensia cynotis*.

strain 1) To overstretch, especially a muscle injury. 2) A particular subtype of an organism. 3) The popular use is to filter or press hard to make something pass through; *see also* TENESMUS.

strangles A highly infectious condition in horses, caused by *Streptococcus equi*; produces constriction of the upper airway.

strangulated Involving restriction of the blood flow, as in a **strangulated hernia**: partial torsion of a hernial sac.

stranguria Slow and painful emission of urine; *see also* CALCULUS.

stratum A layer or anatomical structure, as in the outer layer of the cornea.

stratum basale Base or innermost layer of the skin's epidermis; between the cells are the melanocytes; alternative name is stratum germinativum.

stratum corneum Main layer of outermost skin, consisting of tough, unnucleated cells; modified epidermis but has no blood vessels so repairs more slowly than deeper layers; see also CHELOID.

stratum germinativum The innermost layer of epidermis, which has rapid mitosis to supply skin cells, also known as stratum basale.

stratum granulosum Layer of epidermal cells above the stratum spinosum and below the stratum lucidum, which show signs of flattening and become infiltrated with keratin.

stratum lucidum Layer of the epidermis immediately below the stratum corneum, where cells lose their nuclei.

stratum spinosum Layer of the epidermis immediately above the stratum basale.

strepto- Implies a twisted chain of bodies.

Streptococcus Bacterial genus whose Gram-positive organisms always appear in pairs or in short chains.

streptokinase Fibrinolytic used as an injection in pulmonary thrombosis.

streptomycin An aminoglycoside antibiotic that must be used with caution because of ototoxicity, especially in cats.

stress Physiological state as a result of injury, disease and worry, such as a caged animal in a trap. Stress can be measured by blood pressure changes and cortisol secretion levels apart from behavioural observations.

stress fracture A tiny break in a bone (usually the cannon bone in the horse) causing inflammation in the area of the break.

striated Stripe-marked; in histology, describes the marking on voluntary or skeletal muscle fibres.

striated muscle Name for voluntary skeletal muscle, from its striped appearance when seen with a microscope.

stricture A narrowing of an orifice such as a blood vessel or the oesophagus usually after a foreign body injury.

stridor Louder and harsher than a wheeze; difficult breathing noise from the larynx or trachea; see also LARYNGEAL PARALYSIS.

stringhalt Involuntary flexion of the hock of the horse when walking, giving a 'snatching' action. The cause of this abnormal behaviour is not known. Treatment involves sectioning the lateral digital extensor tendon.

strip graft Pattern for skin grafting where a length of skin is laid across the wound; see also PINCH GRAFT.

strip, mammary A technique used in the treatment of mammary neoplasia in the cat, less popular in the bitch now that individual gland removal and histological sampling is preferred as a less radical alternative to a total excision of all the tissues.

strobila Tapeworm structure arrangement where a chain of proglottids grow away from the head end; a method used for dispersing the tapeworm ova in the host's faeces.

stroke General term for a sudden weakness developing in humans; the result of a reduction in the blood supply to a part of the brain, often from a thrombus, embolism or intracranial haemorrhage. Owners describe a similar sequence in dogs, but they may confuse such attacks with those of vestibular disease. **Heat stroke**: examples of hyperthermia and sudden collapse in animals may be a result of water deprivation and confinement in a closed space such as a walled yard or a car left in the sun.

struck off The removal of a veterinary nurse or surgeon from the RCVS register if they are found guilty of serious or disgraceful misconduct.

struvite calculus Otherwise known as triple phosphate, the commonest calculus found in dogs; also found in cats.

Student Experience Log Record used to monitor skills learned during training; these logs are often electronic repositories held by professional bodies.

stud tail Bare area on the dorsum of the tail seen in breeding animals and

S

short-haired breeds of cat as they grow older; sebaceous gland activity may be detrimental to hair follicle function; also seen in dogs.

stump amputation Description of a limb or tail that has had its distal part removed for surgical reasons.

stupor A state of near unconsciousness with poor response to external stimuli such as noise or light.

stye See HORDEOLUM.

stylet A slender probe, commonly used to stiffen urinary catheters.

styloglossus muscle The muscle that connects the tongue to the stylohyoid bone at the base of the skull. It retracts and raises the tongue as in lapping or in panting.

styloid Pen-shaped or pointed structure, as in **stylohyoid**; used in anatomy.

styptic Something to stop bleeding; assisting blood to clot chemically, e.g. styptic pencil made of anhydrous aluminium sulphate which causes blood vessels to contract on contact.

sub- Prefix meaning 'beneath', 'below'.

subarachnoid The space between the arachnoid membrane and the pia mater; provides a channel for CSF.

subclavian Relating to the area of the axilla or 'under the armpit' or clavicle.

subclinical Describing a disease that is suspected but has not developed with positive symptoms.

subconjunctival Relating to the potential space below the conjunctiva of the eyelid or the sclera that can be used for injection of medications.

subcutaneous (s.c., SC) The most frequently used route for injections in pet practice; the layers beneath the skin are almost painless to approach and have an adequate blood supply.

subcutis Term for the area below the dermis or skin layer, composed of adipose and loose connective tissue; *see also* CELLULITIS.

subfertility State of poor reproductive function so that apparently normal matings produce less than the expected results.

subjective Indicates that it is something experienced by an individual; there may be symptoms not apparent to others.

Subjective, Objective, Assessment, Plan (SOAP) A methodology for recording a hospitalized patient's progress on a daily basis.

sublingual artery One of the available pulse points in an anaesthetized animal – an artery located under the tongue; the adjacent vein may be used as a site for injecting an anaesthetized patient.

sublingual glands Paired salivary glands that are found under the tongue; *see also* RANULA.

subluxation Partial dislocation of a joint where there is still some contact between the bones' articular ends; *see also* LUXATION.

submandibular Relating to the area below the mandibles, subject to swelling after injury or infection.

submandibular lymph nodes Soft nodules that usually can be palpated in the angle of the jaw.

submaxillary Below the eyes, adjacent to the maxilla bone.

submental organ Area of sebaceous glands on the chin of the cat; concerned with scent marking, but cats may develop a sebaceous folliculitis in this area.

submissive urination May occur when the animal is placed in a threatening situation or as a response to a dominating owner; occurs more often in a young dog that is reliably house-clean at other times.

subnormal temperature Body temperature below normal; varies with the species. Temperatures should always be checked a second time before reporting or charting as it can be a sign of a failing metabolism; *see also* TOXAEMIA.

substantia propria The structure that makes up the main thickness of the cornea; it has no blood supply but has sensory nerves.

substrate The substance on which an enzyme reacts. The enzyme increases the speed of the reaction (catalysis) to change the substrate.

sucking Vacuum-assisted means of moving air or liquids into the mouth.

sucking lice One of the two main groups of lice that feed on animals. *Linognathus* is the most common species in the dog.

sucralfate Preparation used in the treatment of gastric irritation; the aluminium sulphate helps to protect the gastric mucosa.

sucrose Cane sugar used medicinally in water to reduce thirst of vomiting dogs; it requires the enzyme sucrase to make the carbohydrate available as a nutrient; *see also* SUGARS.

suction Vacuum apparatus required during surgery to remove fluids and to reinflate the thoracic cavity contents after pneumothorax.

sudoriferous Smelling of sweat.

suffocation Cessation of breathing as a result of drowning or smothering.

sulcus, *pl.* sulci 1) One of the clefts or inward folds of the brain surface. 2) May also be used to describe a groove or furrow in other anatomical structures such as the heart or the penis. The **gingival sulcus** is the groove in the gum where it meets the tooth.

sulpha drugs Those in the sulphonamide group. International form is now moving to 'sulfa', which is also the US form.

sulphonamide One of the first chemotherapeutic groups of drugs used against bacteria, developed before penicillin; the clinical use of this group has decreased in recent years.

sulphosalicylic acid test Original test for protein in the urine; largely superseded by dipstick tests. Positive test is turbidity in the urine sample.

sunburn Inflammation of the skin by ultraviolet rays; severe cases cause skin necrosis, but this is unlikely in breeds that have some amount of natural pigmentation.

sunstroke Heat accumulation is more the result of fluid loss and an inability to replenish by drinking rather than damage to the brain.

summer pasture-associated obstructive pulmonary disease (SPAOPD) Bronchospasm, hypersecretion and airway obstruction that develops whilst horses graze pasture over the warmer months; treatment is based on symptom control and environmental control to remove contact with the trigger.

super- Prefix meaning 'better than', 'excessive' or 'above the normal'.

supernumerary Greater in number than is required or is usual for species; *see also* TEATS.

suppurative In a pus-forming state.

supra- Prefix meaning 'above', 'higher than the rest'.

supravital stains Stains used in the laboratory on living cells to detect inclusions and other cellular material including *Mycoplasma* and *Babesia* species.

surfactant Substance similar to a detergent that is important in the functioning of the lungs; it enables the alveoli to open at birth and reduces surface tension in pulmonary fluid.

surgery 1) The branch of medical work that deals with injuries, growths, deformities and the removal of unwanted parts by operation or manipulation. 2) Used to denote a place – a **veterinary surgery**.

surgical 1) Adjective for anything treated by cutting, freezing, burning, etc. 2) Relating to the work performed by the veterinary surgeon.

surgical anaesthesia A level of anaesthesia sufficient to undertake an act of surgery.

surgical shock Physiological state that develops as a result of trauma during surgery; to some extent should be preventable; *see also* FLUID THERAPY.

surgical team All the staff in the theatre undertaking a surgical procedure; may include surgeons, surgical assistants, scrub nurse, anaesthetist, intensive care nurse and radiographer.

suture 1) Method of assisting the closure of a wound; can also be used to describe the type of material used in stitching. 2) Anatomically, the junction between flat bones.

suxamethonium Drug used to relax voluntary muscles; respiration may then have to be assisted.

Simple interrupted   Vertical mattress

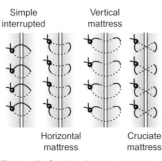

Horizontal mattress   Cruciate mattress

Figure 47. Sample of suture patterns.

swab Pad of absorbent material, may be attached to a stick when used to collect laboratory specimens.

swaged needle Type of needle where the suture material is 'welded into' the metal thus causing no drag when the needle passes through delicate tissues.

sweat glands Known as sudiferous glands; only active on the nose and foot pads of dogs and cats; the horse's glands are active all over the body.

sweet itch Also called allergic dermatitis; the skin of horses becomes very itchy, sometimes resulting in weeping sores in the spring, summer and autumn months. Caused by allergic reaction to midge and insect bites; affected horses will commonly rub their manes and tails.

swimmer Popular term for a puppy that fails to stand on its front legs while still in the nest; may be the result of an overweight puppy with too rapid growth or one of the obscure muscular dystrophy conditions.

SWOT analysis Business tool for analyzing a product or service in terms of its strengths, weaknesses (internal characteristics) and opportunities and threats (external factors that may affect uptake of a product); see also PEST ANALYSIS.

sylvatic rabies The type of rabies found in wildlife, including foxes; woodland animals are no more susceptible than urban-living creatures to the viral infection.

symbiosis A relationship of peaceful coexistence in which there should be mutual aid and benefit.

symblepharon Eyelids adhering to each other and to the eyeball as a result of sticky discharge. Normal state of the newborn puppy or kitten.

sympathetic The part of the autonomic nervous system that works closest to the effects of adrenaline (epinephrine). The 'fright, flight, frolic' response is initiated by the sympathetic nervous system and followed up by the secretion of adrenaline (epinephrine) for a sustained response; see also ADRENALINE.

sympathomimetic Producing the results similar to stimulation of the postganglionic part of the sympathetic nervous system; see also ADRENERGIC, ISOPRENALINE.

symphysis A junction or place where two bones join each other, as in the pelvis.

symptom Subjective indication of a disease, such as fever or lameness.

synapse Junction of two nerves; production of acetylcholine or noradrenaline (norepinephrine) as a neurotransmitter allows the chemical transmission of an electrical impulse in the nerve; see also NEURONE.

synarthrosis Cartilaginous junctions allowing little or no joint movement.

synchondrosis Type of cartilaginous joint that is converted to bone in adult life but remains a point of weakness; see also MANDIBULAR SYMPHYSIS.

synchysis scintillans Small particles seen in the posterior chamber of the eye in older animals; may contribute to a bluish reflective haze from the vitreous but is not considered a cause of blindness; see also ASTEROID HYALOSIS.

syncope Sudden collapse similar to human fainting. May be cardiac in origin with a temporary cerebral anaemia or the result of hypotensive drugs such as acetylpromazine.

syndesmosis Joint that has a fibrous connection, e.g. the suspension of the hyoid apparatus.

syndrome, physiological A group of symptoms that give a clinical picture but not necessarily a disease that can be named; *see also* CUSHING'S SYNDROME, KEY–GASKELL SYNDROME.

synechia An adhesion from the iris to the lens or the cornea; potentially dangerous as a cause of cataract; classified as anterior or posterior depending on the attachment place.

synergism The state of working together; often applied to medication such as the use of two antibiotics simultaneously to enhance the effects of both.

synorchism An adhesion between the two testes so that they are fused into one mass.

synostosis Fusion of bone between joints.

synovial fluid Fluid closely related to plasma but with extra lubrication; it occurs in joint spaces, providing nutrients for the cartilage and lubrication for movement; it has become the subject of research in the prevention of arthritis.

synovitis Inflammation of a synovial membrane; usually the sac becomes filled with serous fluid but there may be infection, with pus present.

synovium Synovial membrane lining joints and the fluid it produces.

synsacrum Fused bones in birds that make up structural support from the sacrum and pelvis.

synthesis Production of a substance in the body or the manufacture of a compound that may be the replica of a natural product.

syringe Surgical tool for introducing a substance into the body or sometimes for withdrawing a fluid such as blood from a vein or other internal site; *see also* HYPODERMIC, BIOPSY.

syringe driver A small infusion pump used to gradually administer small amounts of fluid or medication to a patient from a syringe over an exact period of time.

syrinx An adaptation of the bird's trachea to produce a voice box in the absence of the mammalian larynx.

systemic Affecting the whole body.

systemic circulation The part of the blood flow that takes oxygenated blood to all parts of the body and then returns deoxygenated blood to the heart; *see also* PULMONARY CIRCULATION.

systemic desensitization Using repeated exposure to a stimulus, often starting at a low intensity, to eventually eliminate a response of fear, anxiety or aggression.

systemic lupus erythematosus *See* SLE.

systemic vascular resistance (SVR) This maintains the blood pressure after blood is pumped into the elastic arteries. It is largely controlled by a precapillary sphincter mechanism under the control of the sympathetic nervous system.

systole The contracting phase of the heart, especially when the ventricles force the blood out through the arteries.

systolic murmur Noise produced during the ejection phase of the heart's cycle usually associated with aortic valve incompetence and regurgitation of blood; always potentially dangerous as a cause of dilation of the ventricles and heart failure.

S

tablet Solid drug formulation administered orally. Tablets with enteric coatings should not be broken; the enteric coating either protects the stomach from contact with an irritant drug or prevents degradation of an acid-labile agent.

tachycardia Elevated heart rate; common causes include pain, stress (adrenaline (epinephrine)), hypotension and drugs such as atropine; exercise and excitement are nonmedical causes.

tachypnoea Elevated respiratory rate; common causes include pain, shock, airway obstruction, effusions and pneumonia; panting, exercise and excitement are nonmedical causes.

Taenia A genus of cestodes (tapeworms); endoparasitic worms that infect carnivores. All have an intermediate host, such as mice, where the cysticercus stage develops; adult worms are long and ribbon-like, and eggs are shed in the faeces in packets (proglottids) resembling rice grains; proglottids have a single genital pore. Species include *T. hydatigena*, *T. pisiformis*, *T. ovis*, *T. multiceps*, *T. serialis and T. taeniaeformis*; *see also DIPYLIDIUM CANINUM, ECHINOCOCCUS GRANULOSUS, TAENIA TAENIAEFORMIS.*

Taenia taeniaeformis A cat tapeworm.

tail biting A habit developed by some dogs; may be difficult to control as the tail is awkward to bandage; an Elizabethan collar may be required or a plastic tail guard; severe self-mutilation can necessitate amputation of the tail in persistent cases.

tail-fold pyoderma Infection of the skin fold located at the base of the tail in breeds of dog with a corkscrew tail, such as the bulldog and pug.

tail gland Region towards the base of the tail on the dorsal surface where there are numerous sebaceous glands and the skin tends to be thickened; *see also* CIRCUMANAL GLANDS.

tail-gland hyperplasia Hyperplasia of the sebaceous glands of the tail, with the formation of an oval patch of alopecia; associated with generalized seborrhoea and testicular tumours; *see also* SEBORRHOEA, STUD TAIL.

tail shedding Many species of lizard can voluntarily shed their tail as an escape mechanism, and therefore, the tail should not be used as a means of restraint.

talocrural joint The articulation between the tibia/fibula and the talus; tibiotarsal joint; inaccurately called the hock.

talus One of the bones in the proximal row of tarsal bones; articulates with the tibia and fibula proximally and with the calcaneus laterally (there is little movement at this latter joint).

tamponade Compression of the heart as a result of an increased volume of fluid within the pericardium, e.g. haemopericardium caused by haemangiosarcoma; signs include dyspnoea, tachycardia and muffled heart sounds; may require emergency pericardiocentesis.

tapetal Relating to the tapetum.

tapetum Reflective, nonpigmented part of the retina, just above the optic disc.

tapeworm See TAENIA, DIPYLIDIUM CANINUM, ECHINOCOCCUS GRANULOSUS.

tapioca Cereal food of Asian origin used in specialized diets as a novel single carbohydrate when no wheat gluten protein is used.

tardive A skin disease when hair loss is a prominent symptom.

target Part of the anode (within the X-ray tube head) that is bombarded by the focused, high-energy electron beam to produce X-rays; the target is usually made from a hard-wearing metal, such as tungsten, and rotates at high speed.

target cell Type of red blood cell seen in some anaemic patients, having pigment around the periphery and centrally.

target tissue Site of action of a drug.

tarsal Relating to the tarsus or hock.

tarsal glands Meibomian glands located within the tarsal plate, along the borders of the eyelids.

tarsal plate The thin fibrous layer that gives shape to the eyelid margins.

tarsometatarsal joint Articulation between the distal row of tarsal bone and the metatarsal bones in the hindleg; there is little movement at this level.

tarsorrhaphy Suturing together of the eyelids to protect the cornea, e.g. during ulcer healing.

tarsus The collection of seven bones between the tibia and the metatarsal bones; the talus, calcaneus, central tarsal and first to fourth tarsal bones; the hock; site of spavin in the horse.

tartar The hard deposit that builds up on teeth; dental calculus; *see also* CALCULUS.

taste Sensation produced by molecules reaching the mouth; taste is relayed via the facial (VII) and glossopharyngeal (IX) cranial nerves.

tattooing Permanent means of identifying animals; used in greyhound racing,

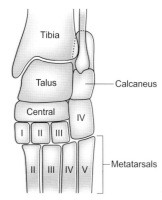

Figure 48. Tarsus: cranial view, left hind.

with a tattoo being placed inside the ear flap.

taurine Amino acid essential in the diet of cats as they cannot synthesize it themselves; signs of taurine deficiency include infertility and central retinal degeneration. The condition is rare now as cat foods have adequate levels of taurine, but deficiency can arise if cats are fed long-term on dog food.

taxonomy The scientific and systematic classification of living organisms into groups.

T cell Thymus-derived lymphocytes that confer cell-mediated immunity.

T connector A disposable connector that can be positioned between an intravenous or arterial catheter and attached tubing to allow medication or fluid to be introduced without disconnecting the tubing.

tears Fluid secreted by the lacrimal gland ventromedial to the eye, which bathes the cornea and conjunctiva; tears then drain via the nasolacrimal duct into the nasal chambers, where they evaporate.

tear staining Discoloration of the coat at the medial canthus of the eye caused by the chronic overflow of tears; *see also* EPIPHORA.

teat Nipple; usually arranged in pairs along the thorax and abdomen.

technetium A radioisotope that emits gamma rays; it can be linked to several different molecules, which are taken up by specific organs; in the veterinary field it is used mainly for bone scans.

tectum A roof-like covering.

teeth Dentition; teeth have one or more roots, a pulp cavity, dentine and a covering of tough enamel. Full dentition comprises incisors, canines, premolars and molars; carnassial teeth are the large crushing first molar on the mandible and fourth upper premolar.

teeth clipping The teeth of rats, mice, gerbils, hamsters and rabbits are open-rooted so the teeth grow continuously. If there is malocclusion, where the upper and lower teeth fail to meet correctly, the teeth will require periodic shortening; hard foods should be provided to minimize the problem; signs that clipping is necessary include drooling saliva, inappetence and pawing at the mouth; incisors are most commonly affected, but it should be remembered that the cheek teeth may also be overgrown.

Tegus lizard Moderately large lizard, related to Caiman lizards, all belong to the Teiidae family.

telangiectasis Dilation of capillaries or end blood vessels.

telencephalon 1) Alternative name for the cerebrum, the forebrain. **2)** The olfactory bulbs, cerebral cortices and basal nuclei constitute the telencephalic part of the brain.

teleost The bony fish, the most common type of fish seen in veterinary practice.

telephone skills Prompt answering of the telephone (within three rings), politeness, accurate message taking and relaying are all part of a good telephone manner.

telogen The resting phase in the hair growth cycle; *see also* ANAGEN.

telogen effluvium Shortening of the anagen (growth phase) of the hair cycle so that many hairs enter the telogen (resting) phase at the same time; these hairs are then shed a few weeks later; this moulting may be part of the normal hair growth cycle or can follow an illness, pregnancy, lactation or drug therapy.

temperament The demeanour of an animal; its character and psychology.

temperature A measure of the degree of heat; measured in degrees centigrade: **room temperature** is taken to be 20–24°C; the incubation of bacterial culture plates is usually performed at 37°C; refrigerators operate at 4°C and freezers at −20°C; *see also* HYPERTHERMIA, HYPOTHERMIA, PYREXIA, APPENDIX 1.

temporal The region overlying the temporal bone, forming the caudodorsal portion of the skull.

temporomandibular joint (TMJ) The joint of the lower jaw, with articulation between the condylar process of the vertical ramus of the mandible and the temporal bone of the skull; the jaw is closed by the action of the temporal, masseter and pterygoid muscles and opened by the digastricus.

tenaculum Surgical instrument for gripping tissues.

tendinitis (tendonitis) Inflammation of a tendon, usually a result of a strain injury; may be chronic or acute; treated with rest and anti-inflammatory drugs, followed by controlled exercise; *see also* STEM CELL THERAPY.

tendon Tough, fibrous band connecting a muscle to a bone.

tenement disease Description of a cat injury specific to those that live in apartment blocks and suffer from a fall with a 'five point landing'.

tenesmus Excessive straining to urinate or defecate; associated with constipation, colitis, urinary calculi and other obstructions.

Tenon's capsule The dense fibrous connective tissue of the periorbita, surrounding the rectus and retractor muscles.

tenorrhaphy The sutured repair of severed tendons; appropriate suture patterns include Bunnell, Bunnell–Mayer, horizontal mattress and Kessler locking loop.

tenosynovitis Inflammation of a tendon and its tendon sheath.

tenotomy Surgical sectioning of a tendon to correct a defect caused by shortening of the tendon.

tension band wire Orthopaedic technique used to secure fragments internally that

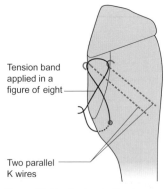

Tension band applied in a figure of eight

Two parallel K wires

Figure 49. Tension band wiring for fixation of avulsed tibial crest.

tend to distract under the pull of muscles and tendons; *see also* WIRING.

tensor Any muscle that acts to create tension in a body area, e.g. **tensor fascia lata** muscle contracts to increase the tension in the fascial planes over the thigh.

tentorium cerebelli A folding in of the dura mater that divides the cerebral hemispheres and the cerebellum; *see also* MENINGES.

teratogen A substance that causes abnormal development and malformation of a fetus.

teratoma A tumour of embryonic origin consisting of cells that would not normally be found at the tumour location; most commonly affects the ovaries and testes.

teres Usually a round anatomical structure such as the teres muscle of the shoulder or the teres ligament in the hip joint.

test tube Basic laboratory apparatus; a glass vial in which chemical reactions can be carried out.

testicle *See* TESTIS.

testis, *pl.* testes The male reproductive gland, in most mammals located within the scrotal sac; sometimes known as the testicle; *see also* GONAD.

testosterone An androgenic, steroid-type hormone formed by the Leydig (interstitial) cells of the testes but also in small amounts by the ovaries; causes the development of male characteristics, libido and secondary sexual organs.

tetanus Disease affecting many species, caused by *Clostridium tetani*; characterized by progressive tetanic (sustained) muscle contractions caused by the effect of bacterial neurotoxin on the CNS; the organism enters via accidental wounds, bites, surgical sites, etc. Treatment is with antitoxin and antibiotics, but the prognosis is guarded, with death caused by respiratory or cardiac failure. Vaccine is used routinely in humans, and staff working with animals should ensure that they have in-date cover. Symptoms are caused by the exotoxin tetanospasmin, cats are more resistant than dogs to the effects. Horses are particularly sensitive and are routinely vaccinated against the disease.

tetany Protracted muscle spasm; *see also* ECLAMPSIA.

tetra- Prefix meaning 'four'.

tetracycline Broad-spectrum, bacteriostatic antibiotic; may sometimes cause yellowing of the teeth if given to immature animals.

tetralogy of Fallot A serious congenital cardiac abnormality comprising pulmonic stenosis, ventricular septal defect, displaced aorta and right ventricular hypertrophy, resulting in a right-to-left shunt; affected animals are often stunted and have poor exercise tolerance; there is a systolic murmur and ECG changes. The condition is confirmed by ultrasound or angiography; surgical correction may be attempted, but the outlook is guarded.

tetraparesis Weakness affecting all four legs but, the animal is still able to make coordinated stepping movements if its weight is supported.

tetraplegia Paralysis of all four legs, with no stepping movements; *see also* QUADRIPLEGIA.

tetraploid Having four times the haploid number of chromosomes; *see also* DIPLOID, HAPLOID.

thalamus Part of the diencephalon, deep within the brain, surrounding the third ventricle; it acts as the major sensory relay centre for information passing up to the cerebral cortex.

theatre Room suitably equipped and a controlled environment for performing aseptic surgical procedures.

theobromine A methylxanthine derivative; a myocardial stimulant and diuretic; also dilates the coronary arteries and relaxes smooth muscle; occurs naturally in chocolate, and overdose has been reported in dogs, the signs being vomiting, diarrhoea, diuresis and collapse; treatment is symptomatic; *see also* CHOCOLATE POISONING.

theophylline A widely used methylxanthine; a bronchodilator, with positive inotropic and chronotropic effects on the heart; used in the management of congestive heart failure and other cardiogenic pulmonary disease.

therapeutics The science of the use of drugs to treat disease.

thermal burn Burn caused by contact with a heated object, such as fire, boiling water or steam; chemical, electrical and radiation burns can also occur.

thermocautery Electrocautery; use of an electric current to generate heat that controls haemorrhage or can be used to cut through tissue.

thermometer Instrument for measuring temperature.

thermophile A bacterium that thrives at temperatures above 50°C.

thermoplastic Describes material that softens when heated and hardens again as it cools; used as splinting and casting materials.

thermoreceptor Receptor nerve endings sensitive to temperature changes.

thermoregulation Control of body temperature; body temperature is regulated by the hypothalamus. When body temperature drops, skin blood vessels constrict, the coat stands on end and shivering is used to generate heat; conversely, when body temperature rises, peripheral blood vessels dilate to increase heat loss, sweating occurs and animals start to pant; *see also* HEAT STROKE, HYPERTHERMIA, HYPOTHERMIA.

thermotherapy Use of heat treatment to promote vasodilation, thus increasing the blood supply to the affected area. The application of heat relaxes the muscles and increases flexibility and is effective in reducing muscle spasms.

ThermoVent A disposable device that can be connected to an endotracheal tube during anaesthesia or to a tracheostomy tube for humidifying inhaled gases.

thiamin *See* VITAMIN B.

thiaminase An enzyme present in raw fish that breaks down thiamin; animals fed exclusively on raw fish are likely to develop thiamin deficiency.

thiazide diuretics Group of diuretics, e.g. hydrochlorothiazide, that increase urine production and sodium ion excretion.

thiopental sodium An agent commonly used for the induction of general anaesthesia; provided as a powder, which is made up into a 2.5% solution for small animals and 5% for horses using a sterile technique. Administered intravenously, it rapidly crosses the blood–brain barrier, inducing narcosis; there is a period of apnoea; stored in body fat; accidental perivascular injection is irritant because of the high pH; *see also* BARBITURATES.

third eyelid *See* NICTITATING MEMBRANE.

third-intention healing Occurs where wounds are first allowed to granulate before being debrided and sutured at a later date.

thirst The desire to drink and the primary regulator of water intake; the thirst centre is located in the hypothalamus.

Thomas–Schroeder splint A frame used as a means of external fracture support; time-consuming to apply, it has been largely superseded by other casting and splinting materials.

thoracic Relating to the thorax and chest area.

thoracic duct The main route for the return of lymph to the circulation; lymph draining from the viscera and pelvic limbs runs into the cisterna chyli, which in turn becomes the thoracic duct, running alongside the aorta and azygous vein; the duct opens into the left brachiocephalic vein within the thorax.

thoracocentesis Insertion of a needle or catheter into the thoracic cavity to drain off free fluid or air.

thoracolumbar Relating to the loin region over the last few thoracic and first few lumbar vertebrae.

thoracotomy Surgical opening of the thorax; once the thorax is opened the negative pressure is lost and lung tissue will collapse; therefore some form of ventilation is required, e.g. intermittent positive pressure ventilation, use of a ventilator.

thorax The chest cavity; bounded by the ribs, intercostal muscles and the diaphragm, it contains the heart, lungs, great vessels, pleura, thymus and mediastinum.

THR Total hip replacement.

three-way tap A connector with three attachment ports for tubing or syringes that allows one of the ports to be occluded to direct fluid in the direction required.

thrill A palpable vibration accompanying a cardiac murmur.

thrombin The enzyme that converts fibrinogen to fibrin to assist in blood clotting; the liver synthesizes the precursor prothrombin, which circulates as a plasma protein and is activated to thrombin at sites of blood vessel damage.

thrombocyte Blood platelet.

thrombocytopenia Reduction in the number of circulating platelets; may be a result of bone marrow suppression, immune-mediated disease, chronic haemorrhage, DIC, etc.

thromboembolus An embolism arising from a thrombus; *see also* EMBOLISM.

thrombokinase Enzyme concerned with the change from prothrombin to thrombin during blood clotting, triggered by thromboplastin.

thrombolytic An agent that dissolves a thrombus.

thromboplastin Enzyme released by damaged thrombocytes (platelets) that sets off the cascade involved when blood clots; *see also* HAEMOSTASIS.

thrombopoiesis Process of forming blood platelets or thrombocytes.

thrombopoietin Hormone that affects the bone marrow, controlling the output of platelets.

thrombosis The process of thrombus formation.

thrombus A blood clot.

thrush 1) Infection with the yeast *Candida albicans*. 2) A chronic infection of a horse's foot.

thumps Equine hiccups (also known as synchronous diaphragmatic flutter) caused by the diaphragm going into spasm, often after exercise.

thymol A phenolic compound that may be used to preserve urine samples that cannot be examined immediately.

thymoma Benign neoplasm of the thymus, located within the anterior mediastinum;

clinical signs may arise because the neoplasm puts pressure on vital structures such as the trachea or cranial vena cava.

thymus A gland lying within the anterior mediastinum; part of the lymphatic system and most active in the late fetal stages and in neonates; processes T lymphocytes, priming them for their role in cell-mediated immunity.

thyroglobulin The form in which thyroid hormones are stored by the thyroid gland; consists of thyroid hormone linked to a colloid.

thyroglobulin autoantibodies (TGAA) Found in immune-mediated thyroiditis.

thyroid The bilobed endocrine gland in the neck that secretes thyroid hormone (from follicular cells) to control metabolic rate and calcitonin (from the parafollicular C cells) to modulate calcium and phosphate metabolism; *see also* CALCITONIN, GOITRE, HYPOTHYROIDISM, HYPERTHYROIDISM, THYROXINE.

thyroid cartilage One of the main cartilages of the larynx; *see also* ARYTENOID.

thyroidectomy Surgical removal of the thyroid gland, used to treat hyperthyroidism.

thyroid hormones Thyroxine (T_4) and triiodothyronine (T_3); the hormones produced by the thyroid gland; these hormones stimulate cell metabolism, increase heart rate and blood pressure and stimulate gut motility; they are also necessary for growth and reproduction.

thyroid-stimulating hormone (TSH) Hormone produced by the anterior pituitary gland, stimulating the release of thyroid hormones from the thyroid.

thyroxine The main thyroid hormone (T_4).

tibia The main long bone of the distal hindleg, running from stifle to tarsus.

tibial tuberosity The bony prominence at the cranioproximal end of the tibia in the midline; the insertion point for the patellar ligament.

tibiotarsal joint The articulation between the distal tibia and the talus.

tick Arthropod, blood-sucking ectoparasite. Those of veterinary importance are mainly of the genus *Ixodes*; oval body, four pairs of legs and a well-developed beak (capitulum); go through larval and nymph stages and are not generally host-specific. Ticks themselves may cause local irritation and pruritus but they also act as vectors for many diseases, e.g. *Babesia*; ticks can be removed manually but care must be taken to ensure that the mouthparts are totally removed (swabbing with ether first may help).

tick fever Febrile disease caused by biting ticks that carry *Rickettsia* spp. or *Babesia canis*.

tick paralysis Flaccid weakness and paralysis reported in the USA and Australia and caused by neurotoxins injected by some species of tick.

tidal volume The volume of air that passes in and out of the airways during one normal respiratory cycle.

tie Part of the mating process in dogs when the muscles in the vagina of the bitch contract around the penis of the dog so that it cannot be withdrawn. The dog may step over the bitch's back during this stage, so that they stand back-to-back; the tie can last from a few seconds up to an hour, but the animals should not be separated during this time. Device unique to canines to promote fertility, not seen in other animals that live in packs or groups.

Tieman catheter Bitch urinary catheter.

time gain compensation One of the principles of ultrasound examination: the echoes from the acoustic surface close to the transducer are stronger than echoes from more remote structures so a compensatory mechanism is necessary to obtain the best uniform image.

time management Skills allowing the most effective and efficient use of a person's time.

ting points The beginning or ending of a meridian as required in veterinary acupuncture. Points are located along the meridians, and for the horse, all the ting points are on the coronary band of the hoof.

tissue respiration Metabolic process that takes place at cellular level to provide energy; *see also* INTERNAL RESPIRATION.

titre The amount or level of a substance.

TIVA Total intravenous anaesthesia, i.e. without any volatile agent being used.

TLI Trypsin-like immunoreactivity; a test used for the diagnosis of exocrine pancreatic insufficiency.

TMJ Temporomandibular joint; found in the head, cranial to the ear.

toad Amphibious animal that causes an acute response poison reaction if licked or ingested by dogs; usually too bitter for cats to be poisoned.

to-and-fro circuit Type of anaesthetic circuit incorporating a soda lime canister so that gases can be rebreathed. Exhaled air passes through the soda lime into a reservoir bag and is then rebreathed back through the soda lime; the circuit is economical to run but can only be used on animals over 7–10 kg because of the resistance.

tocopherol Vitamin E.

toe The distal digit, comprising the first, second and third phalanges.

toggle Surgical technique for repair of hip luxations, where a synthetic round ligament is passed through a tunnel drilled in the femoral head and anchored on the medial side of the acetabulum using a metal toggle pin.

tolerance Process of acclimatization so the body does not respond so strongly

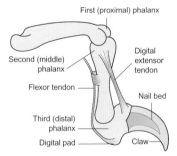

First (proximal) phalanx

Second (middle) phalanx

Flexor tendon

Third (distal) phalanx

Digital pad

Digital extensor tendon

Nail bed

Claw

Figure 50. Toe: feline digit.

after repeated use. The glucose tolerance test is used in monitoring diabetes mellitus.

tongue The muscle mass occupying the oral cavity; used for chewing and swallowing; carries taste buds and caudally directed papillae.

tonic 1) Having tone; used to describe a muscle that is under tension.
2) Medicine said to increase appetite and sense of well-being.

tonicity The osmotic pressure of a solution.

tonometry Measurement of pressure; a tonometer may be used to measure intraocular pressure in suspected glaucoma.

tonsil The paired collection of lymphoid tissue located in the pharynx, caudal to the palatoglossal arch; they are partially covered by the tonsillar fold of the soft palate.

tonsillectomy Surgical removal of the tonsils.

tonsillitis Inflammation of the tonsils.

tooth *See* TEETH.

tooth root abscess A painful inflammatory condition of a tip of tooth root that can cause swelling of the gum/face and fever. It is caused by an infection that is often the result of a broken or cracked tooth; can otherwise be known as a periapical abscess.

tophus A urate plaque deposited in soft tissues, most commonly in periarticular fibrous tissue.

topical Applied locally.

torpor A state of much reduced activity in an animal, which includes a reduction in body temperature and metabolic rate, as in hibernation.

torsion Twisting; *see also* GASTRIC TORSION, VOLVULUS.

torticollis Spasm of cervical muscles so that the head is twisted to one side.

total ear canal ablation (TECA) Surgical removal of both the horizontal and vertical parts of the external ear canal; used to treat severe otitis externa.

total hip replacement Replacement of a diseased hip joint with a prosthetic acetabulum and femoral head.

total lung capacity The total amount of air within the respiratory system; equal to the vital capacity plus the residual volume.

total plasma protein The amount of protein carried in the bloodstream (predominantly albumin, globulins and fibrinogen); as these molecules do not diffuse out of the circulation, plasma proteins are used to assess an animal's state of hydration.

tourniquet A constricting band or bandage applied to control haemorrhage; it must be released every 10–15 minutes to prevent excessive tissue ischaemia and subsequent necrosis; *see also* ESMARCH BANDAGE.

towel clip Self-retaining clamp with two points used to anchor surgical drapes to the patient.

toxaemia Presence of toxins from infectious agents within the bloodstream.

Toxascaris leonina A nematode (roundworm) of the dog and cat; may cause visceral larva migrans in humans; *see also* ASCARID.

toxic Harmful, poisonous.

toxic epidermal necrolysis (TEN) Rare, immune-mediated disorder characterized by the acute onset of severe ulceration of the skin and mucous membranes; most commonly an allergic response to drugs but may also be associated with infections and neoplastic conditions; guarded prognosis.

toxin A poisonous substance, biological in origin.

Toxocara canis Common nematode (ascarid) of the dog, also affects cats; the L2 stage causes ocular larva migrans and visceral larva migrans in humans. Adult worms are round, fleshy and 10–20 cm long; large worm burdens in puppies can cause clinical signs; controlled by regular worming, especially of pregnant bitches and puppies, and by good hygiene.

Toxocara cati Ascarid worm specific to the cat.

toxocariasis Infection with toxocaral nematodes.

toxoid A toxin that has been processed so that it is no longer harmful to the body but retains its antigenicity; used to produce active immunity, e.g. tetanus toxoid.

Toxoplasma gondii A coccidial parasite of the cat that can use many mammals and birds as intermediate hosts; most cats are asymptomatic and may periodically excrete the protozoa; the oocysts take at least 24 hours to become infective and so daily cleaning of litter trays is a useful control measure; in intermediate hosts, the parasite has a predilection for the CNS and muscle, causing diverse neurological signs and cysts; the zoonotic form of the disease can lead to fetal abnormalities, fever and myalgia; diagnosis is confirmed by muscle biopsy (cysts) or demonstrating a rising antibody titre to the organism.

TP Training practice. A designation for a practice or a group that has been approved to provide training for the veterinary nurse qualification.

T plate Bone plate in the shape of a letter T, which is used for some distal radial fractures and carpal arthrodesis.

TPN Total parenteral nutrition. The feeding of a patient entirely via intravenous means.

trabecula, *pl.* trabeculae A network of tissue, e.g. bone.

trace element Mineral required in the diet in small amounts, e.g. iron, copper, zinc, manganese. Cobalt is necessary for the synthesis of vitamin B_{12}.

trachea The windpipe, running from the larynx, down the neck and into the thorax, bifurcating at the level of the base of the heart into the right and left main bronchi. The tube is composed of C-shaped rings of cartilage linked by a tough membrane; lined with mucosa.

tracheal Relating to the trachea.

tracheal collapse Congenital dorsoventral flattening of the tracheal rings, seen most commonly in toy breeds of dog; affected sections of the trachea collapse on inspiration, creating an upper airway obstruction and generating a classical hard, dry cough; if mild, the condition may be managed using bronchodilators, corticosteroids and antitussives; surgery involves supporting the trachea by using prosthetic rings.

tracheal hypoplasia A rare congenital disorder, associated with laryngeal hypoplasia; the prognosis is guarded.

tracheal rupture Trauma to the trachea can lead to rupture of the tracheal membrane; a large tear will cause marked respiratory distress necessitating immediate action; small tears can lead to gradual subcutaneous emphysema and pneumothorax or pneumomediastinum.

tracheal stenosis Rare condition with narrowing of the tracheal lumen; possibly secondary to rough intubation.

tracheal worm *See* OSLERUS OSLERI.

tracheitis Inflammation of the mucous membrane lining the trachea; *see also* KENNEL COUGH.

tracheostomy tube A plastic or metal tube inserted into the hole following a tracheotomy procedure in order to keep the opening patent to allow the patient to breath.

tracheotomy Creation of a temporary opening in the neck into the trachea; may be elective, e.g. to facilitate the reduction and repair of jaw fractures, or may be an emergency measure, e.g. laryngeal foreign body.

tracking responses Test of vision where cotton wool balls are thrown near to the animal to see if it can track them by moving its eyes; cotton wool will not make a noise or generate air currents that the animal may sense instead of seeing.

tract A pathway or route.

traction Application of a drawing force, e.g. to overcome the pull of contracted muscles to allow fracture reduction or correction of a luxation.

trade name Brand name of a drug legally protected by registering the name, for example Metacam; *see also* GENERIC NAME.

trailering (loading) problems Horses that are difficult to load into a lorry or trailer may be conditioned by altering the environment: interior darkness, noise of hoofs on the ramp and any instability of the trailer need to be corrected first.

trait A characteristic.

tranquillizer An ataractic; a drug that calms a patient without sedating; in practice, most tranquillizers have some degree of sedative effect.

trans- Prefix meaning 'across' or 'through'.

transcription The conversion of the genetic code from a length of DNA into mRNA.

transcutaneous electrical nerve stimulator (TENS) Analgesic device that delivers small electric pulses via pads placed over a painful focus; the current blocks the pain message from the area before it is perceived by the brain.

transdisciplinary The sharing of roles, information and communication across all aspects of clinical and nonclinical functions to provide holistic patient care.

transducer A device that converts a specific form of energy into a different specific form of energy; e.g. converting a pulse into an electrical signal; also a device used for ultrasonography.

transect To cut across.

transfection The introduction of DNA into a cell by chemical gene transfer methods; used in molecular endocrinology.

Transfer of Undertakings (Protection of Employment) Regulations 1981 (TUPE) Regulation to ensure that staff are able to maintain their rights and privileges of employment on the transference of the owner of a business.

transformer Part of the X-ray machine that converts the alternating mains current into a direct current.

transfusion Transfer of whole blood, plasma or platelets from a donor animal to a recipient.

transfusion reaction Response to an incompatible blood transfusion; signs include salivation, restlessness, vomiting, abdominal cramps, jaundice, DIC, pyrexia and collapse.

transit time The time taken from ingestion to the appearance in the faeces.

transitional cell carcinoma Malignant tumour of transitional epithelial cells.

transitional epithelium A region of epithelium bridging two different types, e.g. changing from squamous to columnar epithelium.

transitional vertebra Rare abnormality where a vertebra has some of the characteristics of vertebrae from an adjacent region, e.g. L7 having transverse processes that are fused to the pelvis (a characteristic of sacral vertebrae).

transketolase An enzyme found in all organisms; it requires thiamine diphosphate as a cofactor; transketolase activity in RBCs is reduced in thiamine deficiency.

transmissible Able to be passed from one individual to another.

transmissible venereal tumour (TVT) A sexually transmitted granulomatous tumour of the penis, prepuce, vulva or vagina in the dog; extremely rare in the UK.

transplacental Able to pass across the placenta.

transponder The active part of a microchip.

transtentorial herniation Severe injury after head trauma, the brain is pushed caudally in the skull. The midbrain is squashed and the cerebellum is pushed into the foramen magnum; see also MENINGES, TENTORIUM CEREBELLI.

transudate Fluid that has passed through cells or across a membrane into a body cavity or onto the skin, the direction of transfer depending on the osmotic pressure on either side.

transverse At right angles to the long axis.

trauma Physical or mental injury. The state of shock will be present to a greater or lesser extent; emergency care requires an order of priority in actions; see also GOLDEN HOUR.

travel sickness Motion sickness; common in animals transported by car, etc.; acepromazine has a central effect to reduce travel sickness.

Travers retractor Pattern of self-retaining surgical retractor for joint and muscle exposure.

treadmill A piece of equipment used to exercise horses and dogs in order to assess their musculoskeletal, cardiac and respiratory systems in a controlled environment; used for measuring exercise tolerance, studying gait and lameness and for ECG recording during controlled exercise.

tree frog Brightly coloured neotropical frogs of *Hyla* species; very agile; have disc-like protuberances on each digit to facilitate climbing.

trematode Flatworm endoparasites, e.g. fluke.

tremor Repetitive, involuntary movement.

trephine A surgical instrument used to remove a circle of bone to allow access to the brain, nasal sinuses, etc.

treponematosis A sexually transmitted venereal infection caused by the spirochete *Treponema paraluis-cuniculi.*

TRH Thyroid-releasing hormone.

triage The action of prioritizing patients according to the severity of their injuries, so that life-threatening conditions are treated before less-serious injuries. A skilled but rapid assessment is needed in all injured animals, often to establish priorities in treatment and other actions.

triceps Muscle mass caudal to the humerus, the main action of which is to extend the elbow.

trichiasis The presence of aberrant hairs around the eye, e.g. on prominent skin folds, which irritate the corneal surface; require surgical removal.

trichobezoar A hairball.

Trichodectes canis The common biting louse of the dog; an intermediate host for *Dipylidium caninum.*

trichomoniasis Disease caused by infection with a *Trichomonas* protozoal parasite; a common disease in pigeons, with inappetence, diarrhoea and respiratory signs; antiprotozoal agents can be given in the drinking water, but poor hygiene and overcrowding should also be addressed.

Trichophyton A genus of fungi causing ringworm; may affect dogs, cats, humans, etc.; do not generally fluoresce under ultraviolet light; *see also MICROSPORUM.*

Trichuris vulpis The dog whipworm.

tricuspid Having three cusps; describes the heart valve between the right atrium and ventricle.

trigeminal neuralgia Pain resulting from irritation of the trigeminal (V) cranial nerve.

triglyceride Glycerol molecule with three attached fatty acid chains.

trigger points Used in acupuncture; are associated with myocardial pain; they can be found in any muscle and are associated with common orthopaedic problems; a tender point, often a hyperirritable locus with a taut band of skeletal muscle or associated fascia abnormalities.

trigone The triangular region at the neck of the bladder.

triiodothyronine The thyroid gland hormone commonly known as T_3. Liothyronine is used as a synthetic source.

trismus An early sign of tetanus; inability to open the mouth resulting from spasm of the masseter muscles; *see also* TETANUS.

trocar A sharp metal probe that fits into a sleeve.

trochanter A bony prominence; there are greater, lesser and third trochanters on the proximal femur.

trochlea A smooth, articular surface of bone.

Trombicula autumnalis Harvest mites; only the larval stage is parasitic and affects dogs, cats and humans; can cause seasonal pruritus in the summer and autumn.

trypsin Digestive enzyme that breaks down protein; secreted as trypsinogen by the exocrine pancreas.

trypsin-like immunoreactivity Test commonly used to assess exocrine pancreatic insufficiency; *see also* PANCREAS.

trypsinogen Precursor enzyme from the acinar cells of the pancreas that becomes active trypsin after enterokinase acts as an enzyme.

TSH Thyroid-stimulating hormone.

TTA Tibial tuberosity advancement; surgical procedure used to repair ruptured cruciate ligaments in dogs.

TTD Time to diagnosis; a measure of a clinician's success in identifying the causes of a disease presented by the patient.

tube feeding Method of force-feeding anorexic patients or animals that cannot eat and swallow normally; techniques include nasogastric, pharyngostomy, gastrostomy and PEG tubes.

tuber calcis The proximal prominence of the calcaneus; the point of the hock.

tubercle 1) A small bony eminence.
2) A granulomatous nodule.

tuberculosis Disease caused by *Mycobacterium tuberculosis*; typical lesions are granulomatous nodules with a necrotic centre, which can occur in any tissues; rare – cats are more frequently infected by the oral route than dogs.

tuberosity A bony prominence.

tubule A small tube.

tularaemia Rare zoonotic disease of cats and rabbits caused by *Francisella tularensis*; clinical signs include pyrexia, depression, anorexia, splenomegaly and lymphadenopathy.

tulle A material for wound dressing; a gauze mesh impregnated with paraffin wax.

tumefy To swell.

tumor (L.) 'swelling'; one of the signs of inflammation; *see also* CALOR, DOLOR, RUBOR.

tumour Means 'swelling', is usually a neoplasm or 'growth'; may be benign or malignant; caused by the unchecked, abnormal proliferation of cells; *see also* NEOPLASM.

tunica A coat or covering.

tunica adventitia The outermost layer of blood vessels; made up of collagen and elastic fibres; more elastic as the outermost layer of the artery and less elastic in the vein.

tunica albuginea Part of the coat of the testis in the scrotum.

tunica intima The endothelial lining forming the inner layer of the blood vessel; helps to form the valves in the veins.

tunica media The middle layer of the blood vessel, composed of smooth muscle and elastic fibres.

tunica mucosa The innermost lining of the intestine with the mucosal layer; *see also* BRUSH BORDER.

tunica muscularis The central layer of the intestines, largely smooth muscle.

tunica serosa The outer layer of the intestines; forms part of the peritoneum.

TUPE *See* TRANSFER OF UNDERTAKINGS (PROTECTION OF EMPLOYMENT) REGULATIONS 1981.

turbid Cloudy, as in a fluid sample, etc.

turbinate Scroll-shaped bones within the nasal chambers.

twitch A nerve-stimulating device, such as a looped length of cord attached to a pole that, when applied to the top lip of the horse and tightened, can assist in restraint and immobilization; an involuntary muscle movement; *see also* CHOREA.

tympanic bulla Bony ventral extension of the petrous temporal bone; may become involved in middle ear disease.

tympanic membrane The membrane at the end of the horizontal ear canal, separating the external ear from the middle ear; *see also* EAR DRUM.

tympany Gaseous distension of the abdomen or a hollow organ, also known as bloat.

type II cells Lining cells of the alveoli that secrete surfactants that help to keep airway open.

tyrosine An amino acid.

Tyzzer's disease Disease of rats, mice, rabbits, gerbils, etc. caused by *Bacillus piliformis*; causes sudden death, diarrhoea and lethargy; highly contagious; antibiotics and supportive treatment can limit the disease in contacts; attention to hygiene is also important. In the horse, it is seen mainly as an infection of foals and produces neurological symptoms.

T

U

Uberreiter's syndrome Traditional name for the eye disease that has a breed specificity in German shepherd dogs; seen as a chronic superficial keratitis or pannus; *see also* PANNUS.

ulcer A full-thickness crater or erosion defect in the surface of the skin or mucous membrane, often surrounded by a zone of inflammation. A **corneal ulcer** is a defect in the corneal epithelium; stains with fluorescein. A **decubitus ulcer** is a pressure sore ulcer on the point of the elbow; *see also* BED SORE. A **gastric ulcer** is seen after endoscopy or radiography; may be treated with ranitidine or cimetidine to protect the mucosa. An **indolent ulcer** is a nonhealing ulcer, particularly a corneal ulcer. A **rodent ulcer** is a specific condition of the cat's nasal area; *see also* EOSINOPHILIC, RODENT ULCER.

ulcerative colitis Medical condition, usually in the larger breeds of dog; *see also* COLITIS.

ulcerative glossitis Painful condition of the cat's mouth with ulcers on the tongue surface, usually caused the herpesvirus feline calicivirus. It is associated with the feline lymphocytic gingivitis stomatitis complex; *see also* GINGIVITIS.

Ulcerative pododermatosis *See* SORE HOCKS.

ule- (ulo-) 1) Scars, scar tissue. **2)** The gums.

ulnar Relating to the smaller of the two bones of the forearm or the medial aspect.

ulnectomy Surgical procedure to remove a piece of the ulna bone in the growing puppy as a treatment for elbow joint disease.

ultra- Prefix meaning 'beyond', 'in excess of' or 'on top of'.

ultracentrifuge Method of removing particles using a high centrifugal force, perhaps assisted by a vacuum.

ultrafiltration The type of filtration in the nephron that removes waste material.

ultramicroscopic Describes particles too small to be visualized with the highest power light microscope; *see also* VIRUS, PRION.

ultrasonic Describes sound waves too high for the human ear to be aware of them; increasingly used for diagnostic imaging, cleaning teeth, cleaning surgical instruments, etc.

ultrasound Sound waves of extremely high frequency, over 20 000 Hz real time, that are produced by a scanning machine and used to create and record images of internal anatomical structures; used as a diagnostic and surgical intervention tool.

ultraviolet High-frequency but short-wavelength invisible rays beyond the normal spectrum of visible light; can cause skin damage but may be used for bacterial sterilization; *see also* VITAMIN D, WOOD'S LAMP.

umbilical cord The connection of the fetus to its placenta and then to the mother.

umbilical hernia Point of weakness in the midline where fat or other viscera may bulge outwardly from inside the abdomen with a skin 'lump'; may have a hereditary basis caused by incomplete fusion in the midline.

umbilical infection The patent umbilicus of the newborn can easily become infected; peritonitis and septicaemia may result.

umbilicus The area of connection of the fetus to its placenta and its mother; *see also* NAVEL ILL.

unciform Shaped like a sickle or a hook.

Uncinaria One of the two genuses of hookworm found in the UK.

Uncinaria stenocephala Nematode that infects dogs; unusual in that it may cause skin lesions on the feet through larval migration. Sometimes known as the northern hookworm.

unconditioned response Any response that is evoked by a stimulus without it having to be first taught and learned. Sometimes called unconditioned 'reflexes'.

unconscious A state of deep sleep-like unawareness of surroundings with reduced responses to external stimuli; often the result of a head injury or administration of anaesthetic agents; *see also* COMA.

underdevelopment 1) In X-ray developing, a fault recognized by the greyish, flat background in place of the normal black of exposed parts of the film. **2)** May mean poor growth, as found in the ovaries or testes of late-maturing animals.

under his/her care A term used by the Veterinary Medicine Regulations defined by the RCVS as that the veterinary surgeon has been given the responsibility for the health of animals treated, the animal must have been seen immediately or recently before prescribing and the veterinary surgeon must maintain clinical records of the herd/flock/individual.

undershot jaw Condition of the mandible where the incisor teeth of the lower jaw are placed in front of those in the upper jaw.

under-training Where there is insufficient training involving different circumstances, too few repetitions to develop a habit or a 'learned behaviour'.

undescended testis The visible defect may be bilateral or unilateral, where the normal migration of the testis into the scrotum soon after birth fails for a genetic or hormonal reason; *see also* CRYPTORCHID.

undifferentiated Error of development when a primitive feature still remains; is important in biopsy cell diagnosis of malignancy.

undulant fever Name formerly used for human brucellosis infection.

ungual Relating to the hooves, nails or claws.

uni- Prefix meaning 'single' or 'one of a kind'.

unicellular Having a one-cell structure; typical of bacteria and of protozoa.

unilateral Involving one side of the body.

union Coming together or forming a junction; *see also* FRACTURE.

uniparous Giving birth to a single offspring; more typical of human reproduction than of pet animals; sometimes called primiparous, as in a pregnancy that produces one young capable of survival.

unmyelinated Describes nerve axons that have no myelin sheath.

unsaturated Describes fats that have a structure with one or two double bonds in their carbon chain structure; they are considered beneficial in some skin and circulatory disorders.

unsocial behaviour Any behaviour pattern that offends the human keeper of animals but in some cases may be a perfectly natural occurrence, e.g. urine marking as an expression of 'normal behaviour'.

unstriated The type of muscle that moves involuntarily, as in smooth muscle of the viscera or the more specialized cardiac muscle.

ununited Refers to the nonhealing fracture or when an epiphysis does not join with a diaphysis. Common in osteochondrosis of the elbow where part of the anconeal process fails to fuse with the main head of the ulna; *see also* OSTEOCHONDROSIS.

upper Above, but sometimes words such as cranial, rostral or oral may have a similar usage.

upper motor neurones Efferent neurones with cell bodies in the brain and axons that run down the spinal cord to synapse with the lower motor neurones. They initiate and control muscle movements.

upper respiratory tract The nose, paranasal sinuses, nasopharynx and larynx.

U

upsaliensis A type of *Campylobacter* infection that has become recognized as a common cause of dog diarrhoea; named from the Swedish veterinary centre at Uppsala.

urachus The part of the umbilical cord that connects to the bladder; usually a solid fibrous cord at birth, but sometimes it will remain open and dribble urine, when it is known as a 'pervious urachus'.

uraemia Elevated levels of urea in the blood, usually associated with kidney disease; the harmful effects of urea are not as great as some of the other products retained; *see also* AZOTAEMIA.

uraemic fits Convulsions may result from many causes but in advanced renal failure, often accompanied by hepatic failure, toxic products such as ammonia have deleterious effects on brain function.

uranoschisis An alternative name for a cleft palate.

urate Salt of uric acid; Dalmatians normally excrete high levels of urate as part of their metabolism; a salt with ammonia sometimes forms in acid urine and may be one of the types of calculi found.

urea Nitrogenous compound produced in the liver as a less toxic substance than the ammonia that results from protein metabolism. Commonly measured in the laboratory as a simple indicator of renal function.

urease Enzyme that will break down urea; a constituent of one of the stick tests for measuring blood urea. Many bacteria produce a urease. A test for *Helicobacter pylori*, which colonizes the stomach, is the urease test.

ureter A tube that connects the pelvis of the kidney to the neck of the bladder. An **ectopic ureter** is a misplaced tube that drains directly into the vagina and is a possible cause of incontinence in the 'difficult-to-house-train' puppy.

ureteral Relating to the ureter.

ureteral calculus One of the concretions causing dysuria; *see also* CALCULUS.

ureteral fibroepithelial polyp (UFEP) Benign neoplasm or the result of chronic inflammation; often associated with urinary incontinence.

ureteral obstruction Caused by a combination of an obstructing body and a spasm of the smooth muscle.

ureterocolostomy Surgical method of connecting the ureter to the colon to bypass the bladder; the operation is a form of ureteroenterostomy.

ureteropyelography Method of radiographic examination of the kidneys and ureters using an intravenous contrast medium.

ureterovaginal fistula Passage between the ureter and the vagina; an abnormality said to be produced by incautious spaying surgery.

urethra Tube from the bladder to the exterior – short in the female and longer and narrower in the male.

urethral Relating to the urethra.

urethral calculus Small stone or concretion causing a total or partial obstruction to the flow of urine; most frequently found at the point where the urethra is restricted by the shape of the os penis and less frequently where the urethra curves round from the floor of the pelvis.

urethral obstruction A calculus is the most common obstruction, but trauma or scar tissue may have a similar effect.

urethral plug More typical of feline urolithiasis syndrome when small calculi form an obstruction with mucilaginous protein.

urethral stricture A narrowing of the urethra, often a sequel to calculus damage or a previous urethrotomy.

urethritis Inflammatory condition of the urethra, may be associated with calculi.

urethrorectal fistula Passage between the urethra and the rectum; the result of a developmental defect in producing a cloaca or sometimes after a birth canal trauma by a tear of the vaginal roof; *see also* FISTULA.

urethrostomy Permanent hole after a surgical incision into the lumen of the urethra, usually to relieve an obstruction and help in the passage of calculi out of the bladder. A **perineal urethrostomy** is an incision made between the anus and the scrotum. A **scrotal urethrostomy** is an incision made at the level of the scrotum, sometimes accompanied by castration; *see also* STOMA.

urethrotomy The surgical incision into the urethra when a temporary opening is created.

-uria Suffix relating to a condition of urine; *see also* POLYURIA.

uric acid Naturally produced end-product of purine breakdown, found especially in bird excrement; may be one cause of calculi in the urinary tract.

uricotelic Excreting uric acid as a white paste via deamination; excretion by lizards, snakes and birds.

urinalysis The testing of urine for diseases such as diabetes, nephrosis, etc.

urinary Relating to the urine production and excretion mechanisms.

urinary calculus 'Stones' in the tract anywhere between the kidney and the tip of the penis.

urinary energy (UE) The loss of energy in urine from food and the breakdown of endogenous metabolized proteins.

urinary incontinence Some failure of the mechanism that allows urine to be stored in the bladder until the appropriate time for bladder emptying.

urinary territory marking Behaviour mechanism that allows urine to be emptied from the bladder in any appropriate place to show that an individual animal has visited the spot.

urination The controlled and periodic emptying of the bladder through the urethra; applies equally to males and females; *see also* MICTURATE.

urine Complex solution of excreted products produced by the kidneys and the major route of nitrogen excretion.

urine marking Usually occurs as cats spraying by backing up to a vertical object or male dogs leg-lifting at any vertical marking post. Should be differentiated from normal bladder emptying by the different body posture adopted.

urine output A measurement of the total volume of urine produced over a given period of time. A number of metabolic and renal diseases can be indicated by changes in urine output.

urine scald Skin inflammation similar to a burn caused by urine that has soaked into the skin; often caused by urinary incontinence or poor husbandry.

urinogenital Relating to the tracts involved in reproduction as well as the excretory system for urine.

urinometer Laboratory instrument formerly used for estimating the specific gravity of urine.

uroabdomen Condition where urine leaks into the peritoneal cavity, often the result of a tear in the bladder wall.

urobilin Pigment substance formed by the oxidation of urobilinogen.

urobilinogen Product of the breakdown of bilirubin when bacteria act in the intestine; some may be absorbed back into the bloodstream then excreted by the kidneys.

urochrome One of the colouring agents of urine, produced from bile pigments.

urogenital Relating to both systems; *see also* URINOGENITAL.

urography Radiographic examination of the urinary tract; *see also* PNEUMOCYSTOGRAM.

urolith A stone in the bladder or urethra; common materials are struvite, ammonium urate, calcium oxalate, silicate and cystine.

urolithiasis The state of producing calculi in the urinary tract.

URT Upper respiratory tract.

urticaria Allergic response; involves oedema and a vascular response to mast cell degradation; *see also* NETTLE RASH.

uterine Relating to the breeding organ of the female.

uterine adenocarcinoma Neoplasia of the uterus; one of the commonest causes of death in unneutered female rabbits.

uterine horn The part of the uterus leading to the ovary as two tubes running cranial to the main body; especially important in multiple birth animals. Birds have two, but only the left one is functional.

uterine milk Used for the internal secretion of mucoid, milk-like fluid that surrounds the fertilized egg before implantation.

uterine prolapse Eversion of the uterus so it reaches the exterior through the vulva; often a sequel to a difficult birth and the expulsion of fetal membranes.

uterine stump granuloma Chronic inflammation and discharge as a result of a hysterectomy where part of the cervix remains in place as a focus of infection; often associated with unabsorbed ligature material.

U

uterine tube The connection between the fimbriae and the uterine horn; the site of fertilization of the ova; *see also* FALLOPIAN TUBE, OVIDUCT.

uteroverdine A green vulval discharge seen 2 hours before birth is due; *see also* WHELPING.

uterus Found in the female as an important hollow organ; during pregnancy functions first for the development of the fetus and later the surrounding smooth muscle of the uterine wall is used to propel the developed offspring to the outside world; *see also* DELIVERY.

UTI Urinary tract infection.

utricle A little sac-like cavity. **1)** In the ear where the macula responds to the position of the head with respect to the pull of gravity. **2)** The cavity in the prostate gland used for fluid storage that connects with the urethra.

uvea Term used for those vascular and pigmented structures occupying the middle part of the eyeball within the outer sclera: ciliary body, lens suspension, iris and choroid.

uveal tract Name for the vascular area of the eye: choroid, ciliary body and iris.

uveitis Inflammation of the uvea; may be an important cause of blindness; *see also* IRIDOCYCLITIS.

uvula Pendulous structure at the back of the soft palate, not evident in domestic animals.

vaccinate Administer a vaccine.

vaccination Inoculation of an individual with antigenic material to stimulate artificial active immunity; vaccination protocols usually consist of two primary injections (although only one may be required with live vaccines), followed by regular boosters; see APPENDIX 10.

vaccination reaction Anaphylactic reaction following the administration of a vaccine; rare; see also ANAPHYLACTIC SHOCK.

vaccine Any preparation of antigenic material that will stimulate an immune response, e.g. bacterial wall proteins, killed bacteria, attenuated virus or toxoid.

vacuole Fluid-filled cavity within the cytoplasm of a cell; surrounds material that is being digested by the cell.

Vacutainer Blood collection system consisting of a tube sealed under a vacuum, a holder and a needle; the apparatus allows blood sampling without the operator coming into contact with the blood; tubes are available containing a range of anticoagulants.

vacuum A space containing either no gas or gas at a very low pressure.

vagina Part of the female reproductive tract; a muscular tube extending from the cervix to the vulva; see also TIE.

vaginal smear A smear made from the cells lining the vagina, which may be used to determine the stage of oestrus cycle in the bitch. Red blood cells appear in the smear during prooestrus, while keratinized epithelial cells predominate during oestrus; vaginal mucus may also be sampled for pregnancy diagnosis in the bitch, the ferning pattern of the mucus having a characteristic formation during pregnancy.

vaginate Enclosed in a sheath.

vaginitis Inflammation of the vagina.

vaginoplasty Removal of congenital fibrous bands that may be the cause of problems at mating; see also WHELPING, EPISIOPLASTY.

vaginoscope Speculum for dilating the vulva and vagina to facilitate examination and urinary catheterization.

vaginovesical Relating to the vagina and the urinary bladder.

vagolytic A drug inhibiting the effects of the vagus nerve.

vagomimetic A drug whose effects mimic the actions of the vagus nerve.

vagus Cranial nerve X; it is both motor and sensory to the pharynx, larynx, lungs and digestive tract, controlling important autonomic functions such as swallowing and digestion.

valency Measure of the ability of elements to combine with others during formation of molecules, based on that of hydrogen, which has a valency of 1.

valgus Angular limb deformity with outward rotation of the foot away from the midline.

valproate Anticonvulsant medication used in the treatment of epilepsy.

valve A flap-like structure or fold of a membrane within a vessel to limit the flow to one direction only, e.g. the mitral (bicuspid) valve, which prevents blood flowing back from the left ventricle into the atrium, vein valves.

vane Structure of the bird's wing composed of the barbs and barbels; separated into inner and outer webs by the central shaft.

vaporizer The part of an anaesthetic circuit where the liquid volatile agent is converted to a vapour; the more modern vaporizers are temperature and pressure compensated to provide a controlled and accurate percentage of anaesthetic agent in the gaseous mix, irrespective of changes in flow rate and cooling.

vapour permeable film Skin dressing used to aid moist wound healing and act as a barrier to protect an open wound.

V

varicosis Dilation of a vein.

varus Angular limb deformity with inward rotation of the foot towards the midline.

vas deferens, *pl.* **vasa deferentia** Part of the male reproductive tract; one of a pair of vessels that carry spermatozoa from the epididymis to the urethra.

vascular Having a blood supply; tissues that become avascular, e.g. as a result of trauma, are nonviable.

vascular ring anomaly Developmental abnormality where a ring of intrathoracic blood vessels constricts the oesophagus, leading to difficulty swallowing, regurgitation and megaoesophagus cranial to the constriction; *see also* PERSISTENT RIGHT AORTIC ARCH.

vasculitis Inflammation of the walls of blood vessels; *see also* MENINGITIS.

vasculogenic shock Imbalance between circulating blood volume and tissue oxygen requirements because of excessive vasoconstriction.

vasectomy Surgical transection of the vasa deferentia, rendering the male sterile; *see also* VAS DEFERENS.

vasoactive Having an effect on the tone and diameter of a blood vessel.

vasoconstriction Narrowing of blood vessels caused by the contraction of smooth muscle in the vessel wall.

vasodilatation Widening of the lumen of a blood vessel caused by relaxation of smooth muscle in the vessel wall.

vasodilator Agent or drug that causes dilation of blood vessels.

vasomotor Able to constrict and dilate, thus changing diameter; term is applied to blood vessels.

vasomotor centre Nerve control centre in the medulla oblongata that regulates blood pressure by vasoconstriction and vasodilation.

vasopressin Antidiuretic hormone (ADH); produced by the posterior pituitary gland; increases water resorption by the kidneys.

VD Ventrodorsal; term used in X-ray positioning.

vector An invertebrate animal such as a tick or a mite that carries a parasite from one vertebrate host to another.

vecuronium bromide A nondepolarizing neuromuscular blocking agent.

vegetans Describes a granulomatous type of dermatitis; *see also* PEMPHIGUS.

VEGF Vascular endothelial growth factor; a protein factor that promotes angiogenesis.

vein A thin-walled blood vessel carrying deoxygenated blood towards the heart (NB: the pulmonary vein carries oxygenated blood to the heart from the lungs).

Velpeau sling A foreleg bandage that may be used to prevent weight bearing, e.g. after reduction of an elbow luxation.

velvet (golden rust disease) Flagellate infection of fish that makes them appear covered in a gold dust, caused by *Oodinium* spp.

Venables plate Metal bone plate with circular screw holes, used for internal fixation of fractures.

venae cavae The great veins; the **cranial vena cava** is formed by the union of the right and left brachiocephalic veins and carries deoxygenated blood back to the heart from the head, neck, forelimbs and cranial thorax; the **caudal vena cava** is formed by the union of the common iliac veins and brings blood to the right atrium of the heart from the caudal thorax, abdomen and hindlimbs.

venepuncture *See* VENIPUNCTURE.

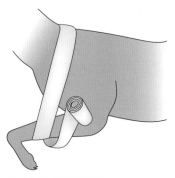

Figure 51. Velpeau sling.

venereal disease A disease that is transmitted at mating; *see also* TRANSMISSIBLE VENEREAL TUMOUR.

venipuncture Puncture of a vein with a needle to obtain a blood sample or inject a solution.

venography Radiographic study where positive contrast media are injected into a vein; for example, ionic contrast media may be injected into the hepatic portal vein to demonstrate a portosystemic shunt.

venom Poisonous substance produced by many snakes, scorpions, etc.; antisera to specific venoms may be available.

venom gland A gland that produces and stores venom.

venous sinus Normal dilations and enlargements of veins, e.g. the venous sinuses around the spinal cord beneath the dura mater.

vent *See* CLOACA.

vent gleet Inflammation of the avian vent, with a characteristic smell, caused by a herpesvirus infection; it is contagious and affected birds should be culled.

ventilate Provide with oxygen during anaesthesia; an anaesthetized patient may be ventilated if necessary by squeezing the reservoir bag or by using a mechanical ventilator; *see also* VENTILATOR.

ventilation–perfusion mismatch Any imbalance between alveolar ventilation and the pulmonary blood flow, resulting in hypoxia.

ventilator Mechanical apparatus to supply oxygen automatically to a patient, e.g. Manley, Minivent Blease, which have now been superseded by electronic ventilators; the respiratory rate and tidal volume are set so that ventilation is adequate; essential when muscle relaxants have been given as part of the anaesthetic protocol.

ventral Towards or near the lower body surface or belly; includes the undersurface of the neck and tail.

ventral slot Surgical technique that involves a ventral approach to the cervical spine and the removal of a rectangular area of bone and intervertebral disc material from two adjacent vertebrae, thus relieving pressure on the spinal cord; a surgical option for some cases of cervical disc prolapse and wobbler syndrome.

ventricle A chamber, e.g. ventricles of the heart, ventricles of the brain or laryngeal ventricles.

ventricular Referring to ventricles, usually of the heart.

ventricular arrhythmia Any irregularity in the pattern of cardiac ventricular contractions.

ventricular fibrillation Life-threatening cardiac arrhythmia where the ventricles fail to contract in a coordinated fashion but quiver instead; inadequate blood volume is supplied to the brain, resulting in rapid loss of consciousness and death if the normal rhythm is not restored rapidly.

ventricular septal defect (VSD) Any defect (usually congenital) in the muscular wall between the right and left ventricles. A VSD allows blood to move from the left (high-pressure) side of the heart into the right (low-pressure) ventricle, leading to right ventricular overload and pulmonary congestion. A murmur is often audible, and the defect is found in association with other cardiac abnormalities such as tetralogy of Fallot and pulmonic stenosis.

ventrodorsal In a direction from the ventral surface towards the spine.

venule Small vessel receiving deoxygenated blood from a capillary.

vera Means 'true' or 'real'; **polycythaemia vera** is a neoplastic condition with increased red cell formation.

vernier scale A scale that accurately measures small distances; the vernier scale on the stage of a microscope is

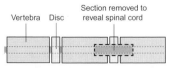

Figure 52. Ventral slot.

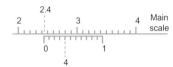

Reading 2.44

Figure 53. Vernier scale.

used to pinpoint the exact position of an object so that it can be relocated; a reading is obtained by seeing which mark on the main scale is closest to the zero on the short scale and the next decimal place is obtained by seeing where the marks on the two scales align.

vertebra, *pl.* vertebrae Bone of the spinal column; cervical, thoracic, lumbar, sacral and caudal (coccygeal).

vertebrate An animal having a spine made up of vertebrae.

vertical transmission Transmission of a disease from one generation to the next, usually passed from mother to offspring.

vesical Relating to a bladder, usually the urinary bladder.

vesicle A fluid-filled blister.

vesicovaginal Relating to the bladder and vagina.

vestibular disease Disease of the vestibular apparatus of the inner ear, leading to head tilt, circling and ataxia.

vestibule A space leading to the entrance to a canal.

vestibulocochlear nerve The eighth cranial nerve, the vestibular component providing information concerning the orientation of the head and the cochlear division mediating hearing; lesions along the nerve give rise to symptoms such as head tilt, ataxia, nystagmus and deafness.

Veterinary Medicines Directorate (VMD) A UK government body sponsored by DEFRA and charged with promoting animal health and welfare by assuring the safety, quality and efficacy of veterinary medicines.

Veterinary Surgeons Act 1966 Parliamentary act that governs the veterinary profession and restricts the right to practise to members of the RCVS; Schedule 19 restricts the practice of veterinary surgery to registered members but Schedule 3 permits veterinary nurses to perform certain duties as defined by the Schedule 3 Amendment Order 2002.

veterinary technician The American equivalent of a qualified veterinary nurse; they will have undertaken a period of academic study, participated in on-the-job training and passed state-administered examinations.

vibrissa, *pl.* vibrissae Stiff sensory hairs located on the muzzle of many species.

villus, *pl.* villi Finger-like projection of tissue found in the small intestine and the placenta; the projections greatly increase the surface area over which diffusion and absorption of molecules can occur.

Vinca rosea Periwinkle plant, now grown commercially to source vincristine as a chemotherapeutic agent.

vincristine An antineoplastic alkaloid used in the treatment of lymphosarcoma and leukaemia; *see also* CYTOTOXIC.

viper Alternative name for the British poisonous snake *Vipera berus*. Also known as the adder.

viraemia Having virus particles in the bloodstream.

virile Possessing male characteristics and able to reproduce.

virulence A measure of the power of a pathogen to cause disease.

virulent Highly pathogenic and able to cause disease.

virus An infectious agent that is smaller than a bacterium and incapable of growth or reproduction outside a living host cell; viruses contain either RNA or DNA but not both.

visceral gout Disease of birds where kidney failure leads to the deposition of urates in internal organs.

visceral larva migrans (VLM) A syndrome in humans caused by the migration of *Toxocara canis* larvae through the tissues; symptoms depend on the location of the larvae but include fever, jaundice and ocular disturbances.

viscous Sticky, thick, glutinous.

viscus, *pl.* **viscera** Any organ within the pleural, pericardial and peritoneal cavities.

vision The ability to see.

vital capacity The volume of air that can be expelled after taking a maximally deep breath.

vitamin A dietary component other than fat, protein, carbohydrate and inorganic salts; present in small amounts in the food but essential for growth, reproduction and good health. Species differ in their vitamin needs.

vitamin A Retinol, a fat-soluble vitamin used in the synthesis of rhodopsin and in cell division and differentiation. Foods with high vitamin A content include liver and fish; deficiency leads to reproductive failure, night-blindness and xerophthalmia and is rare in all species other than terrapins; hypervitaminosis A (e.g. in cats fed solely on fish or liver) accelerates bone remodelling and leads to the formation of exostoses; widespread exostoses may limit movement in the spine so animals may have difficulty grooming themselves; exostoses around the optic nerves may impair vision.

vitamin B A water-soluble complex of substances (thiamine, riboflavin, niacin, pyridoxine, pantothenic acid, folic acid and biotin) that are important coenzymes in many cell metabolic processes; toxicities are rare as any excess is readily excreted; deficiency causes anaemia, etc.

vitamin C Ascorbic acid; water-soluble vitamin found predominantly in fresh fruits and vegetables; adequate vitamin C is manufactured in the liver of most animals other than primates and guinea pigs and is not therefore required in the diet.

vitamin D A steroidal calciferol complex formed by the action of sunlight on precursor molecules; fat-soluble; important for bone and teeth formation; excess vitamin D leads to elevated blood calcium levels and results in calcification of soft tissue, anorexia and weight loss; deficiency causes rickets and osteomalacia.

vitamin E Alpha-tocopherol; fat-soluble vitamin important as an antioxidant; deficiency causes muscular dystrophy and pan-steatitis.

vitamin K A fat-soluble factor necessary for the biosynthesis of prothrombin and therefore important in clotting; deficiency results in clotting disorders; used as part of the treatment for warfarin poisoning.

vitiligo A skin condition characterized by the appearance of depigmented patches; thought to have an underlying autoimmune mechanism.

vitreous Resembling glass or having the colour of glass.

vitreous humour Fluid that fills the posterior chamber of the eye; normally of a stiff jelly composition.

vivarium Container often used for housing reptiles and other exotic species, literally means 'cage of life'.

viviparous Giving birth to live young.

vivisection Scientific experimentation using animal models.

VMD *See* VETERINARY MEDICINES DIRECTORATE.

VMP Veterinary Medicinal Product.

VMR Veterinary Medicine Regulations; regulations introduced in 2005 and implemented by the VMD; rules governing the provision of veterinary drugs, categories now Prescription Only Medicine – Veterinarian (POM–V), Prescription Only Medicine – Veterinarian, Pharmacist, Suitably Qualified Person (POM–VPS), Non-Food Animal – Veterinarian, Pharmacist, Suitably Qualified Person (NFA–VPS), Authorised Veterinary Medicine – General Sales List (AVM–GSL)

vocal fold Membranes covering the vocal chords; the folds project into the larynx and are used to produce sound.

vocational Practical training for a profession or occupation; *see also* NATIONAL COUNCIL FOR VOCATIONAL QUALIFICATIONS.

volar On the undersurface of a fore- or hindfoot; *see also* PALMAR, PLANTAR.

volatile A substance that evaporates readily.

Volkmann canal The network of canals within bone that carry blood vessels from the surface to the haversian systems.

Volkmann curette A small, spoon-shaped curette used for obtaining cancellous bone graft material.

voltage The electrical potential difference between two points.

voluntary Under the conscious control of an individual.

voluntary consent An owner's decision to consent or not to consent to treatment of their pet must be made by the owner without pressure or undue influence from veterinary professionals or others.

voluntary muscle Muscles under conscious control; *see also* STRIATED MUSCLE.

volvulus Obstruction of a hollow organ caused by twisting, e.g. **gastric volvulus**.

vomeronasal organ A structure at the base of the nasal septum; thought to play a role in olfaction.

vomit Expel stomach contents through the mouth.

vomiting Autonomic reflex where stomach contents are ejected via the mouth; sometimes confused with regurgitation; *see also* REGURGITATION.

vomitus The material expelled during vomiting.

von Willebrand factor A clotting factor essential for platelet adhesion and aggregation.

von Willebrand's disease An inherited bleeding disorder, endothelial in origin, transmitted as an autosomal trait. Haemorrhage may occur spontaneously, e.g. epistaxis, or it may follow routine surgery such as spaying; an autosomal dominant characteristic; has been reported in more than 50 different breeds, including particularly Dobermann and German shepherd dogs.

voracious Greedy appetite, characterized by very rapid eating.

V-plasty Surgical technique for the repair of full-thickness eyelid defects; a V-shaped section, encompassing the defect, is removed, and the conjunctiva and skin are then closed in two separate layers.

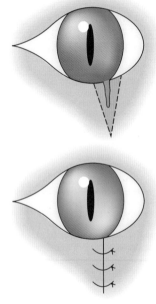

Figure 54. V-plasty (eyelid).

Wallerian degeneration The degeneration that occurs to the portion of a nerve fibre distal to the point of injury; characterized by demyelination and resorption of the axon.

Walpole's solution Low pH; used to help dissolve struvite calculi plugs that may form in the male cat's urethra.

warfarin Potent anticoagulant used as a rodenticide; also used therapeutically in some prothrombotic disorders, such as DIC. The accidental consumption of warfarin by pets should be treated with vitamin K and emetics; *see also* COAGULATION DISORDERS.

warm-blooded Able to thermoregulate and maintain a body temperature higher than that of the external environment.

wart Verrucose benign growth, often caused by papillomavirus infection.

washing machine murmur Splashing sounds due to gas and fluid in the pericardial sac.

washing soda Sodium carbonate; may be used as an emergency measure to induce vomiting if an animal has recently ingested a nonirritant poison; *see also* EMETIC.

waste, clinical All waste materials generated by a business, such as a veterinary practice, that may be contaminated with animal matter (e.g. bedding, bandages, swabs), plus drug packaging; has to be disposed of in labelled yellow bags via a licensed clinical waste carrier.

waste, pathological Animal tissue such as excised tumours, uteri, etc. generated by a business.

waste transfer note (WTN) Legal document that must be completed and accompany any transfer of waste between different holders. Notes have to be kept for proof of transfer of waste to a licensed carrier and to demonstrate to inspectors that waste has been disposed of correctly.

water Chemically, H_2O; liquid consisting of hydrogen and oxygen; a major constituent of all animal and vegetable tissues; vital to sustain life. Animals require access to water at all times unless specifically contraindicated for short periods, e.g. prior to general anaesthesia or during water deprivation tests.

Waters canister Part of a rebreathing anaesthetic circuit; a canister packed with soda lime where exhaled carbon dioxide is reabsorbed; *see also* SODA LIME.

WBC *See* WHITE BLOOD CELL.

wean Put on to solid food and remove access to maternal milk (gradual is best).

web The sheet of tissue bridging the space between each of the toes.

wedge ostectomy Surgical technique used to correct an angular limb deformity; a wedge of bone is removed from the region of greatest curvature and the fracture reduced using a bone plate or external fixation device; the technique results in some shortening of the limb, although this is not usually of functional significance.

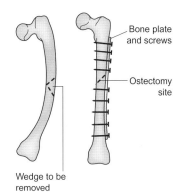

Figure 55. Wedge ostectomy.

weight The force exerted on a body by the gravity of the earth. Body weight or heaviness is usually measured in kilograms (kg). **Atomic weight** is the mass (in grams) of 1 mole (6×10^{-3}) of atoms of an element. **Molecular weight** is the sum of the atomic weights of the atoms in a molecule.

weight loss Reduction in body weight; may be desirable in obese animals or may be associated with many disease states; body weight will reduce if calorific intake is below the metabolic requirement or if metabolic needs increase, e.g. burns, postsurgery.

Weil's disease Disease caused by *Leptospira icterohaemorrhagiae*; characterized by pyrexia and jaundice; *see also* ICTERIC, JAUNDICE.

welfare Well-being of the animal; an important responsibility of all people caring for animals. The Animal Welfare Act 2006 brought together and updated 20 pieces of animal welfare legislation and defines the duty of care to animals.

West Nile Virus Flavivirus transmitted by mosquitoes that can affect horses in warm climates across Europe, Middle East, Africa, Asia and America; clinical signs include fever and neurological abnormalities arising from encephalitis; a vaccine is available in the US.

West's retractors Self-retaining retractors with curved teeth; used for holding soft tissues out of the surgical field.

Wesselsbron disease Caused by a *flavivirus,* a disease mainly of farm livestock in Sub-Saharan Africa; notifiable disease in Australia.

wet tail A common condition in recently weaned hamsters, characterized by profuse diarrhoea; possibly caused by stress and *Escherichia coli* infection.

wheal An area of reddened, oedematous skin; part of the classic inflammatory response (pain, redness, heat, swelling and loss of function); also spelled weal.

wheat-sensitive enteropathy Allergy to the gluten in ingested wheat products, resulting in malabsorption, weight loss and chronic diarrhoea; mainly reported in Irish setters and West Highland white terriers; treatment involves feeding a gluten-free diet.

wheeze Audible whistling sound made during dyspnoeic breathing.

whelp 1) Give birth to puppies. 2) Unweaned puppies – **whelps**.

whipworm *Trichuris* sp. nematode; endoparasite that may occasionally cause diarrhoea in dogs but is of more clinical significance in warmer climates; adult worm is about 7 cm long with a slender anterior portion; eggs are barrel shaped with a plug at each end.

whirlpool bath Form of hydrotherapy involving partial immersion of the patient in a bath with jets of warm water.

white blood cell (WBC) Leukocyte; any cell formed by the reticuloendothelial system: neutrophils, eosinophils, basophils, small and large lymphocytes and monocytes.

white blood cell count Laboratory technique for counting the number of WBCs per unit volume of blood; process may be mechanized or can be carried out using a counting chamber; having ascertained a total WBC count, a differential count can then be done by counting 100 WBCs in a smear.

white matter Areas of the brain and spinal cord that appear white as they contain nerve axons wrapped in myelin sheaths; *see also* GREY MATTER.

white muscle disease Muscular dystrophy resulting from a lack of vitamin E; rare but used to be seen in calves and lambs.

white spot External disease of fish caused by the parasite *Ichthyophthirius multifiliis*; white areas appear, especially around the gills but may break out over much of the fish; proprietary treatments are available based on malachite green solution.

whorl Circular patch of hair.

Willebrand's disease *See* VON WILLEBRAND'S DISEASE.

Willis, circle of Ring of arterial blood vessels within the cranium at the base of the brain; formed by the paired internal carotid arteries and vertebral arteries; supplies blood to the mid- and forebrain.

windgalls Fluid distension of the fetlock joints or tendon sheaths of horses.

wind-sucking Contraction of upper neck muscles in the horse, causing air to be sucked into the upper oesophagus and resulting in a gulping sound (also known as aerophagia).

Winslow, foramen of *See* EPIPLOIC FORAMEN.

wiring A technique for fracture fixation; may be used as a modified means of stabilization in birds. **Cerclage wiring** is an internal fixation technique where wire is wrapped tightly around two bone fragments to hold them together; cannot be used as the sole method of fixation but is a useful adjunct for long spiral fractures that are inherently stable. In **hemicerclage wiring,** a wire suture is anchored through a drill hole in one bone fragment and wrapped around the external circumference of the second fragment. A **K wire** is a thin metal pin that may be used to anchor fracture fragments; may be used as cross pins or used to hold fragments temporarily while other fixation devices are applied; useful fixation technique for some epiphyseal fractures in young animals where the fracture line may cross a growth plate; also used in tension band wiring to hold the figure-of-eight wire in position. **Tension band wiring** is an internal fixation technique for bony fragments that are likely to avulse or distract, such as the tibial crest; the fragment is secured with two parallel K wires and wire is then wrapped around the pins and through a hole drilled in the bone in a figure-of-eight.

withdrawal reflex Normal protective response with flexion of the limb joints away from a painful stimulus; may be elicited by pinching the toes or the webbing between the toes; as the stimulus is increased, the more proximal limb joints should also be flexed; used to assess neurological function and responses during anaesthesia.

withers The top of the shoulders in horses. This is the point used to measure the height of a horse.

wobbler syndrome Cervical spondylopathy; a neurological condition characterized by progressive ataxia and neck pain. **1)** Particularly common in young great Danes and older Dobermann pinschers; caused by pressure on the cervical spinal cord from unstable discs, deformed vertebrae or hypertrophied spinal ligaments; may be managed conservatively but many affected dogs require surgery such as ventral slotting or cervical fusion. 2) Equine wobbler syndrome is also characterized by ataxia (most commonly in young horses) caused by malformations or compression of the spinal cord. Treatments include corrective surgery, drug therapy, controlled exercise regimens and nutritional management.

Wolff's law The law describing the normal response of bone to the stresses placed upon it: bone remodels constantly such that it is deposited in areas that are subjected to stress and is removed from regions that do not experience stress; therefore bone is resorbed when a limb is immobilized.

wolf teeth Small teeth that may be present in front of the first molar in the horse, often removed if they interfere with the action of the bit.

womb Uterus.

Wood's lamp Ultraviolet lamp used to detect fluorescent hairs in the coat infected with *Microsporum* spp. of ringworm; fluorescence is typically an apple-green or yellow and is most commonly seen on the ears, around the face and on the paws.

wool eating Behavioural disorder of dogs and cats that can rapidly become a habit; may be associated with early weaning and sucking reflexes. Similar behaviour may be seen in rabbits that make nests with their own and other rabbits' fur.

Working Time Directive A directive from the European Union that gives EU workers the right to a minimum number of holidays each year, rest breaks, a maximum average 48-hour week, etc. as excessive working hours can be a major cause of stress and illness; hours should be stipulated in a contract of employment (in the UK, more than 48 hours can be worked in a week in some professions and with the signed agreement between employer and employee as long as the average does not go over 48 over any 17-week period).

work-up Term used to describe the logical and thorough diagnostic approach to a case, including the rational use of tests

W

such as radiography, laboratory tests and electrodiagnostic testing.

worm Common endoparasite of all animals and humans; various roundworm and tapeworm species inhabit the gastrointestinal tract. The stages of the life cycle may involve migration through body tissues; worms may target lung tissue (e.g. *Aelurostrongylus abstrusus*), the urinary tract (e.g. *Capillaria putorii*) or blood vessels (e.g. *Dirofilaria immitis*). Although generally controlled by routine worming and good hygiene measures, a number of worms cause serious zoonotic diseases (*see* APPENDIX 4); appropriate worming preparations should be used for the specific worms in question.

wound Trauma to the body resulting in tissue damage and a break in continuity; includes surgical wounds, incised wounds (made by sharp objects) and puncture wounds (opening is small compared with the depth of the wound).

wrist Lay term for the carpus.

wrymouth Lateral displacement of the mandible and teeth – a show fault in dogs.

wryneck *See* TORTICOLLIS.

WVAG Western Veterinary Acupuncture Group. The association, which was founded in 2000, applies scientific principles in the use of acupuncture in practice. The European School of Veterinary Postgraduate Studies offers a General Practitioner Certificate in Western Veterinary Acupuncture and Chronic Pain Management.

xanthine oxidase Enzyme involved in the production of uric acid; the inhibitor allopurinol has been used in the treatment of urolithiasis where uric acid forms calculi; *see also* UROLITHIASIS.

xanthochromic Yellow-coloured; deposition of yellow pigments is commonly associated with jaundice; *see also* JAUNDICE.

xanthoma Benign granulomatous lesion of the skin; caused by deposition of cholesterol to form fatty, yellow plaques and nodules.

X chromosome The sex chromosome present in both the sexes, males being heterozygous (XY) and females being homozygous (XX).

xenograft Tissue/organ grafting technique where the donor and recipient are from different species; *see also* HETEROGRAFT.

xerophthalmia Dryness of the conjunctiva and cornea, resulting from vitamin A deficiency; can predispose to corneal ulceration.

xiphisternum *See* XIPHOID PROCESS.

xiphoid cartilage Cartilaginous (distal) portion of the xiphoid process, where the linea alba and rectus abdominis muscle insert.

xiphoid process Xiphisternum; the most caudal sternebra; continues as a cartilaginous projection and is the insertion for the abdominal muscles.

X-linked Describes a trait carried by a gene on the X (female) chromosome; if the gene results in disease, all males will be affected as they have one X and one Y chromosome; females may be affected or carriers, depending on whether they have one or both X chromosomes with the gene.

X-radiation Invisible ionizing radiation that is part of the electromagnetic spectrum; it has a shorter wavelength than visible light, penetrates tissue and affects photographic film; produced in the X-ray tube head by bombarding a metal target (usually tungsten) with high-speed electrons. The absorption of X-radiation by tissue depends on the density and atomic weight of the material; chronic exposure to radiation is damaging to tissues; *see also* RADIATION.

X-ray film Light-sensitive film used to produce a radiographic image.

X-ray tube head Part of the X-ray machine housing the target where the X-rays are produced; *see also* TARGET.

xylazine A sedative/hypnotic that is used as a premedicant or in combination with ketamine to provide anaesthesia; may also be used to induce vomiting in cats.

xylose A five-carbon sugar; poorly absorbed from the small intestine and so is used in some specialized tests for intestinal function.

Y chromosome Sex chromosome only present in males.

yeast Unicellular fungus; in the diet it can be a source of B vitamins; a commensal of the skin and oral cavity but also associated with ear infections, stomatitis, dermatitis and enteritis if present in high numbers, e.g. in immunocompromised patients; *see also MALASSEZIA.*

yellow fat disease A disorder of cats metabolism caused by a deficiency of selenium and/or vitamin E; *see also* PANSTEATITIS.

Yersinia Genus of enteropathogenic Gram-negative rods that cause enteritis, colitis and diarrhoea; possibly zoonotic; affect dogs, cats, chickens, horses and cattle.

Yersinia pseudotuberculosis Organism causing pseudotuberculosis, a rare disease characterized by lethargy, weight loss and chronic diarrhoea.

Y-fracture A combination of an intercondylar and a supracondylar fracture of the distal humerus or femur, resulting in three fracture fragments; more commonly seen affecting the humerus, where there is separation of the two sides of the condyle through the articular surface and the supratrochlear foramen; also known as a T-fracture; requires prompt internal fixation to ensure joint mobility and function are restored.

yolk sac Structure within the embryo that contains yolk, the nutritive material for the developing fetus.

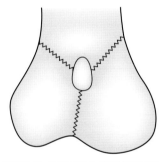

Figure 56. Y-fracture in distal humerus.

Ziehl–Neelsen stain Bacteriological staining method where the fixed smear is flooded with red Ziehl stain and heated for 1 minute, followed by decolouration in acid–alcohol and counterstaining with methylene blue; acid-fast organisms, such as *Mycobacteria* spp., stain red; *see also* ACID-FAST.

Zimmer splint A light finger splint made for humans consisting of a thin aluminium strip lined with a layer of foam padding; available in several widths and easily cut to length, although sharp metal ends should be rounded off. Useful as a first aid splinting material or can be included within the layers of a support bandage to provide additional external support; only suitable for cats and small dogs.

zinc A metallic dietary mineral and trace element necessary as a cofactor for a number of metalloproteases and other enzymes; deficiency is rare as dietary sources are generally adequate, but some animals may have poor uptake and respond to supplementation.

zinc oxide tape Nonelastic, adhesive tape used for anchoring dressings.

zinc-responsive dermatosis Hyperkeratotic skin disorder, characterized by crusty lesions around the eyes and mouth, thought to be caused by a defect in zinc uptake; treatment is to provide a zinc supplement in the diet.

zona pellucida The membrane initially surrounding the fertilized ovum.

zonary placentation Type of placentation found in the dog and cat where the villi from the allantochorion form a discrete broad band across the placenta – this is in contrast to other species where the villi are diffuse (mare, sow) or concentrated at sites known as cotyledons (ruminants).

zonule of Zinn Small zone on the anterior face of the vitreous body of the eye, consisting of fine ligamentous strands that run from the ciliary processes to the equator of the lens and hold the latter structure in place.

zonulysis A technique in cataract surgery to free the lens, to make it easier to remove.

zooeyia The positive benefits to human health from interacting with animals, focussed on the companion animal (the inverse of zoonoses).

zoogamy Reproduction using the fusion of two gametes.

Zoo Licensing Act 1981 Parliamentary act governing all zoos and open collections of nondomestic animals.

zoology The study of the biology of animals.

zoonosis A disease that can be communicated between animals and humans, *see also* APPENDIX 4.

Z-plasty Surgical technique for relieving tension on a skin incision by making two parallel incisions and joining them to create two triangular skin flaps, which are then rotated and sutured.

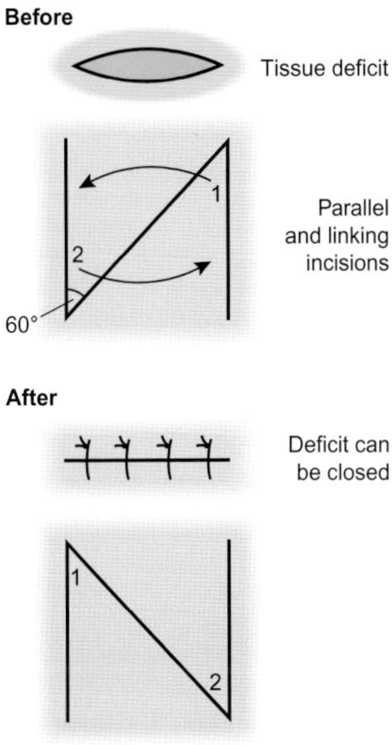

Before

Tissue deficit

Parallel
and linking
incisions

60°

After

Deficit can
be closed

Figure 57. Z-plasty.

zygapophysis Alternative name for the articular process on a vertebra.

zygomatic arch Cheekbone.

zygote The fertilized ovum, formed by the fusion of two haploid gametes, thus restoring the usual diploid number of chromosomes.

zymogen cells Found in the fundus of the stomach; secrete pepsinogen; *see also* CHIEF CELLS.

Appendices Contents

Appendix 1

1.1 Temperature, pulse and respiratory rates for different species

Species	Temperature °C (°F)	Pulse rate (beats/min)	Respiratory rate (breaths/min)
Cat	38.0–38.5 (100.4–101.6)	100–140 (170–220 in clinic)	20–30
Chicken	40.6–43.0 (105.0–109.4)	250–300	30–40
Degu	36.0–38.0 (96.8–100.4)	100–150	75–120
Dog	38.3–38.7 (100.9–101.7)	60–120	15–30
Gerbil	38.0–39.0 (100.4–102.2)	100–150	40–80
Guinea pig	39.0–40.0 (102.2–104.2)	130–190	90–150
Hamster	36.0–38.0 (98.0–101.0)	300–600	33–127
Horse	38.0–38.5 (100.4–101.6)	30–40	8–10
Rabbit	37.0–39.4 (99.0–103.0)	220	38–65
Rat	37.5–38.0 (99.8–100.5)	260–450	70–150

Appendix 2

2.1 Biochemistry parameters for dogs, cats, rabbits and horses

Test	Units	Normal range for adults			
		Dog	Cat	Rabbit	Horse
Alanine aminotransferase (ALT)	U/L @ 30°C	<25	<70	25–65	Not liver-specific
Albumin	g/L	25–37	26–41	27–50	31–38
Alkaline phosphatase (ALP)	U/L @ 30°C	<80	<70	10–70	70–220
Ammonia	µmol/L	<50	<100		
Amylase	U/L @ 30°C	1800	2500	166.5–314.5	198–476
Aspartate aminotransferase (AST)	U/L @ 30°C	<25	0–20	14–113	
B$_{12}$, vitamin	pmol/L	>140	>120		
Bile acids (fasting)	µmol/L	<5	<5		
Bile acids postprandial	µmol/L	<15	<15		
Bilirubin (total)	µmol/L	<16	<10	3.4–8.5	
Calcium	mmol/L	2.3–3.0	2.0–2.5	3.2–4.2	2.71–3.1
Chloride	mmol/L	99–105	117–140	92–112	
Cholesterol	mmol/L	3.8–7.0	2.5–6.0	10–80	
Cortisol (basal)	nmol/L	<130	<200		
Cortisol (post-adrenocorticotrophic hormone stimulation)	nmol/L	<550	<475		
Cortisol (post-dexamethasone suppression test 8 h)	nmol/L	<40			
Creatinine	µmol/L	<106	80–180	45–230	121–194
Creatine kinase (CK)	U/L @ 30°C	<190	<151	133–738	
Folate	nmol/L	11–30	9.0–25		
Gamma glutamyltransferase (GGT)	U/L	5–34			
Globulin (total)	g/L	23–52	26–51	15–28	16–30
Glucose	mmol/L	2.5–5.0	3.0–7.5	4.2–7.8	
Insulin (fasting)	µU/mL	5.0–20			
Phosphorus	mmol/L	0.8–1.6	1.0–2.0	4.0–6.9	
Potassium (K)	mmol/L	3.5–5.6	4.0–5.0	3.6–6.9	2.4–4.9
Protein (total)	g/L	54–77	54–78	54–78	50–64
Sodium (Na)	mmol/L	135–154	145–160	131–155	141–147
Sodium/potassium (Na/K) ratio		27–38	32–41		
Sorbitol dehydrogenase	U/L	1.8–6.7			
Thyroid-stimulating hormone (TSH)	ng/mL	<0.45			
Thyroxine (free)	pmol/L	5.0–30	9.0–33		
Thyroxine (total)	nmol/L	15–28	15–40	1.0–4.0	
Urea (BUN)	mmol/L	1.7–7.4	3.5–10.5	6.1–8.4	2.8–5.8
Urea/creatinine ratio		<0.07	<0.07		

2.2 Normal parameters for urine for dogs, cats and rabbits

Species	pH	Specific gravity (SG)	Isosthenuria (SG of urine = SG of blood)	Urine protein/ creatinine ratio
Dog	5.5–7.5	1.018–1.045	1.007–1.015	<1
Cat	5.5–7.5	1.020–1.040	1.007–1.015	<1
Rabbit	8.2	1.003–1.036		<0.6

2.3 Urine crystals

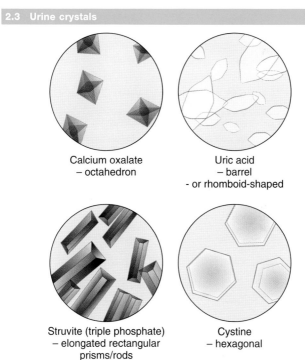

Calcium oxalate
– octahedron

Uric acid
– barrel
- or rhomboid-shaped

Struvite (triple phosphate)
– elongated rectangular
prisms/rods

Cystine
– hexagonal

Figure 58.

Appendix 3

Dictionary of Veterinary Nursing

Appendices

3.1 Haematology parameters for dogs, cats, rabbits and horses

Test	Units	Normal range for adults			
		Dog	Cat	Rabbit	Horse
Red blood cells	× 10^{12}/L	5.0–8.5	5.5–10.0	5.1–7.9	5.5–9.5
Haemoglobin (Hb)	g/100 mL (g%)	12–18	9–17	10.0–17.4	8–14
Packed cell volume (PCV or haematocrit)	(%)	37–57	27–50	33–50	24–44
MCV (mean corpuscular volume)	fL	60–77	40–55	57.8–66.5	34–59
MCH (mean corpuscular haemoglobin)	pg	19–23	13–17	17.1–23.5	12.3–20.5
MCHC (MCH concentration)	g/100 mL (g%)	31–34	31–34	29–37	31–38.6
White blood cells	× 10^9/L	6–15	4–15	5.2–12.5	5.4–14.3
Mature neutrophils	× 10^9/L	3.6–10.5	2.5–12.5		2.3–8.6
	%	60–70	45–75	20–75	
Band neutrophils	× 10^9/L	0–0.3	0–0.45		
	%	0–2	0–3		
Lymphocytes	× 10^9/L	1–4.8	1.5–6.5		1.5–7.7
	%	12–30	25–33	30–85	
Eosinophils	× 10^9/L	0.1–1.5	0.1–1.8		0–1
	%	2–10	4–12	1–4	
Monocytes	× 10^9/L	0.18–1.5	0–0.6		0–1.5
	%	3–10	0–4	1–4	
Basophils	× 10^9/L	Rare	Rare		0–0.3
	%	Rare	Rare	1–7	
Platelets	× 10^9/L	200–500	200–600	250–650	100–600

4.1 Zoonotic diseases

Disease	Causative agent	Symptoms in humans
Aspergillosis	*Aspergillus spp.*	Mainly respiratory symptoms, in immune-compromised people or those with other lung conditions
Bird 'flu'	Avian influenza virus (some strains)	Flu-like symptoms
Brucellosis	*Brucella abortus*, from infected cattle	Undulant fever
Campylobacter	*Campylobacter spp.*	Diarrhoea
Cat scratch fever	*Bartonella spp.*	Cellulitis at site of scratch or bite, fever, septicaemia
Cheyletiella	Surface-living mite	Skin irritation
Chlamydophila (formerly *Chlamydia*) *psittaci*	Intracellular parasite causing psittacosis; passes to humans by inhaling *Chlamydophila* in air-borne dust or cage contents of infected birds	Psittacosis: fever, dry cough, muscle pain and headaches Pneumonia: can be fatal; condition responds to tetracycline or erythromycin
Clostridium difficile	Anaerobic bacterial infection that has the potential to be transmitted via many complex routes; high risk for immunosuppressed individuals	Usually foul-smelling, watery diarrhoea
Cryptosporidiosis	Protozoa infection, transmitted via contaminated faeces	Watery diarrhoea
Ebola	Viral infection of humans, primates; possibly contracted via contact with infected blood and body fluids from bats but source remains unclear	Severe fever, diarrhoea, sore throat, vomiting, haemorrhage and death
Echinococcus granulosus	Cestode found in intestines of dogs and sheep	Hydatid cyst can develop in liver, lungs or brain; treated by anthelminthics, drainage of cyst and surgical removal of cyst wall, which is a hazardous procedure; in the worst case, malignant cyst tumours can develop in humans
Erysipeloid	*Erysipelothrix rhusiopathiae* infection, contracted from direct contact with animals with skin lesions	Erythematous skin infections
E. coli	Gram-negative bacterium *Escherichia coli*	Diarrhoea
Fleas	*Ctenocephalides felis* and *C. canis* from cats and dogs, respectively	Rarely live on humans but can cause severe irritation from bites

(Continued)

4.1 Zoonotic diseases—cont'd

Disease	Causative agent	Symptoms in humans
Giardiasis	Protozoal infection from dogs, cats, birds; drinking contaminated water, direct contact with infected animal, ingestion of contaminated food	Range of symptoms from asymptomatic to vomiting, fatigue, fever, diarrhoea, and anorexia
Hendra, Nipah and Menangle viruses	Paramyxoviridae (Australia) with Flying Foxes (fruit bats) as their reservoir host. Can be transmitted via close contact with the infected animal.	Respiratory syndrome, encephalitis
Leptospirosis/ Weil's Disease	Gram-negative spirochaetal bacteria *Leptospira canicola* and *L. icterohaemorrhagiae* found in dog and rodents	Symptoms include fever, jaundice, meningitis and renal failure
Listeriosis	*Listeria monocytogenes*	Meningitis
Lymphocytic choriomeningitis viral infection	Rodents (hamsters, mice, guinea pigs) monkeys and humans; infected via excreted virus in urine, faeces and saliva	Mild influenza-like symptoms
Lyssa virus	Lyssa is a virus within the same group of viruses as rabies, which is present within the Australian bat population; can be transmitted via human contact with infected bats; infected bats may appear normal	Symptoms include severe flu-like symptoms, difficulty swallowing, neurological issues, seizures and death
Melioidosis	Bacterial infection (*Burkholderia pseudomallei*) of horses; transmitted by inhalation of contaminated dust	Cholera-like symptoms (fever, chills) skin lesions, enlarged lymph nodes, septicaemia and pneumonia
Methicillin-resistant Staphylococcus aureus (MRSA)	Resistant bacterial infection, transmitted from direct contact with infected tissues/fluid into a human open wound/broken skin	Various infections
Newcastle disease	Newcastle disease virus affects many avian species. Humans become infected by direct contact with faeces and respiratory discharges or by contaminated food, water, equipment and clothing	Mild flu-like symptoms and conjunctivitis
Orf	Orf virus, mainly from sheep and cattle	Fever and skin granulations
Poxvirus	Viral infection through direct skin contact with lesions of infected animals – nonhuman primates, swine, cattle, horse and birds	Localized lesions, rash, fever, lethargy, encephalitis
Q fever	*Coxiella burnetii*, spread by inhalation of the organism from placental fluid of sheep, goats, cattle and native (Australian) species; the affected animals can appear normal	Severe flu-like symptoms that last months

Disease	Causative agent	Symptoms in humans
Rabies	Rhabdovirus in dogs and cats, will pass through cuts and abrasions or by a bite; carried in saliva	Hydrophobia, malaise, fever, difficulty in breathing, salivation and painful muscle spasms in throat; convulsions and death follow; injection of rabies vaccine and antiserum may prevent the disease from developing; notifiable: police must be contacted immediately; humans can be vaccinated by initial course and regular boosters
Ringworm	Dermatophytes: *Microsporum*, *Trichophyton* and *Epidermophyton* passed by direct contact with dogs, cats, rabbits or guinea pigs	Circular lesions causing intense irritation; treated by antifungal agents taken orally or applied locally
Salmonellosis	Gram-negative bacteria *Salmonella spp.* that inhabit intestines of animals and humans	Food poisoning, gastroenteritis and septicaemia
Sarcoptic mange	Burrowing mites *Sarcoptes scabiei var. canis;* spread by direct contact with infected dogs; foxes are a possible source	In humans, the lesions are small and self-limiting; a separate type of *Sarcoptes* causes scabies in humans
Strongyloidiasis	Nematode parasitic infection from dogs, cats and monkeys via handling infected faecal material	Human symptoms include abdominal pain, diarrhoea and rash
Toxocara canis and *T. cati*	Nematode found in dogs and cats; passed to children by poor hygiene when handling animals or coming into contact with animal faeces	Toxocariasis or 'visceral larva migrans'. Larvae migrate through body; can cause blindness if they come to rest in retina
Toxoplasmosis	Protozoal parasite *Toxoplasma gondii* affecting mammals and birds; passed to humans by eating infected meat or accidentally swallowing sporulated oocysts from cat faeces	Flu-like symptoms and malaise; can lead to blindness, brain defects and death. In pregnant women, can result in abortion or fetal abnormalities
Tuberculosis (TB)	Multiple strains of *Mycobacterium spp.*	Chronic cough, granulomas
Trichinellosis	Infection with *Trichinella spp.*; contracted by eating undercooked or raw meat	Initially gastrointestinal symptoms, followed several weeks later by fever, muscle pain, headaches and weakness
Tularaemia	*Francisella tularensis,* from hares and rabbits	Slow fever and weight loss
Yersiniosis	*Yersinia enterocolitica* bacterium spread through faeces, being shed by dogs, cats and pigs and can be ingested via uncooked pork	Gastrointestinal disease in humans and systemic granulomatous disease in cats

Appendix 5

5.1 Biological data for smaller pets

Type of pet	Average life expectancy (years)	Age at maturity	Size of litter	Age at weaning	Body temperature (°C)
Chicken	5–10	4–6 months	Variable	NA	40.6–43.0
Chinchilla	10–15	8 months	1–4	6–8 weeks	38.0–39.0
Degu	7	6 months	6–8	4 weeks	36.0–38.0
Ferret	5–7	9–12 months	2–10	6–7 weeks	38.8–39.0
Gerbil	1.5–2.5	10–12 weeks	3–6	3–4 weeks	38.0–39.0
Guinea pig	4–7	4–10 weeks	2–6	3–3.5 weeks	39.0–40.0
Hamster	1.5–2	6–10 weeks	3–7	3–4 weeks	36.0–38.0
Mouse	1–2.5	3–4 weeks	5–7	3–4 weeks	37.5
Rabbit	6–8	31 months	2–7	6 weeks	37.0–39.4
Rat	3	5 weeks	6–12	3–4 weeks	37.5–38.0
Sugar glider	4–9	8–14 months	1–2		

5.2 Ferret normal values

Parameter	Data
Physiological data	
Adult weight*	
Male	1000–2000 g
Female	600–950 g
Daily food intake†	50–75 g
Daily water intake	75–100 mL/kg
Rectal temperature	39°C
Heart rate	180–250 beats/min
Blood pressure	
Systole	140 ± 35 mmHg
Diastole	110 ± 3 mmHg
Respiratory rate	33–36 breaths/min
Biochemical data	
Serum protein	5.1–7.4 g/dL
Albumin	2.6–4.1 g/dL
Globulin	2.5–4.8 g/dL
Glucose	62.5–207 g/dL
Blood urea nitrogen	10–45 mg/dL
Creatinine	0.2–0.9 mg/dL

5.2 Ferret normal values—con't

Parameter	Data
Total bilirubin	<1 mg/dL
Cholesterol	64–296 mg/dL
Sodium	137–162 mmol/L
Potassium	4.3–7.7 mmol/L
Calcium	8.0–11.8 mg/dL
Phosphorus	4.0–9.1 mg/dL
Alanine aminotransferase	82–289 U/L
Aspartate aminotransferase	28–248 U/L
Alkaline phosphatase	9–120 U/L
Breeding data	
Puberty	9–12 months
Gestation	38–44 days (average 42)
Average litter size	8
Birth weight	7–10 g
Weaning age	6–7 weeks
Haematological data	
Erythrocytes	$6.77–13.2 \times 10^6/mm^3$
Packed cell volume	36–61%
Haemoglobin	12–18.2 g/dL
Platelets	$297–910 \times 10^3/mm^3$
Reticulocytes	0–3%
Leukocytes	$2.5–19.1 \times 10^3/mm^3$
Neutrophils	11–84%
Lymphocytes	12–69%
Eosinophils	0–9%
Monocytes	0–9%
Basophils	0–2.9%
Blood volume	70 mL/kg
Safe volume of single bleed	7 mL/kg
Urinalysis	
Volume produced in 24 h	
Male	8–48 mL
Female	8–140 mL
pH	6.5–7.5
Protein	
Male	7–33 mg/dL
Female	0–32 mg/dL
Ketones	+

*Both sexes show a periodic weight fluctuation of 30–40%. Fat is laid down in the autumn and lost in the winter.
†Dry carnivore pelleted diet. This should be fed soaked in hot water to form a paste for ferrets.
Reproduced from Lloyd M. Veterinary care of ferrets 1. Clinical examination and routine procedures, 2002. In: Practice 24:90–95, by kind permission of the Editor and Dr. Maggie Lloyd.

5.3 Rabbit normal values

Parameter	Data	Comment
Physiological data		
Adult weight	1–7 kg	Varies with breed
Daily food intake*	50–75 g	
Daily water intake	50–100 mL/kg	Varies with diet
Rectal temperature	37–39.5°C	
Heart rate	130–150 beats/min	Increases to 325 if handled or frightened
Respiratory rate	33–36 breaths/min	
Faecal volume	Up to 175 hard pellets by day. Caecotrophs (soft) variable in amount	In pet rabbits, caecotrophs may never be seen if passed at night or in morning
Biochemical data	See Appendix 2 for normal range†	
Breeding data		
Puberty	4–7 months	
Gestation	28–32 days	
Litter size	2–12	Average 7
Weaning age	7–8 weeks	
Lifespan	5–12 years	

*Levels may vary with dietary intake and types of food supplied.
†Individual laboratories should supply normal data for their range of test.

5.4 Biological data for caged birds

Bird	Lifespan (years)	Age at sexual maturity (months)	Bodyweight (g)
Budgie	10–20	6–12	50–60
Cockatiel	10–15	6–12	40
Canary	6–20	12	15–25
African grey parrot	50	48–72	360–560
Cockatoo	40	44–72	450–750

5.5 Physiological data for caged birds

Bird	Heart rate (bpm)	Respiration rate (bpm)
Budgie	600–750	55–75
Cockatiel	450–604	30–40
Pigeon	90–95	15–25
Parrot	120–780	10–20

Appendices

Dictionary of Veterinary Nursing

Appendix 6

6.1 Obstetrical information for different species

Species	Gestation period (days)	Other information
Cat	63	Induced ovulator; oestrus cycle every 14 days; seasonally polyoestrous (Feb. to Sept.)
Chicken	21 days	Continuous breeding cycle, although egg production will reduce as daylight hours reduce. A cockerel must be present for eggs to be fertile. Naturally, hens may sit on eggs for the three weeks to hatching. Otherwise, an incubator is needed, to keep the eggs at 37.5°C and 45–50% humidity. Eggs need to be turned and incubator should be thoroughly disinfected between batches.
Degu	90	Seasonally polyoestrous
Dog	63	Continuous breeding season; two oestrus cycles each year
Gerbil	24	Continuous breeding season; oestrus cycle every 4–6 days
Guinea pig	59–72	Continuous breeding season; oestrus cycle every 13–20 days
Hamster	15–21	Continuous breeding season; polyoestrous all year round
Horse	340	Polyoestrous, with 21-day cycles through the spring and summer
Rabbit	31–32	Induced ovulator; oestrus cycle every 4–5 h; continuous breeding season but less active in winter
Rat	21–23	Continuous breeding season; oestrus cycle occurs for 12 h every 4 days

Appendix 7

7.1 Information on caring for smaller animals

Type of pet	Amount of care needed	Special needs
Rabbits and guinea pigs	Roomy hutch and outside run; unlimited hay, commercial diet and limited vegetables; fresh water always available; plenty of straw for bedding	Keep dry; clean out regularly; watch for diarrhoea and fly-strike; clip nails and teeth; myxomatosis and VHD vaccines available; enjoy company
Rats and mice	Roomy cage, sawdust or shredded paper; commercial diet, vegetables, fruit and seeds; fresh water always available	Clean out once a week; handle carefully
Gerbils and hamsters	As for rats and mice; hygiene is important	As for rats and mice; watch for wet-tail in hamsters
Chinchillas	Large cage with ledges and dust-bath; commercial pellet diet, hay, fruit, vegetables and seeds; fresh water always available	Clean out regularly; best kept in pairs; long-lived when well cared for
Degu	Large cage with ledges and dust-bath, nest box; commercial chinchilla or guinea pig pellet diet (not rabbit food), hay, fruit, vegetables and seeds; avoid sugary foods; fresh water always available	Degus need space/toys to exercise. Keep at moderate room temperature (as they cannot sweat)
Ferrets	As for rabbits and guinea pigs; eat meat, eggs and milk; can buy frozen carcasses; fresh water always available	Need lots of attention and exercise; clean out regularly; distemper vaccine available, but care needed with dosages
Birds (e.g. budgies, canaries, parrots)	Roomy cage with space to stretch wings; toys to prevent boredom and access to fly out of cage; commercial seed diet, fruit, cuttlefish, etc.; fresh water always available	Clean out weekly; handle carefully; beaks and claws need clipping; best kept in pairs or groups; parrots enjoy human company
Reptiles/ amphibians	Adequate space in glass tanks with gravel/sand; diet of frozen carcasses, fish, crickets, locusts, fruit and vegetables; fresh water always available	Temperature, humidity and lighting very important; good hygiene also essential; research further into preferred species
Fish	Roomy glass tank or aquarium with gravel, ornaments and plants; commercial food; take care not to overfeed	Clean out weekly or more often if large numbers; do not overcrowd; filters needed for large tanks; research further into preferred type, especially for tropical fish
Invertebrates	Roomy tanks with leaves, foliage, fruit and vegetables; spiders will need insects, etc.	Similar to reptiles; temperature/ humidity/hygiene important; further research into preferred species essential

8.1 Mathematical formulae for use in veterinary nursing

Temperatures

Converting °F to °C	$°C = (°F - 32) \times 5/9$
Converting °C to °F	$°F = °C \times 9/5 + 32$

Radiography

New mA with a grid	mA normally used × grid factor
New mA with new FFD* (inverse square law)	Old mA × new FFD^2/old FFD^2
New mA with nonscreen film	Old mA (using screen film) × screen factor or intensification factor
If kV increased by 10	mA halved, to keep exposure the same
If kV decreased by 10	mA doubled, to keep exposure the same

Surgical

Anaesthetic flow rate	Minute volume × circuit factor
Percentage solution, e.g. 1 in 100 = 1%	5 g thiopental in 200 mL water = 2.5%

*FFD, film–focal distance

8.2 Fluid therapy calculations

There are three areas that need to be considered when calculating fluid therapies
Replacement, maintenance and ongoing losses

1) Replacement

Based on level of dehydration via clinical assessment of the patient

Replacement = % dehydration × bodyweight (kg) × 10

Calculation is based on replacement of deficit over a 24-h period

2) Maintenance

Maintenance fluid therapy is the basic fluid requirements an animal needs. For adult patients: 50 mL/kg/24hrs or 2 mL/kg/hr.

Paediatric, geriatric and small-sized animals (toy breeds) may have altered maintenance fluid requirements.

3) Ongoing losses

Ongoing losses are based on predicting losses which are more than maintenances losses. These losses can be from vomiting, diarrhoea, wounds, drains, etc.

Ongoing losses = amount per loss (mL/kg) × body weight (kg) × no. of losses

This is then added to the maintenance rate fluid therapy

Requirement per hour (mL/hr) = requirement per day (mL/24hours) ÷ 24 hours

Requirement per minute (mL/min) = requirement per hour (mL/hr) ÷ 60 minutes

Requirement per second (mL/s) = requirement per minute (mL/min) ÷ 60 seconds

Drops per second = requirement per second (mL/s) × giving set factor

8.3 Converting body weight in kilograms or pounds into body surface area in metres squared

kg	lb	m²	kg	lb	m²
2	4.4	0.15	28	61.6	0.92
4	8.8	0.25	30	66.0	0.96
6	13.2	0.33	32	70.4	1.01
8	17.6	0.40	34	74.8	1.05
10	22.0	0.46	36	79.2	1.09
12	26.4	0.52	38	83.6	1.13
14	30.8	0.58	40	88.0	1.17
16	35.2	0.63	42	92.4	1.21
18	39.6	0.69	44	96.8	1.25
20	44.0	0.74	46	101.2	1.28
22	48.4	0.78	48	105.6	1.32
24	52.8	0.83	50	110.0	1.36
26	57.2	0.88			

8.4 Common fluids

Fluid therapy number	Name	Constituents	Indications
1	Sodium chloride/saline 0.9%	Sodium Chloride	Dehydration Sustained vomiting cases – metabolic alkalosis
3	Sodium chloride/saline 0.9% + 5 % dextrose	Sodium Chloride Glucose	Same indications as for No. 1, but with added glucose 5%, for when the patient's blood glucose is not maintaining adequately enough
6	D5W	Dextrose 5% in water	Normally only used in small amounts to dilute certain drugs
11	Compound sodium lactate/ Hartmann's	Sodium Chloride Sodium lactate Potassium chloride Calcium chloride dihydrate	Most widely used crystalloid fluid: Dehydration Hypovolaemia Corrects many electrolyte abnormalities, for instance, hyponatraemia, hyperkalaemia, etc. Only contains a small amount of potassium
18	Sodium chloride 0.18% Glucose 4%	Sodium chloride 0.18% Glucose 4%	Hypernatraemia Caution must be used due to reduced sodium levels in the solution, can cause hyponatremia
20	Hypertonic saline	Sodium Chloride 7.2%	Hypertonic solution used to draw fluid from intracellular to extracellular: Hypovolaemia Hyponatraemia Raised intracranial pressure *Must be used with extreme caution – can cause severe hypernatraemia – leading to seizures and death*

Appendix 9

9.1 Infectious diseases of the dog, cat, rabbit, horse and birds

Disease	Causative agent	Incubation period
Dog		
Canine distemper	Morbillivirus	7–12 days
Infectious canine hepatitis (ICH)	Adenovirus 1 (CAV-1)	5–9 days
Leptospirosis	Gram-negative bacteria, Leptospira canicola, L. icterohaemorrhagiae	5–7 days
Canine contagious respiratory disease (CCRD)	CAV-1, CAV-2, canine parainfluenza virus (CPIV), canine herpesvirus (CHV), reovirus	5–7 days
Parvovirus	Canine parvovirus 1 and 2 (CPV-1, CPV-2)	3–5 days
Rabies	Rhabdovirus	2 weeks to 4 months
Cat		
Feline panleukopenia	Parvovirus	4–5 days
Feline upper respiratory tract disease (FURD)	Feline calicivirus (FCV), feline herpesvirus 1 (FHV-1)	2–10 days
Feline infectious peritonitis (FIP)	Coronavirus	Months
Feline pneumonitis	Chlamydia spp.	4–10 days
Feline leukaemia virus	Retrovirus	Months/years
Feline immunodeficiency virus (FIV)	RNA retrovirus	Months/years
Rabbit		
Myxomatosis	Type of poxvirus	5–14 days
Viral haemorrhagic disease (VHD)	Calicivirus	1–2 days
Horse		
Equine encephalomyelitis (sleeping sickness)	EE virus	4–10 days
Equine influenza	Equine-1/equine-2 flu virus	1–3 days
Equine rhinopneumonitis	Herpesvirus	2–20 days
West Nile Virus (not UK)	Mosquito-borne virus	7–14 days
Rabies, viral (not UK)	Rhabdovirus	1–2 months but can vary from one week to several years
Strangles	Streptococcus equi	7–14 days
Potomac horse fever (not UK)	Neorickettsia risticii	10–18 days
Equine infectious anaemia (EIA)	Retrovirus	10–45 days
Equine viral arteritis	Arteriviruses	1–8 days

(Continued)

9.1 Infectious diseases of the dog, cat, rabbit, horse and birds—con't

Disease	Causative agent	Incubation period
Chicken		
Bacterial respiratory infection	*Mycoplasma gallisepticum*	4–21 days
Avian Rhinotracheitis (ART)	Pneumovirus of Paramyxoviridae family	5–7 days
Infectious Bronchitis (IB)	Coronavirus	24–48 hours
Infectious Laryngotracheitis (ILT)	Herpesvirus	6–12 days
Avian Coccidiosis	Eimeria	4–7 days
Marek's Disease Virus (MDV)	Alpha-herpesvirus	4–12 weeks
Avian Leukosis Virus (ALV)	Leukosis virus	4–6 months
Avian Pathogenic E.coli (APEC)	*E. coli*	1–3 days
Avian Influenza (AIV, 'bird flu')	Influenza virus	2–8 days
Campylobacter infection	*Campylobacter jejuni*	within 3 days
Salmonellosis	*Salmonella enterica*	12–72 hours but may be subclinical

Appendix 10

10.1 Current vaccination schedules for dogs, cats, rabbits, horses and chickens

Disease	Type of vaccine	Schedule
Dog		
Canine distemper	Modified live vaccine	First vaccine from 6 weeks of age, second dose at 12 weeks; boosted annually or as advised (some vaccines have 3-year duration)
Infectious canine hepatitis (ICH)	Live CAV-2 (canine adenovirus 2) vaccine	As for canine distemper
Canine leptospirosis	Killed serotypes of *Leptospira canicola* and *L. icterohaemorrhagiae*	As for canine distemper for initial course, then annual boosting essential as immunity is short-lived
Canine parvovirus	Live vaccine	As for canine distemper
Canine contagious respiratory disease (CCRD)	Live vaccines available against *Bordetella bronchiseptica*, CAV and canine parainfluenza virus (CPIV)	CPIV as for canine distemper; *Bordetella* vaccine given intranasally, booster every 6 months; ideally give 10–14 days prior to kennelling
Rabies	Inactivated vaccine	Initial vaccination involves a single injection from 3–4 months and regular boosters
US vaccination protocols	Core vaccines are parvovirus, distemper, canine hepatitis and rabies. Other vaccines include *Bordetella bronchiseptica*, *Borrelia burgdorferi*, *Leptospira* and canine parainfluenza	Vaccine intervals vary by region/state Rabies vaccine given at 12 weeks or older (depending on state), then annually
Australian vaccination protocols	Parvovirus, distemper, hepatitis, canine cough	Normally given at 6–8 weeks followed by 12 weeks, then annually
Cat		
Feline panleukopenia	Killed and modified live vaccines available	Initial vaccine from 6 weeks, second injection at 12 weeks; booster annually
Feline upper respiratory disease (FURD)	Injectable and intranasal vaccines available; intranasal is modified live vaccine; dead vaccine used in pregnant queens	Initial vaccine includes 2 injections at 9 and 12 weeks; intranasal protection achieved within 5 days; occasionally mild signs of the disease will follow; booster annually
Feline pneumonitis (*Chlamydia*)	Modified live vaccine; not for use in pregnant queens	Initial course starts at 9 weeks, second given 3–4 weeks later; booster annually

(Continued)

10.1 Current vaccination schedules for dogs, cats, rabbits, horses and chickens—con't

Disease	Type of vaccine	Schedule
Feline leukaemia (FELV)	Genetically engineered vaccine	Initial course 2 injections given 2–3 weeks apart; booster annually; ideally test cats for the disease before vaccinating
Rabies	Inactivated vaccine	As for dogs, see above
US vaccination protocols	The Advisory Panel of the American Association of Feline Practitioners (AAFP) recommends that feline panleukopenia (FPV), feline herpesvirus-1 (FHV-1) and feline calicivirus (FCV) as core vaccines. Noncore vaccines include rabies, feline leukemia virus (FeLV), feline immunodeficiency virus (FIV), *Chlamydophila felis*, *Bordetella bronchiseptica*, feline infectious peritonitis (FIP) and dermatophyte vaccines	
Australian vaccination protocols	Feline infectious enteritis, feline calicivirus, feline viral rhinotracheitis	Initial doses at 8 weeks, 12 weeks, 16 weeks then annually
Rabbit		
Myxomatosis	Live vaccine	Initial vaccine from 6 weeks; booster annually, or every 6 months in rabbits likely to be heavily challenged by disease
Viral haemorrhagic	Inactivated vaccine disease (VHD)	Initial vaccine from 10 weeks; booster annually; take care not to self-inject as causes intense vascular spasm; seek urgent medical help
Horse		
Equine influenza	Inactivated vaccine	Initial dose from 4 months, second dose 4–6 weeks later with a third dose after 6 months; annual booster
Tetanus	Tetanus toxoid	Initial dose from 4 months, second dose 4–6 weeks later with a third dose after 6 months; booster every 24 months, available as combined vaccine with flu
US vaccination protocols	American Association of Equine Practitioners recommends core vaccination against Tetanus, Eastern Equine Encephalitis/Western Equine Encephalitis (EEE/WEE), West Nile Virus (WNV) and Rabies. Risk-based vaccination against anthrax, botulism, Equine Herpes Virus (EHV), Equine Viral Arteritis (EVA), equine influenza, Potomac horse fever, rotaviral diarrhea and strangles	
Australian vaccination protocols	Tetanus, strangles, equine herpes virus infection (rhinopneumonitis) – EHV1 and EHV2, salmonella	
Chickens	Marek's disease, infectious bronchitis (IB), avian rhinotracheitis (ART), *Mycoplasma gallisepticum* (MG), salmonella. The need for vaccination depends on many factors, such as health status of flock, whether birds are being brought in, etc.	

11.1 Average weights for certain breeds of dog

Breed	kg	lb
Afghan hound	22–27	48.5–59.5
Airedale terrier	21–24	46.3–52.9
Alaskan malamute	44–48	97–105.8
Anatolian shepherd dog	54–57	119–125.6
Basenji	9–11	19.8–24.2
Bassett hound	19–22	41.8–48.5
Beagle	9–14	19.8–30.8
Bearded collie	20–22	44–48.5
Bedlington terrier	9–10	19.8–22
Bernese mountain dog	50–60	110.2–132.2
Bichon Frisé	4–9	8.8–19.8
Bloodhound	40–55	88.1–121.2
Border collie	19–24	41.8–52.9
Border terrier	5–7	11–15.4
Borzoi	34–41	74.9–90.3
Boston terrier	8–11	17.6–24.2
Boxer	26–31	57.3–68.3
Briard	34–39	74.9–85.9
Bull terrier	20–30	44–66.1
Bulldog	22–25	48.5–55.1
Bullmastiff	45–55	99.2–121.2
Cairn terrier	5–7	11–15.4
Cavalier King Charles spaniel	5–7	11–15.4
Chihuahua	1–3	2.2–6.6
Chow Chow	25–27	55.1–59.5
Clumber spaniel	29–36	63.9–79.3
Cocker spaniel	12–14	26.4–30.8
Curly coat retriever	32–35	70.5–77.1
Dachshund	4–10	8.8–22
Dalmatian	25–27	55.1–59.5
Deerhound	30–47	66.1–103.6
Dobermann	33–38	72.7–83.7
English pointer	25–29	63.5–66
English setter	27–29	59.5–63.9
Flat coat retriever	29–30	63.9–66.1
German shepherd	29–37	63.9–81.5
German short-haired pointer	24–30	52.9–66.1
Golden retriever	29–34	63.9–74.9
Great Dane	45–62	99.2–136.6
Greyhound	23–36	50.7–79.3
Hovawart	30–35	66.1–77.1
Hungarian Vizsla	22–30	48.5–66.1

(Continued)

11.1 Average weights for certain breeds of dog—con't

Breed	kg	lb
Irish setter	26–31	57.3–68.3
Irish terrier	11–12	24.2–26.4
Irish wolfhound	50–70	110.2–154.3
Italian greyhound	2–4	4.4–8.8
Jack Russell terrier	5–8	11–17.6
Japanese Akita	45–55	99.2–121.2
Keeshond	18–20	39.6–44
King Charles spaniel	4–6	8.8–13.2
Labrador retriever	28–31	61.7–68.3
Lakeland terrier	7–8	15.4–17.6
Lhasa Apso	5–8	11–17.6
Mastiff	67–78	147.7–171.9
Newfoundland	52–67	114.6–147.7
Norfolk terrier	5–7	11–15.4
Norwich terrier	5–7	11–15.4
Old English sheepdog	29–37	63.9–81.5
Papillon	2–3	4.4–6.6
Pekinese	4–6	8.8–13.2
Pomeranian	2–3	4.4–6.6
Poodle (miniature)	5–7	11–15.4
Poodle (standard)	25–40	55.1–88.1
Poodle (toy)	4–5	8.8–11
Pug	5–8	11–17.6
Pyrenean mountain dog	40–60	88.1–132.2
Rhodesian ridgeback	32–37	70.5–81.5
Rottweiler	38–50	83.7–110.2
Rough collie	18–30	39.6–66.1
Saint Bernard	68–75	149.9–165.3
Saluki	19–24	41.8–52.9
Samoyed	20–30	44–66.1
Schnauzer (giant)	30–40	66.1–132.2
Schnauzer (miniature)	4–8	8.8–17.6
Schnauzer (standard)	13–18	28.6–39.6
Scottish terrier	7–10	15.4–22
Sealyham terrier	8–10	17.6–22
Shar-Pei	15–22	33–48.5
Shetland sheepdog	8–13	17.6–28.6
Shih-Tzu	5–9	11–19.8
Siberian husky	15–25	33–55.1
Springer spaniel (English/Welsh)	18–25	39.6–55.1
Staffordshire bull terrier	13–15	28.6–33
Tibetan spaniel	5–7	11–15.4
Tibetan terrier	8–13	17.6–28.6
Weimaraner	22–27	48.5–59.5
Welsh corgi	10–12	22–26.4
West Highland white terrier	7–9	15.4–19.8
Whippet	10–12	22–26.4
Yorkshire terrier	1–3	2.2–6.6

12.1 Calculating nutritional needs for dogs and cats

Basal energy requirement = 30 × (body weight in kg) + 70
For dogs <2 kg or >25 kg, use 70 × (kg) × 0.75
Basal requirement × adjustment factor = Maintenance energy requirement (kcal/day)

Adjustment factors	Dog	Cat
Cage rest	1.25	1.1
After surgery	1.3	1.12
Trauma	1.5	1.2
Sepsis	1.7	1.28
Severe burns	2	1.4

Appendix 13

13.1 Anaesthetic factors for dogs and cats

Species	Respiratory rate (breaths/min)	Tidal volume (ml/kg)	Minute volume (ml/kg/min)	O_2 consumption (ml/kg/min)
Dog >30 kg	15.0–20.0	12.0–15.0	150–250	5.8
Dog <30 kg	20.0–30.0	16.0–20.0	200–300	6.2
Cat	20.0–30.0	7.0–9.0	180–380	7.3

13.2 Arterial blood gas values

Test	Dog	Cat
P_aO_2 (partial pressure of oxygen) (mmHg)	85–100	85–100
P_aCO_2 (partial pressure of carbon dioxide) (mmHg)	35–45	35–45
HCO_3 (bicarbonate) (mmol/l)	21–27	21–27
pH	7.35–7.45	7.35–7.45

Appendix 14

14.1 Gas cylinder colour coding (UK only)

Name of gas	Symbol	Colour of cylinder body	Colour of valve where different from body
Oxygen	O_2	Black	White
Nitrous oxide	N_2O	Blue	–
Cyclopropane	C_3H_6	Orange	–
Carbon dioxide	CO_2	Grey	–
Ethylene	C_2H_4	Violet	–
Nitrogen	N_2	Grey	Black
Oxygen and carbon dioxide mixture	$O_2 + CO_2$	Black	White and grey
Oxygen and helium mixture	$O_2 + He$	Black	White and brown
Oxygen and nitrous oxide mixture	$O_2 + N_2O$	Blue	Blue and black
Air, medical	AIR	Grey	White and black

14.2 Oxygen cylinder size and content

Size	E	F	G	J
O_2 content (lbf/in^2)	680	1340	3400	6800

Appendix 15

15.1 Blood tube and Vacutainer colours

Blood tube colour	Vacutainer colour	Anticoagulant	Type of sample	Application
White	Red	None	Clotted blood/serum	Biochemistry, serology
Orange	Yellow/green	Heparin	Whole blood/plasma	Biochemistry, lead, glutathione peroxidase (GXH-Px) for measuring selenium and transketolase
Pink	Lavender	EDTA	Whole blood	Haematology
Yellow	Grey	Fluoride oxalate	Whole blood	Glucose
Purple	Light blue	Sodium citrate	Whole blood/plasma	Coagulation tests
N/A	Dark blue	None	Clotted blood/serum	Trace elements

16.1 Dog breeds and coat colours

Breed	Coat colour/markings
Afghan hound	Domino, black masked red, brindle, black, black tan, cream/white, blue
Airedale terrier	Black/tan
Alaskan malamute	Various colours, light grey through to black, sable, red
Anatolian shepherd dog	Various colours, including pinto, white, and brindle, but fawn with a black mask is common
Basenji	Chestnut red; pure black; tricolour (pure black and chestnut red); or brindle (black stripes on a background of chestnut red); all with white feet, chest and tail tip; white legs, blaze and collar optional
Bassett hound	Classic tricolour pattern of black, tan, and white or open red and white (red spots on a white coat), closed red and white (solid red with white feet and tail), or lemon and white.
Beagle	Tricoloured
Bearded collie	Slate, brown, blue and fawn; all these colours occur in combination with white
Bedlington terrier	Predominantly white, but the Bedlington comes in several colours and combinations: blue, sandy, liver, blue and tan, sandy and tan, and liver and tan
Bernese mountain dog	Black background colour enhanced by a uniform pattern of white and rich dark-tan markings on the head, chest, legs and tail
Bichon Frisé	Solid white, cream, grey or apricot
Bloodhound	Black and tan, liver and tan, and red
Border collie	Black and white
Border terrier	Red, blue and tan, grizzle and tan, or wheaten (pale yellow or fawn)
Borzoi	Various
Boston terrier	Black, seal, or brindle, all with a white muzzle, face blaze and chest
Boxer	Fawn and brindle, sometimes white
Briard	Tawny, black, and grey
Bull terrier	Variety of colours; white or white with head, ear or eye markings; brindle, black brindle, tricoloured, red and fawn dogs typically with white muzzle, front and socks
Bulldog	Normally made up of several colours, red brindle, other shades of brindle, white, solid red, fawn, piebald
Bullmastiff	Red, fawn or brindle
Cairn terrier	Many colours, including red, brindle, black, sand and grey
Cavalier King Charles spaniel	White/chestnut, black/tan, ruby, tricoloured

(Continued)

Breed	Coat colour/markings
Chihuahua	Range of colours and markings; from solid colours – black, white, fawn, chocolate, grey, silver – to tricolour (chocolate, black, or blue with tan and white), brindle, spotted, merle and a variety of other markings; shades can be very pale to very dark for all the colours
Chow Chow	Red, black, blue, cinnamon and cream
Clumber spaniel	Primarily white, usually with lemon or orange markings around the eyes and on the head or ears
Cocker spaniel	Black, liver, red golden
Curly coat retriever	Black or liver
Dachshund	Variety of colours/patterns: red, cream, black and tan, black and cream, chocolate and tan, chocolate and cream
Dalmatian	Most commonly black or brown (liver) spots on a white background
Deerhound	Dark blue-grey
Dobermann	Black/tan, red
English pointer	Liver (dark brown), black, orange, or lemon, with or without a white background; tricoloured
English setter	Blue belton, orange or lemon belton, blue belton and tan, and liver belton
Flat coat retriever	Solid black or solid liver, a deep reddish-brown colour
German shepherd	Black & red, black & tan, black & cream, black & silver, black (solid black), sable (grey), blue, liver and white
German short-haired pointer	Solid liver or a combination of liver and white
Golden retriever	Blonde, yellow or gold
Great Dane	Black, blue, harlequin, mantle, fawn and brindle
Greyhound	Fawn, black, red, blue, grey or white
Hovawart	Black and gold, black or blond
Hungarian Vizsla	Rusty gold
Irish setter	Burnished mahogany or rich chestnut red
Irish terrier	Bright red, golden red, red wheaten or wheaten (pale yellow or fawn)
Irish wolfhound	Grey, brindle, red, black, white or fawn
Italian greyhound	Fawn, cream, red, blue, or black, either solid or with white markings
Jack Russell terrier	White, white with black or tan markings, or tricolour (white, black and tan)
Japanese Akita	Black, white, chocolate, a combination of colour and white, or brindle
Keeshond	Cream, black and grey
King Charles spaniel	King Charles (black and tan), Prince Charles (white with black and tan patches), Blenheim (white with red patches), Ruby (red)
Labrador retriever	Black, yellow, chocolate, polar white, fox red
Lakeland terrier	Solid blue, black, liver, red and wheaten
Lhasa Apso	Many colours including honey, black, white, slate or particoloured
Mastiff	Fawn, apricot or brindle
Newfoundland	Several colours, including solid black, brown, grey or Landseer, a white coat with black markings

Breed	Coat colour/markings
Norfolk terrier	Red, wheaten, black and tan, or grizzle
Norwich terrier	Red, grizzle (a mixture of black or red hairs with white hairs), wheaten (pale yellow or fawn), or black and tan
Old English sheepdog	Grey, grizzle, blue, blue grey, blue merle, grey with white markings or white with grey markings
Papillon	Particoloured, white with patches of any colour
Pekinese	Any colour or have any markings, including black and tan, fawn or red brindle, and particoloured, which is white with another colour
Pomeranian	Variety of coat colours and patterns including red, orange, white, cream, blue, brown, black, black and tan, wolf sable, orange sable, brindle and particoloured
Poodle	Blue, black, white, grey, silver, brown, café-au-lait, apricot and cream
Pug	Fawn-colored or black
Pyrenean mountain dog	White or white with markings that can be badger, tan, grey or reddish-brown
Rhodesian ridgeback	Light wheaten to red wheaten, with raised crest along dorsum
Rottweiler	Black with markings that are rust to mahogany in colour
Rough collie	Sable, tricolour (black with white markings and tan shadings), blue merle (silvery blue and black) and white
Saint Bernard	Red with white or white with red
Saluki	White, cream, fawn, golden, grizzle and tan, black and tan, and tricolour (white, black, and tan).
Samoyed	Pure white, white and biscuit, cream or biscuit
Schnauzer (giant, miniature, standard)	Black, white, salt and pepper and black and silver
Scottish terrier	Grey or steel, brindle or wheaten
Sealyham terrier	White
Shar-Pei	All solid colours and sables
Shetland sheepdog	Varying amounts of white and/or tan markings, sable, black, blue merle (blue-grey with black)
Shih-Tzu	Black, black and white, grey and white, or red and white
Siberian husky	Variety of colours and markings, from black to pure white with coloured markings on the body that include reds and coppers
Springer spaniel (English/Welsh)	Several colour combinations, black, liver, white

Appendix 17

17.1 Cat breeds and coat colours

Breed	Coat colours
Shorthair	
Abyssinian	Ruddy (usual), red, blue
American short hair	White, black, blue, red, cream, chinchilla, shaded silver, shell cameo (red chinchilla), shaded cameo (red shaded), black smoke, blue smoke, cameo smoke (red smoke), classic tabby, mackerel tabby, patched tabby, brown-patched tabby, blue-patched tabby, silver-patched tabby, silver tabby, red tabby, brown tabby, blue tabby, cream tabby, cameo tabby, tortoiseshell, calico, dilute calico, blue–cream, bicoloured (e.g. black and white)
American wire hair	As for American short hair, excluding patched tabby, brown-patched tabby, blue-patched tabby, silver-patched tabby
Bombay	Black
British short hair	Blue-eyed white, orange-eyed white, odd-eyed white, black, blue, cream, blue–cream, silver tabby, red tabby, brown tabby, mackerel tabby, black smoke, blue smoke, spotted, tortoiseshell, tortoiseshell and white, bicoloured
Burmese	Brown, blue, chocolate, lilac, red, brown (normal), tortoiseshell, cream, blue tortie, chocolate tortie, lilac tortie (lilac–cream)
Colourpoint short hair	Red point, cream point, seal lynx point, chocolate lynx point, blue lynx point, lilac lynx point, red lynx point, seal–tortie point, chocolate-cream point, blue–cream point, lilac–cream point
Exotic short hair	As for American short hair
Egyptian Mau	Silver, bronze, smoke
Foreign short hair	Lilac, white, black
Havana brown	Brown
Japanese bobtail	White, black, red, black and white, red and white, mike (tricoloured), tortoiseshell
Korat	Silver–blue
Manx	As for American short hair, excluding shell cameo, shaded cameo, cameo smoke, cameo tabby
Oriental short hair	White, ebony, blue, chestnut, lavender, red, cream, silver, cameo, ebony smoke, blue smoke, chestnut smoke, lavender smoke, cameo (red) smoke, classic tabby, mackerel tabby, spotted tabby, ticked tabby, ebony tabby, blue tabby, chestnut tabby, lavender tabby, red tabby, cream tabby, silver tabby, cameo tabby, tortoise- shell, blue–cream, chestnut–tortie, lavender–cream
Oriental spotted tabby	Brown, blue, chocolate, lilac, red, cream
Rex (Cornish/Devon)	As for Manx
Russian blue	Blue
Scottish fold	As for American wire hair
Siamese	Seal point, chocolate point, blue point, lilac point, tabby point, tortie point, red point, cream point
Somali	Ruddy/red

17.1 Cat breeds and coat colours—cont'd

Breed	Coat colours
Long hair	
Balinese	Seal point, blue point, chocolate point, lilac point
Birman	As for Balinese
Himalayan/colourpoint long hair	Seal point, chocolate point, blue point, lilac point, flame point, tortie point, blue–cream point, chocolate solid colour, lilac solid colour
Maine Coon	White, black, blue, red, cream, chinchilla, shaded silver, shell cameo (red chinchilla), shaded cameo (red shaded), black smoke, blue smoke, cameo smoke (red smoke), classic tabby, mackerel tabby, silver tabby, red tabby, brown tabby, blue tabby, cream tabby, cameo tabby, tabby and white, tortoiseshell, tortie and white, calico, dilute calico, blue–cream, bicoloured
Persian	As for Maine Coon including patched tabby, brown-patched tabby, blue-patched tabby, silver-patched tabby, chinchilla golden, shaded golden, shell tortie, shaded tortie, smoke tortie, lilac, lilac–cream, Persian van bicoloured, peke-face red, peke-face red tabby, pewter, chocolate, chocolate tortie, but excluding tortie and white and tabby and white
Turkish angora	White, black, blue, black smoke, blue smoke, classic tabby, mackerel tabby, silver tabby, red tabby, brown tabby, blue tabby, calico, bicoloured

Appendix 18

18.1 Rabbit breeds and coat colours

Breeds	Fur type	Coat colour
Angora	Long, fluffy coats requiring regular grooming	White, black, chocolate, blue lilac
Dutch	Short, smooth fur	White around the shoulder area with white stripe down the nose; colour from the waist down and around the eyes Black, blue, chocolate, grey, steel and tortoise
Dwarf Lop	Very dense and thick, which is glossy in appearance with medium-length fur	Many colours
English and English Lop	Short coat; unusual markings with a stripe down the dorsal spine, nose and ears that coloured, with spots to the flank area	There are several different colours, with black the most common colour
French Lop	Short coat	Many colours
Himalayan	Short coat	White with markings in black, blue, chocolate or lilac
Lionhead and Lionhead lop	Fur around the face that can resemble a lion's mane; they often have tufts around tail with short body fur; they vary in fluffiness; regular grooming required Lionhead lop is the same but have lop ears	Black, blue, chocolate, lilac
Netherland Dwarf	Short coat	Self, shaded, agouti, tan, pattern and many more
New Zealand	Thick, dense coat needs grooming	Normally white-albino with pink eyes; black and grey are now very rare
Polish	Short coat that requires minimal grooming	Various colours, most common are sable, smoke pearl, and Himalayan pattern
Rex	Rex breeds have very dense fur that looks and feels like velvet	Many different colours which include amber, black, blue, broken tri-colour, Californian, castor, chinchilla, chocolate, lilac, lynx, opal, otter (black, blue, chocolate, and lilac), red, sable, seal and white
Sussex	Thick and dense coat	Gold (teddy bear colour) and cream

19.1 Horse coat colours

Breeds	Coat colour
Appaloosa	Solid body colour with dark or light spots
Bay	Brown body with black mane, tail and lower legs
Black	Black body colour with black mane and tail
Brown	Brown body colour with brown mane and tail
Buckskin	A pale bay due to the cream dilution gene; body is a yellow/gold; mane, tail and lower limbs are black
Champagne	Diluted colour derived from the action of the champagne gene on the red, black, bay or brown colours
Chestnut	Solid red body colour, with the same colour or lighter mane and tail; also called 'sorrel' (US)
Cremello	Light crème coat colour due to the effect of homozygous cream genes working on a chestnut body colour
Dapple grey	Light patches of grey against a darker background
Dun	Diluted coat colour giving a lighter body with a darker mane and tail, with a dorsal stripe
Flea-bitten grey	Grey body colour with many small darker patches ('flea bites')
Grey	Black skin with a white coat
Liver chestnut	Dark chestnut/red
Paint	A distinct American breed of horse of Thoroughbred and Quarter Horse descent, not a colour
Palomino	Golden body colour with a white (flaxen) mane and tail due to the effect of the cream dilution gene working on a chestnut body coat
Piebald	Black body colour with white patches that may spread down the legs and into the mane and tail
Pinto	Coloured horse with a dark body colour and irregular patterns of white in Tobiano or Overo distribution (US)
Roan (red roan, bay roan, blue roan, etc.)	Even distribution of white hairs throughout a solid colour body coat; head and legs are usually the solid base colour
Skewbald	Any non-black body colour with white patches
Tricolour	Bay body colour with white patches
Sorrel	See Chestnut

Appendix 20

20.1 Veterinary qualifications: interpretation of letters after names

AIMVT – VTS: Academy of Internal Medicine for Veterinary Technicians, Veterinary Technician Specialist (cardiology, neurology, oncology, small animal internal medicine, large animal internal medicine and nutrition)

AVBT – VTS: Academy of Veterinary Behavior Technicians, Veterinary Technician Specialist (behaviour)

AVCPT – VTS: Academy of Veterinary Clinical Pathology Technicians, Veterinary Technician Specialist (clinical pathology)

AVDT – VTS: Academy of Veterinary Dental Technicians, Veterinary Technician Specialist (dentistry)

AVECCT – VTS: Academy of Veterinary Emergency Critical Care Technicians, Veterinary Technician Specialist (emergency & critical care)

AVST – VTS: Academy of Veterinary Surgical Technicians, Veterinary Technician Specialist (surgical)

AVTA – VTS: Academy of Veterinary Technician Anesthetists, Veterinary Technician Specialist in Anesthesia

AVZMT – VTS: Academy of Veterinary Zoological Medicine Technicians, Veterinary Technician Specialist (zoo)

BSc: Bachelor of Science; most universities award a science nonveterinary BSc

BSc (Hons) (Vet Nursing): Bachelor of Science Veterinary Nursing (nonclinical)

BSc (Vet Pathology): Bachelor of Veterinary Pathology

BSc (Vet Sci): Bachelor of Veterinary Science (London)

BVBiol: Bachelor of Veterinary Biology

BVetMed: Bachelor of Veterinary Medicine (London)

BVetSts: Honorary Bachelor of Veterinary Studies

BVM: Bachelor of Veterinary Medicine (Nottingham, overseas)

BVMSci: Bachelor of Veterinary Medicine and Science (Surrey)

BVMedSci: Bachelor of Veterinary Medical Sciences (Nottingham)

BVM&AH: Bachelor of Veterinary Medicine and Animal Husbandry (overseas)

BVMS: Bachelor of Veterinary Medicine and Surgery (Glasgow)

BVM&S: Bachelor of Veterinary Medicine & Surgery (Edinburgh)

BVS: Bachelor of Veterinary Science (Nottingham)

BVSc: Bachelor of Veterinary Science (Bristol, Liverpool, overseas)

BVSc&AH: Bachelor of Veterinary Science and Animal Husbandry (overseas)

CertBR: Certificate in Bovine Reproduction (RCVS)

CertCHP: Certificate in Cattle Health and Reproduction (RCVS)

CertEM (IntMed): Certificate in Equine Medicine (internal medicine) (RCVS)

CertEM (StudMed): Certificate in Equine Medicine (stud medicine) (RCVS)

CertEMS: Certificate in Equine Stud Medicine (RCVS)

CertEO: Certificate in Equine Orthopaedics (RCVS)

CertEP: Certificate in Equine Practice (RCVS)

CertES (Orth): Certificate in Equine Surgery (orthopaedics) (RCVS)

CertES (Soft Tissue): Certificate in Equine Surgery (soft tissue) (RCVS)

CertFHP: Certificate in Fish Health and Production (RCVS)

CertLAS: Certificate in Laboratory Animal Science (RCVS)

CertPM: Certificate in Pig Medicine (RCVS)

CertPMP: Certificate in Poultry Medicine and Production (RCVS)

CertSAC: Certificate in Small Animal Cardiology (RCVS)

CertSAD: Certificate in Small Animal Dermatology (RCVS)

CertSAM: Certificate in Small Animal Medicine (RCVS)

CertSAO: Certificate in Small Animal Orthopaedics (RCVS)

CertSAS: Certificate in Small Animal Surgery (RCVS)

CertSHP: Certificate in Sheep Health and Production (RCVS)

CertSVM: Certificate in State Veterinary Medicine (RCVS)

CertVA: Certificate in Veterinary Anaesthesia (RCVS)

CertVC: Certificate in Veterinary Cardiology (RCVS)

CertVD: Certificate in Veterinary Dermatology (RCVS)

CertVOphthal: Certificate in Veterinary Ophthalmology (RCVS)

CertVPH (MH): Certificate in Veterinary Public Health (meat hygiene) (RCVS)

CertVR: Certificate in Veterinary Radiology (RCVS)

CertVRep: Certificate in Veterinary Reproduction (RCVS)

CertWel: Certificate in Animal Welfare Science, Ethics and Law (RCVS)

CertZooMed: Certificate in Zoological Medicine (RCVS)

DBR: Diploma in Bovine Reproduction (Liverpool)

DCHP: Diploma in Cattle Health and Production (RCVS)

DEO: Diploma in Equine Orthopaedics (RCVS)

DER: Diploma in Equine Reproduction (Liverpool)

DESM: Diploma in Equine Study Medicine (RCVS)

DESTS: Diploma in Equine Soft Tissue Surgery (RCVS)

DipACVECC: Diploma – American College of Veterinary Emergency and Critical Care

DipACVIM: Diploma – American College of Veterinary Internal Medicine

DipAH: Diploma in Animal Health

DipAnGen: Diploma in Animal Genetics

DipAVN: Diploma in Advanced Veterinary Nursing (RCVS)

DipAVN(Med): Advanced Veterinary Nursing Diploma (medical) (RCVS)

DipAVN(Surg): Advanced Veterinary Nursing Diploma (surgical) (RCVS)

DipECVD: Diploma – European College of Veterinary Dermatology

DipECVIM – CA: Diploma – European College of Veterinary Internal Medicine – Companion Animals

DipHECVN: Diploma of Higher Education Clinical Veterinary Nursing (Myerscough)

DipIEMVT: Diploma in Tropical Veterinary Medicine and Animal Husbandry

DipVetMed: Diploma in Large Animal Medicine

DipVetPath: Diploma in Veterinary Pathology (overseas)

DipVMS: Diploma in Veterinary Medical Studies (overseas)

DipVS: Diploma in Veterinary Surgery (overseas)

DLAS: Diploma in Laboratory Animal Science (RCVS)

DPM: Diploma in Pig Medicine (RCVS)

DPMP: Diploma in Poultry Medicine and Production (RCVS)

DPVM: Diploma in Preventive Veterinary Medicine

DSAO: Diploma in Small Animal Orthopaedics (RCVS)

(Continued)

DSAM: Diploma in Small Animal Medicine (RCVS)

DSAS (Orth): Diploma in Small Animal Surgery (orthopaedics) (RCVS)

DSAS (Soft Tissue): Diploma in Small Animal Surgery (soft tissue)

DSc: Doctor of Science

DSHP: Diploma in Sheep Health and Production (RCVS)

DTVM: Diploma in Veterinary Tropical Medicine (Edinburgh)

DVA: Diploma in Veterinary Anaesthesia (RCVS)

DVC: Diploma in Veterinary Cardiology (RCVS)

DVD: Diploma in Veterinary Dermatology (RCVS)

DVM: Doctor of Veterinary Medicine (overseas)

DVOphthal: Diploma in Veterinary Ophthalmology (RCVS)

DVPH (MH): Diploma in Veterinary Public Health (meat hygiene) (RCVS)

DVetMed: Doctor of Veterinary Medicine (London)

DVM&S: Doctor of Veterinary Medicine and Surgery

DVR: Diploma in Veterinary Radiology (RCVS)

DVRep: Diploma in Veterinary Reproduction (RCVS)

DVSc: Doctor of Veterinary Science

DVSM: Diploma in Veterinary State Medicine (Edinburgh)

DWEL: Diploma in Animal Welfare, Science, Ethics and Law (RCVS)

DZooMed (Reptilian): Diploma in Zoological Medicine (reptilian) (RCVS)

EVN: Qualified Equine Veterinary Nurse (RCVS)

FPH: Fellow in Poultry Husbandry

FRAgS: Fellow of the Royal Agricultural Societies

FRC (Path): Fellow of the Royal College of Pathologists

FRCVS: Fellow of the Royal College of Veterinary Surgeons (RCVS)

FRS: Fellow of the Royal Society

GradDipVN: Graduate Diploma in Professional and Clinical Veterinary Nursing

GVSc: Graduate in Veterinary Science

Hon Assoc RCVS: Honorary Associate of the RCVS

Hon FRCVS: Honorary Fellow of the RCVS

MAnimSc: Master of Animal Science

MRCVS: Member of the RCVS

MRes: Master in Research

MSc (Veterinary Physiotherapy): Master of Science in Veterinary Physiotherapy

MSc (Wild Animal Health): Master of Science in Wild Animal Health

MVB: Bachelor of Veterinary Medicine (Dublin, Ireland)

MVD: Doctor of Veterinary Medicine (overseas)

MVM: Master of Veterinary Medicine

MVetMed: Master of Veterinary Medicine (London)

MVSc: Master of Veterinary Science

PhD: Doctor of Philosophy (all universities, higher degree)

QHVS: Queen's Honorary Veterinary Surgeon

RVN: Registered Veterinary Nurse

VetMB: Bachelor of Veterinary Medicine (Cambridge)

VSD: Veterinary Surgeons Diploma (overseas)

Animal Health Trust, Lanwades Park, Kentford, Newmarket, Suffolk CB8 7UU, Tel: 01638 751000; Fax: 01638 750410; website: www.aht.org.uk

Animal and Plant Health Agency (previously Animal Health and VI Centres), Woodham Lane, Addlestone, Surrey, KT15 3NB, Tel: 01932 341111; email: apha.corporatecorrespondence@apha.gsi.gov.uk

Animal Welfare, University Federation (UFAW), The Old School, Brewhouse Hill, Wheathampstead, St Albans, Herts AL4 8AN, Tel: 0158 2831818; Fax: 0158 2831414; website: www.ufaw.org.uk

Blue Cross Animal Welfare, Shilton Road, Burford, OX18 4PF, Tel: 0300 777 1897; Fax: 0300 777 1601; website: www.bluecross.org.uk

British Equine Veterinary Association (BEVA), Mulberry House, 31 Market Street, Fordham, Ely, Cambridgeshire CB7 5LQ, Tel: 01638 723 555; Fax: 01638 724 043; website: www.beva.org.uk

British Horse Society, The (BHS), Abbey Park, Shareton, Kenilworth, Warwickshire, CV8 2XZ, Tel: 02476840500; Fax: 02476840501; website: www.bhs.org.uk

British Small Animal Veterinary Association (BSAVA), Woodrow House, 1 Telford Way, Waterwells Business Park, Quedgeley, Gloucester GL2 4AB, Tel: 01452 726700; Fax: 01452 726701; website: www.bsava.com

British Veterinary Association (BVA), 7 Mansfield St, London W1M 0AT, Tel: 0207 636 6541; Fax: 0207 79086349; website: www.bva.co.uk

British Veterinary Hospitals Association (BVHA), BVHA Office, c/o Station Bungalow, Main Rd, Stocksfield, Northumberland NE43 7HJ, Tel: 07966 901619; Fax: 07813 915954; website: www.bvha.org.uk

British Veterinary Nursing Association (BVNA), 82 Greenway Business Centre, Harlow Business Park, Harlow, Essex CM19 5QE, Tel: 01279 408644, Fax: 01279 408645; website: www.bvna.org.uk

Brooke, The, 5th Floor, Friars Bridge Court, 41–45 Blackfriars Road, London SE1 8NZ, Tel: 020 3012 3456; website: www.thebrooke.org/

Canine Partners, Mill Lane, Heyshott, Midhurst GU20 OED, Tel: 08456 560480; website: www.caninepartners.co.uk

Cats Protection, National Cat Centre, Chelwood Gate, Haywards Heath, East Sussex RH17 7TT, Tel: 0300 012 1212; website: www.cats.org.uk

Cinnamon Trust, 10 Market Square, Hayle, Cornwall TR27 4HE, Tel: 01736 757900; Fax: 01736 757010; website: www.cinnamon.org.uk

College of Animal Welfare, Headland House, Chord Business Park, London Road, Godmanchester, Cambridgeshire PE29 2BQ, Tel: 01480 422060; Fax: 01480 422089; website: www.caw.ac.uk

Department of Environment, Food and Rural Affairs (DEFRA), 17 Smith Square, London SW1P 3JP, Tel: 03459 33 55 77; website: www.defra.gov.uk

Dogs for Good, The Frances Hay Centre, Blacklocks Hill, Banbury OX17 2BS, Tel: 01295 252600; Fax: 01295 252668; website: www.dogsforgood.org

Dogs Trust (formerly the National Canine Defence League), 17 Wakley Street, London EC1V 7LT, Tel: 0207 837 0006; Fax: 0207 833 2701; website: www.dogstrust.org.uk

(Continued)

European College of Veterinary Surgeons, Veterinär-Chirurgische Klinik, Winterhurer Strasse 260, CH-8057, Zurich, Switzerland, Tel: 0041 446358408; Fax: 0041 443 13 03 84; website: www.ecvs.org

Governing Council of the Cat Fancy (GCCF), 5 King's Castle business park, The drove, TA6 4AG, Tel: 01278 427575; website: www.gccfcats.org

Guide Dogs for the Blind Association (GDBA), Head Office, Hillfields, Burghfield Common, Reading RG7 3YG, Tel: 0118 983 5555; Fax: 0118 983 5433; website: www.guidedogs.org.uk

Hearing Dogs for Deaf People, Training Centre, The Grange, Wycombe Road, Saunderton, Princess Risborough HP27 9NS, Tel: 01844 348100; Fax: 01844 348101; website: www.hearingdogs.org.uk

International Cat Care (formerly Feline Advisory Bureau (FAB)), Taeselbury, High Street, Tisbury, Salisbury SP3 6LD, Tel: 01747 871872; Fax: 01747 871873; website: www.icatcare.org

Irish Society for the Prevention of Cruelty to Animals (ISPCA), Derryglogher Lodge, Keenagh, Co. Longford, Ireland, Tel: 0035 043 33 25035; Fax: 0035 0433325024; website: www.ispca.ie

Kennel Club, 1–5 Clarges St, Piccadilly, London W1Y8AB, Tel: 01296 318540; Fax: 0207 518 1058; website: www. the-kennel-club.org.uk

Medical Detection Dogs, 3 Millfield, Greenway Business Park, Winslow Rd, Great Horwood MK12 0NK Tel: 01296 655888; email: operations@ medicaldetectiondogs.org.uk; website: www.medicaldetectiondogs. org.uk

National Animal Welfare Trust, Tylers Way, Watford By-Pass, Hertfordshire WD25 8WT, Tel: 0208 950 0177; website: www.nawt.org.uk

National Fox Welfare Society, 135 Higham Rd, Rushden, Northants NN10 6DS, Tel: 01933 411996; Fax: 01933 411996; website: www.nfws.org.uk

People's Dispensary for Sick Animals (PDSA), Head Office, Whitechapel Way, Priorslee, Telford, Shropshire TF2 9PQ, Tel: 0800 9172509; website: www.pdsa.org.uk

Petlog (Database for microchip numbers), The Kennel Club, 4A Alton House, Gatehouse Way, Aylesbury, Bucks HP193ZH, Tel 01296 336579

Poisons information, Further details of the Veterinary Poisons Information Service are available from: Veterinary Poisons Information Service (VPIS) 13 St Thomas Street, Mary Sheridan House SE1 9RY; Tel: 0207 188020 (24h); website: www.npis.org;

Royal College of Veterinary Surgeons (RCVS), Belgravia House, 62–64 Horseferry Rd, London, SW1P 2AF, Tel: 0207 222 2001; Fax: 0207 222 2004; website: www.rcvs.org.uk

Royal Society for the Prevention of Cruelty to Animals (RSPCA), Head Office, Wilberforce Way, Southwater Horsham RH13 9RS, Tel: 0300 123 4999; website: www.rspca.org.uk

Royal Veterinary College (RVC), Hawkshead Campus, Hawkshead Ln, North Mymms, Hatfield, Herts AL9 7TA, Tel: 01707 666333; Fax: 01707 652090; website: www.rvc.ac.uk

Scottish Society for the Prevention of Cruelty to Animals (SSPCA), Kingseat Rd, Halbeath, Dunfermline. Fife KY11 8RY, Tel: 0300 099 9999; website: www.scottishspca.org

Society for Companion Animal Studies (SCAS), Airport Business Centre, 10 Thornbury Rd, Estover, Plymouth PL6 7PP, Tel: 0845 6012207; website: www.scas.org.uk

Society for Practising Veterinary Surgeons (SPVS), The Governor's House, Cape Rd, Warwick, Warwickshire CV34 5DL, Tel: 01926 410454; Fax: 01926 411350; website: www.spvs.org.uk

St Tiggywinkles Wildlife Hospital, Aston Rd, Haddenham, Aylesbury, Bucks HP17 8AF, Tel: 01844 292292; Fax: 01844 292640; website: www.sttiggywinkles.org.uk

Support Dogs, Head Office, 21 Jessops Riverside, Brightside Ln, Sheffield S9 2RX, Tel: 01142 617800; website: www.support-dogs.org.uk

Ulster Society for the Prevention of Cruelty to Animals (USPCA), Unit 6, Carnbane Industrial Estate (East), Newry, Co. Down, BT5 6QH, Tel: 02830 251000; Fax: 02890 381911; website: www.enquiries@uspca.co.uk

University College Dublin, Faculty of Veterinary Medicine, Ballsbridge, Dublin 4, Ireland, Tel: 0035 317167777; Fax: 0035 316 687878; website: www.ucd.ie/vetmed

University of Bristol, Department of Clinical Veterinary Science, Langford House, Langford, Bristol BS40 5DU, Tel: 0117 928 9280; Fax: 0117 928 9505; website: www.vetschool.bris.ac.uk

University of Cambridge, Department of Clinical Veterinary Medicine, Madingley Rd, Cambridge, CB3 0ES, Tel: 01223 337600; Fax: 01223 337610; website: www.vet.cam.ac.uk

University of Edinburgh, Royal (Dick) School of Veterinary Studies, Summerhall, Edinburgh EH9 1QH, Tel: 0131 650 1000; Fax: 0131 650 6577; website: www.vet.ed.ac.uk

University of Glasgow, Veterinary School, Bearsden Rd, Bearsden, Glasgow G61 1QH, Tel: 0141 330 2000; Fax: 0141 942 7215; website: www.gla.ac.uk/vet

University of Liverpool, Faculty of Veterinary Science, Neston CH64 7TE, Tel: 0151 794 4281; Fax: 0151 794 4279; website: www.liv.ac.uk/vets

University of Nottingham, School of Veterinary Medicine and Science, Sutton Bonington Campus, Sutton Bonington, Leicestershire LE12 5RD, Tel: 01159516116; Fax: 0115 951 6415; website: www.nottingham.ac.uk/vet

University of Surrey, School of Veterinary Medicine. Duke of Kent Building, Level 5, University of Surrey, Guildford, Surrey GU2 7XH Tel: 01483 689165 Fax: 01483 689551; website: www.surrey.ac.uk/vet

Veterinary Defence Society, 4 Haig Court, Parkgate Estate, Knutsford, Cheshire WA16 8XZ, Tel: 01565 652737; Fax: 01565 751079; website: www.veterinarydefencesociety.co.uk

Veterinary Practice Management Association, 76 St John's Rd, Kettering Northants NN15 5AZ, Tel: 0700 0782324; Fax: 08708 362250; website: www.vpma.co.uk

Wildlife Licensing Unit, (Dept of Environment),Natural England,1st floor Temple Quay House, 2 The Square, Bristol BS1 6EB, Tel: 0845 601 4523; Fax: 0845 601 3438; email: wildlife@naturalengland.org.uk

World Horse Welfare, (formerly International League for the Protection of Horses (ILPH)), Anne Colvin House, Snetterton, Norwich NR16 2LR, Tel: 01953 498682; Fax: 01953 498373; website: www.ilph.org

World Society for the Protection Of Animals (WSPCA), 5th Floor, 222 Greys Inn Rd, London WC1X 8HB, Tel: 0207 239 0500; Fax: 0207 239 0653; website: www.wspa.org.uk

World Veterinary Association, Avenue de Tervueren 12, B-1040 Bruxelles Belgium, Tel: + 32 2 533 70 20; website: www.worldvet.org

World Wildlife Fund (WWF), The Living Planet Centre, Rufford House, Brewery Rd, Woking Surrey GU21 4LL, Tel: 01483 426444; Fax: 01483 426409; website: www.wwf.org.uk

Zoology, Institute of, Zoological Society of London, Regents Park, London NW1 4RY, Tel: 0207 449 6670; Fax: 0207 586 1457; website: www.zsl.org/science

22.1 Reporting adverse drug reactions

Veterinary Medicines Directorate (VMD) Pharmacovigilance Unit is the body for any reporting of adverse drug reactions

- Adverse drug reaction in an animal (licenced, unlicenced and human medicines used to treat animals)
- Human adverse reaction to a veterinary medicinal product
- Lack of efficacy of a drug

When reporting an adverse drug reaction, the following will be required:

- The name of the product which you think caused the adverse reaction or lack of efficacy
- The animal(s) or person(s) in which the adverse reaction or lack of efficacy occurred
- The signs observed of the adverse reaction or lack of efficacy that is suspected
- Your contact details as the reporter of the adverse reaction or lack of efficacy

The VMD now also monitors reports of adverse events following microchipping of companion animals

The reporting form is available online and can be found at:

https://www.vmd.defra.gov.uk/adversereactionreporting

Pharmacovigilance team on 01932 338427

General principles

Initial contact with veterinary surgeries about poisoned animals is usually made by telephone.

Take a good history, covering:

- The animal (age, breed, sex, weight, past medical history)
- The 'agent' or poison (product name, ingredients, amounts, units)
- The incident/exposure (route of exposure, time of incident, how it occurred)
- Clinical course (any clinical effects, onset/duration, severity)

Management of poisoning – Decontamination – removing the animal from the poison and the poison from the animal

Remember to protect yourself and owners!

Consider obtaining samples for analysis

Gastric decontamination – emetics

- Prevent absorption if poison ingested recently
- Time limit a matter of debate
- Not suitable in horses, ruminants, rodents, rabbits
- Use of emetics contraindicated if:
  - Animal is depressed, unconscious or has poor swallow reflex
  - Convulsing or showing premonitory signs of so doing
  - Caustic or corrosive materials have been ingested
  - Volatile materials, particularly petroleum distillates and essential oils, have been ingested

Gastric decontamination – by using emetics or gastric lavage

Apomorphine

Xylazine

Other agents

Washing soda crystals – (sodium carbonate)

(Hydrogen peroxide – 3%)

(Mustard)

NOT salt

Gastric lavage

Usually performed on anaesthetized animals

Labour-intensive

Use of cuffed endotracheal tube to minimize aspiration

If corrosives or caustics are ingested, there may be risk of perforation of oesophagus/gastric wall

Adsorbents

Adsorption = the physical binding of a poison to an unabsorbable carrier which is then eliminated in the faeces

Considered the preferred method of gastric decontamination for many poisons

Most effective for large, nonpolar molecules. Ionized compounds less well adsorbed, i.e. ineffective for some poisons such as iron, lithium and other metals; cyanide; ethanol; ethylene glycol/methanol; metaldehyde; sodium chloride; petroleum distillates; anticoagulant rodenticides

May reduce the efficacy of orally administered antidotes

Repeat doses may be useful for agents that undergo enterohepatic cycling

Dictionary of Veterinary Nursing   Appendices

23.2 Toxic agents

Type	Causes	Effects	Treatment
Poisonous fruits and vegetables			
	Fruits of the *vitis vinifera* – grapes, raisins, sultanas, currants	Toxic mechanism unknown Onset: usually between 6–24 hours Initially, effects may be GI, 24–72 hours later renal function starts to deteriorate. Some dogs have shown signs of pancreatitis	Induce vomiting (up to several hours). Repeat doses of activated charcoal every 4 hours may be of benefit. Aggressive IV fluid therapy (e.g. twice the normal maintenance rate) for at least 48 hours. Monitor renal function and electrolytes for at least 72 hours
	Fruits containing cyanogenic glycosides; *Malus* species (apples), *Prunus* species (cherry, plum, almond, peach, nectarine, etc.); often found in the stones/pips of some fruits	Onset is variable, can be rapid or delayed. Death can occur within several minutes of ingestion. Animals may develop ataxia, frothing at the mouth, dilated pupils, hyperventilation, dyspnoea, weakness, tremors, hypotension and collapse	Decontamination recommended, systemic support
	Allium species- onions, garlic , leek, shallot, chives	Onset is variable, can be rapid or delayed. Death can occur within several minutes of ingestion. Animals may develop ataxia, frothing at the mouth, dilated pupils, hyperventilation, dyspnoea, weakness, tremors, hypotension and collapse	Decontamination recommended and systemic support
	Avocado (*Persea americana*)	Onset is variable, can take up to several days Generally myocardial degeneration and heart failure Can manifest as generalized oedema and dyspnoea, raised creatine kinase, aspartate aminotransferase and lactate dehydrogenase, leukocytosis and liver and renal impairment	Decontamination recommended and systemic support
	Brassica species – kale, broccoli, cauliflower, cabbage, Brussels sprouts	Haemolytic anaemia, glucosinolate poisoning – metabolized to irritant compounds which can cause diarrhoea and colic, dehydration, salivation and irritation of GI tract	Decontamination recommended and systemic support

Ragwort (*Senicio jacobae*)	Equine – ingestion when little food available. Acute and chronic liver disease, abdominal pain, diarrhoea, constipation, neurological signs, collapse, coma and death	No cure
Xylitol – artificial sweetener found in many chewing gums, diabetic foods, and 'no added sugar' products	Harmless to humans but causes severe hypoglycaemia in animals due to potent stimulation of insulin release in dogs. Liver damage can occur	Decontamination recommended, systemic support, including close monitoring of blood glucose levels
Yew tree (*Taxus baccata*)	Equine – ingestion. All parts of the tree can be poisonous, including dried material. Signs develop rapidly and death can occur suddenly	Physical removal of yew material, cardiorespiratory stimulants, supportive care
Medicines		
ACP misuse	Accidental overdosing with tablets in the house	Induce vomiting if many tablets have been eaten (unlikely, since few surgeons prescribe more than a few tablets for specific occasions)
	Idiosyncratic reaction to the drug	
	Depression or collapse. (Cats may become hyperaesthetic)	Treat symptoms of collapse/shock, heatstroke and epilepsy
	Vasodilatation leads to decreased blood pressure and increased susceptibility to heatstroke on warm days	
	Brachiocephalic dogs are especially likely to suffer	
	Possible increased likelihood of fits in epileptic animals	
Abnormal response (anaphylactic reaction)	Allergic-type response to medication, e.g. vaccination, antibiotics	Swellings may have cold compresses applied
	Depression, occasionally vomiting and diarrhoea, swelling of injection sites	Treat for shock if collapsed and maintain if unconscious
	Severe reactions result in collapse with signs of shock	Prepare corticosteroid injection

(Continued)

Dictionary of Veterinary Nursing   Appendices

23.2 Toxic agents—cont'd

Type	Causes	Effects	Treatment
Non-steroidal anti-inflammatory drugs (NSAIDs)	Owners using human preparations on their animals (dosing their pets with so-called painkillers) Dogs 'stealing' owners' medication Aspirin: particularly toxic in cats Ibuprofen, flurbiprofen and naproxen: may be rapidly fatal in some dogs Phenylbutazone: more toxic to cats than dogs	Aspirin: depression. Gastric irritation, leading to vomiting and anorexia. Cats may show some incoordination Ibuprofen and flurbiprofen: gastric ulceration and perforation in dogs leads to vomiting and haematemesis, followed by diarrhoea with melaena. Kidney damage may cause acute and fatal renal failure. Dehydration due to fluid losses Naproxen: gastric inflammation and ulceration leading to vomiting and melaena Anaemia due to low-grade blood loss Dehydration	Stop medication with the drugs Before symptoms show: induce vomiting as soon as possible If showing symptoms: give absorptive preparations and/or demulcents. Dosing with activated charcoal is vital in cases of aspirin poisoning and should be given immediately after vomiting ceases. Prepare intravenous fluids Prepare cimetidine for intravenous injection in cases of naproxen poisoning
Paracetamol	Owner-administered dose or tablet packet chewed	Dogs tolerate paracetamol well, but cats are easily poisoned by as little as half a 500 mg tablet. Poisoning with paracetamol results in haemoglobin being changed to methaemoglobin, which is incapable of transporting oxygen Signs: cyanosis Depression or excitement Incoordination due to hypoxia Facial swelling	Induce vomiting if no symptoms shown Give absorptive material by mouth but not before consulting veterinary surgeon – if N-acetyl cysteine is to be used, the absorptive material may also prevent the absorption of this antidote Provide oxygen if any sign of cyanosis; ensure that the animal rests as much as possible. Prepare methionine or N-acetyl cysteine (human preparation, Parvolex) for oral administration
Salbutamol	Human preparations that are used to treat asthma and for premature labour	Stimulation of the sympathetic nervous system, causing peripheral vasodilatation and rapid heart rate (tachycardia) Panting respiration Muscle weakness	General first aid treatment but beta-blockers may be needed if the heart rate becomes excessively high

| Calcipotriol | Vitamin D derivative contained in psoriasis creams and ointments, chewed by pups | Similar to vitamin D overdose. Poisoning leads to hypercalcaemia and hyperphosphataemia, causing acute nephritis and damage to gastrointestinal tract. **Signs:** haemorrhagic diarrhoea Polyuria and polydipsia Collapse with or without convulsions Death may occur within 24 hours | Induce vomiting if ingested within 2–4 hours Prepare activated charcoal solution Prepare Hartmann's solution for i.v. administration – it is important to flush the calcium and phosphates through the kidneys to minimize renal damage Prepare furosemide diuretic injection |

Herbicides

Chlorates	Ingestion of weedkillers or drinking from contaminated puddles – this substance does not degrade readily after use	Vomiting and diarrhoea with abdominal pain Cyanosis of mucosa, turning to a muddy brown colour (blood becomes chocolate in colour because poison causes the formation of methaemoglobin – see Paracetamol)	General first aid treatment Prepare methylene blue injection
Dinitro compounds	Ingestion of 2,4-dinitrophenol (2,4-D) or dinitro-orthocresol (2,4,5-T)	Depression, listlessness, muscle weakness Rapid respiration and dyspnoea Hyperthermia with sweating Urine is almost fluorescent yellow/green	General first aid treatment Monitor rectal temperature to detect hyperthermia
Paraquat	Ingesting weedkiller (although this product is rapidly absorbed onto the soil after application, which renders it harmless). Paraquat has been used in malicious poisonings, but most cases are due to accidents.	Inflammation of the mouth and tongue Vomiting and diarrhoea, with abdominal pain Depression and progressive respiratory distress and cyanosis over a period of days, resulting in death	Induce vomiting as soon as ingestion of this chemical is suspected. Even though this is an irritant poison, the effects of the absorbed poison are so severe that treatment is usually hopeless and the only hope is to remove the poison from the alimentary tract as soon as possible. Administering Fuller's earth is also helpful because the poison will bind to the Fuller's earth and be rendered inactive

(Continued)

Dictionary of Veterinary Nursing   Appendices

23.2 Toxic agents—cont'd

Type	Causes	Effects	Treatment
Insecticides			
Borax	Ant killers (e.g. Nippon), which are based on honey and therefore very attractive to dogs	Vomiting and diarrhoea Collapse, convulsions and possible paralysis Poisoning may be fatal	General first aid treatment
Organophosphates	Overdosing with insecticidal sprays, chewing insecticidal collars, etc.	Vomiting and diarrhoea Salivation Constricted pupils Muscular twitching, excitement, followed by weakness, incoordination	General first aid treatment Prepare atropine sulphate for injection
Organochlorines	Woodworm treatments and other insecticides (aldrin, dieldrin, gamma-BHC, etc.). Many products have been withdrawn from sale but old stocks still exist.	Involuntary twitching of muscles, especially facial, fore- and hindlimbs, and convulsions Behavioural changes, e.g. aggression, pacing, apprehension, frenzy	Wash off contamination Administer absorptive material and/or liquid paraffin to decrease absorption Fatty foods and drinks (including milk) **must not be given** as they may increase absorption of the poison Prepare barbiturate injection to control convulsions
Molluscicides			
Carbamate	See Organophosphates	Incoordination leading to hyperaesthesia and convulsions	General first aid treatment
Metaldehyde	Ingestion of slug bait, which some dogs and cats seem to find very palatable	Rapid pulse and respiration and possibly cyanosis	Dosing with liquid paraffin may delay absorption of poison as long as it is given before the patient shows any symptoms (do not dose the unconscious patient) Prepare barbiturate injection to control convulsions

Rodenticides

Alphachloralose	Rat baits and preparations to control pigeon and seabird populations	Poison acts by lowering the body temperature Progressive depression, incoordination and coma with hypothermia	General first aid treatment but warmth is essential
Calciferol anticoagulant preparations	Ingestion of rat baits. Several different compounds come under this heading; warfarin, coumatetralyl, chlorophacinone, difenacoum, brodifacoum, bromadiolone	See Calcipotriol (Medicines) Interference with clotting mechanism results in haemorrhages in the mucosae, bruising and haematomata, swollen joints, etc.	General first aid treatment Prepare injections of vitamin K. Large and repeated dosing may be necessary.

Household chemicals

Alcohol	Ingestion of alcoholic drink or fermenting grain (especially likely with pups)	Hyperaesthesia, incoordination, collapse and even death	Induce vomiting and provide general first aid treatment
Chocolate	Ingestion of large amounts of high-cocoa-content chocolate or cocoa powder. (Not a common poisoning but causes much public concern)	Nervous excitement progressing to fits and coma Tachycardia Panting	Induce vomiting (may not be effective if chocolate ingested because of its sticky consistency). Gastric lavage may be required. Prepare activated charcoal solution Prepare diazepam/phenobarbital to control fits

(Continued)

Dictionary of Veterinary Nursing | Appendices

23.2 Toxic agents—cont'd

Type	Causes	Effects	Treatment
Disinfectants	Household disinfectants, when diluted to correct strength, do not cause a problem but are often used undiluted or incorrectly diluted by overzealous owners **Phenols:** cats are particularly susceptible to poisoning by phenols	These are corrosive poisons with a strong, distinctive odour, e.g. pine disinfectants Convulsions, coma and death in acute poisoning cases Less acute cases may have inflamed mouths (stomatitis) and occasionally ulcers in the mouth	**Do not induce vomiting** General first aid treatment, including thorough washing of contaminated fur
	Licking paws after walking on wet surfaces recently cleaned with undiluted or incorrectly diluted solutions of disinfectant Grooming coat after accidental spraying or splashing with strong disinfectant solutions **Quaternary ammonium compounds:** as for phenols	Animals may also vomit and have diarrhoea and abdominal pain	
		These are also corrosive poisons but are odourless Depression and anorexia Occasionally vomiting Salivation, stomatitis and mouth ulcers, especially on the tongue tip Skin ulcerations if compound not washed off quickly	As for phenols

Ethylene glycol (antifreeze)	Suspected ingestion of liquid drained from car radiators (dogs seem particularly prone to drink this)	Incoordination, depression and rapid breathing. Later animal may become uraemic	General first aid treatment. Ethanol is the specific antidote and intravenous injections may be prepared if available at the surgery. **Do not induce vomiting**
Petroleum products	Usually a problem in cats that have fallen into containers of sump oil drained from cars. Accidental spillages of petrol, paraffin, etc. Caking of tar in the paws	These are very corrosive poisons with a distinctive odour. Depression, vomiting, collapse and death if enough ingested. If submerged in the liquid may also suffer an aspiration pneumonia, which is very severe because of the extremely irritant nature of the inhaled liquid. Inflammation of the in-contact skin and mouth, especially the tongue if the animal has been allowed to groom	General first aid treatment, including giving olive oil by mouth to decrease absorption of the toxins

Modified from Aspinall, Clinical Procedures in Veterinary Nursing, 2003, Butterworth Heinemann

23.3   Poison/toxicologists contact details

Veterinary Poisons Information Service (VPIS)   +44 (0) 207 188 0200
Toxcall 0203 3686298

Appendix 24

24.1 Hazard warning labels

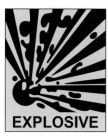
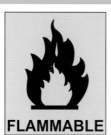
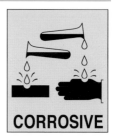

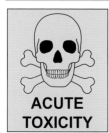
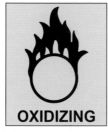
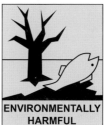

Figure 59. Hazard warning labels. (Contains public sector information published by the Health and Safety Executive and licensed under the Open Government Licence.)

25.1   Anatomical orientation

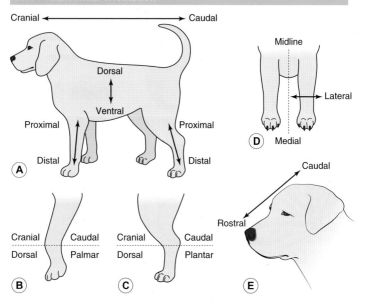

Figure 60. Anatomical orientation. Redrawn with permission from Easton S. Veterinary radiography: a workbook for students. Edinburgh: Butterworth-Heinemann, 2006.

26.1 UK quarantine regulations

All pet dogs, cats and ferrets may enter the United Kingdom provided they fulfil the requirements of the Pet Travel Scheme

From 1 January 2012 all pet dogs, cats and ferrets have been able to enter or re-enter the UK from any country in the world without quarantine provided they meet the rules of the Pet Travel Scheme. Animals that do not meet the requirements will be placed in quarantine and they can be dealt with before an Import Permit can be issued

Entry requirements if entering the United Kingdom from Europe or a listed non-European country such as Australia:

To prepare your dog, cat or ferret:

1. The animal must be microchipped so that it can be permanently identified.
2. The pet must be vaccinated against rabies at least 21 days before the intended entry date. Even if the animal has a current rabies vaccine certificate, it needs injecting again 21 days before entry. Booster vaccines have to be kept up. On second or subsequent entries, the 21-day rule to wait no longer is enforced, provided boosters are up to date.
3. Complete the pet travel documentation – Animals being prepared from Australia will need to obtain an official 'third country veterinary certificate' which can be downloaded from www.defra.gov.uk.
4. Tapeworm treatment: all dogs entering the U K are required to be treated for tapeworms by a veterinary surgeon between 24 hours and 120 hours before the time of entry planned – at present there is no requirement for tick treatment.
5. Arrange for the animal to travel by air or by sea with the appropriate documentation for examination at the Border Inspection Point.
6. Cats from Australia must be accompanied by a certificate showing protection against Hendra disease.

26.2 The importation of dogs and cats to Australia

Pets must meet the Australian Government's BioSecurity regulations. The United Kingdom is listed as rabies-free with other Category 3 countries – Antigua & Barbuda, Argentina, Austria, Bahamas, Belgium, Bermuda, British Virgin Islands, Brunei, Bulgaria, Canada, Canary and Balearic Islands, Cayman Islands, Chile, the Republic of Croatia, the Republic of Cyprus, Czech Republic, Denmark, Finland, France, Germany, Gibraltar, Greece, Greenland, Guernsey, Hong Kong, Hungary, Ireland, Isle of Man, Israel, Italy, Jamaica, Jersey, Kuwait, Latvia, Luxembourg, Macau, Malta, Malaysia (Peninsular, Sabah and Sarawak only), Monaco, Montenegro, the Netherlands, Netherlands – Antilles & Aruba, Norway, Poland, Portugal, Puerto Rico, Qatar, the Republic of South Africa, Reunion, Saipan, Serbia, Seychelles, Slovakia, Slovenia, South Korea, Spain, St Kitts and Nevis, St Lucia, St Vincent & the Grenadines, Sweden, Switzerland (including Liechtenstein), Taiwan, Trinidad and Tobago, the United Arab Emirates, the United Kingdom, the United States (including the District of Columbia, Northern Mariana Islands, Puerto Rico and the US Virgin Islands but excluding Guam and Hawaii, Uruguay).

Category 3 countries are described as approved countries and territories in which rabies is absent or well-controlled and animals from these countries require an import permit to be eligible for import to Australia.

26.2   The importation of dogs and cats to Australia—cont'd

Dogs and cats must be identified by microchips. Australia requires for dogs and cats to enter the country with a minimum of 10 days' quarantine

ISO 11784/11785-compliant ISO microchip: If your pet's microchip is not ISO 11784/11785-compliant, you can bring your own microchip scanner.

Rabies vaccination completed within 1 year of entry

Blood Titre Test (RNATT) no sooner than 180 days prior to entry

Import Permit (This will take about 10 days to process.)

A USDA- (or CFIA-) accredited veterinarian must then complete the Australia Veterinary Certificate for endorsement by the USDA or CFIA if travelling from the United States or Canada. Other requirements apply for other departure countries.

A copy of the Rabies Certificate and Blood Titre Test should also be included for endorsement.

All pets must travel as manifest cargo and will need a health certificate issued within 10 days of travel.

26.3   Exemptions for assistance dogs

Registered assistance dogs may enter without quarantine if the requirements are met with a declaration that the dog has been qualified with the handler and in continuous service for at least 6 months prior to export.

A 'Medical history form for assistance dog handlers', completed by a medical practitioner, and providing evidence of a disability and ongoing dependence on an assistance dog

The 'assistance dog training' form, completed by a representative of a recognized assistance dog training institution and providing confirmation of specialized training. Suitable institutions include member organizations of the International Guide Dog Federation or Assistance Dogs International or that the dog and/or their trainer are accredited under a law of an Australian State or Territory.

In addition, if you are seeking to bring your dog from a category 3 country, you will need to attach the following form:

• The 'Rabies vaccination and rabies neutralizing antibody titre test declaration' form, completed by the Official Government Veterinarian in the country of export, and providing confirmation that the dog has been rabies blood tested at least 6 months prior to export.

26.4   Other exotic species

For further information on the import controls on endangered species, you can contact The CITES Licensing Team in Bristol on 0117 372 8774 or wildlife.licensing@ahvla.gsi.gov.uk or the CITES website

27.1 Action to take when a pet is lost

Lost pet – Owner can call	Local authority	Please check online
	Local dog wardens	
	Local re-homing centres	
	Local practices	Please check online
	Local charity veterinary practices	
	ID chip companies 'Petlog'	0844 4633999
	'Pet Trak'	0800 652 9977
	Anibase	0844 8241235
	RSPCA	0300 1238022
	Local cats protection (if cat)	Please check online
	Online lost/found pet searches databases	http://www.animalsearchuk.co.uk http://www.nationalpetregister.org http://www.petslocated.com

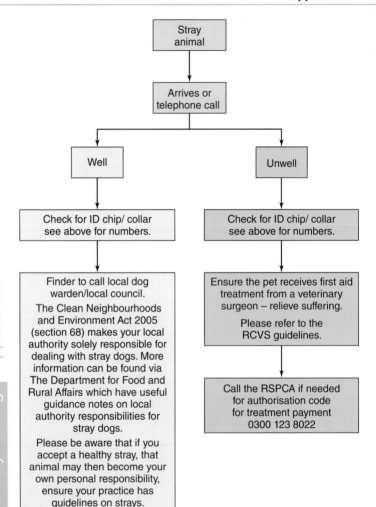

Figure 61. Algorithm for managing stray animals.